Orthopaedic MRI

A TEACHING FILE

Stephen J. Pomeranz, MD

The Christ Hospital
Cincinnati, Ohio

Illustrations by L. Eugene Arrington, MD

J. B. Lippincott Company Philadelphia
New York London Hagerstown

Acquisitions Editor: Dean Manke
Assistant Production Manager: Lori J. Bainbridge
Production: P. M. Gordon Associates
Compositor: Achorn Graphic Services
Printer/Binder: Arcata Graphics/Halliday

6 5 4 3 2 1

Library of Congress Cataloging-in-Publication Data

Pomeranz, Stephen J.
Orthopaedic MRI : a teaching file / Stephen J. Pomeranz.
p. cm.
Includes index.
ISBN 0–397–51105–1
1. Magnetic resonance imaging. 2. Orthopedics—Diagnosis.
I. Title.
[DNLM: 1. Extremities—atlases. 2. Joint Diseases—diagnosis—atlases. 3. Joint Diseases—physiopathology—atlases. 4. Magnetic Resonance Imaging—atlases. WE 17 P785o]
RD734.5.M33P66 1991
617.5′807548—dc20
DNLM/DLC
for Library of Congress 91–10086
CIP

Any procedure or practice described in this book should be applied by the practitioner in accordance with professional standards of care used with regard to the unique circumstances that apply in each practice situation. Care has been taken to confirm the accuracy of information presented and to describe generally accepted practices. However, the authors, editors, and publisher cannot accept any responsibility for errors or omissions or for consequences from application of the information in this book and make no warranty, expressed or implied, with respect to the contents of the book.

Every effort has been made to ensure drug selections and dosages are in accordance with current recommendations and practice. Because of ongoing research, changes in government regulations, and the constant flow of information on drug therapy, reactions, and interactions, the reader is cautioned to check the package insert for each drug for indications, dosages, warnings, and precautions, particularly if the drug is new or infrequently used.

Orthopaedic MRI *A TEACHING FILE*

This book is dedicated to my loving wife, Penny, and to my five children: Christy, Corbin, Taylor, Jory, and Kellen. Their support and good humor has made the task of writing this book enjoyable.

PREFACE

The idea for *Orthopaedic MRI: A Teaching File* came from many of my predecessors who have designed similar texts in the neural axis. The goal of this textbook is to emphasize relevant radiologic anatomy and disease processes, especially in the knee and shoulder, not to provide anatomic and systematic evaluations of every body part and disease. A few unusual disease entities are included in the text; however, the emphasis is on the common, clinically relevant disease and problems encountered in MR skeletal imaging.

The more frequently a problem or diagnostic dilemma arises, the more it is examined in this text. Questions often appear in quiz format since this form of teaching helps emphasize specific issues and allows the physician or student to better remember the point being made. While I emphasize the MR appearances and characteristics of various injuries and disease processes, time is also spent discussing relevant pathology, anatomy, clinical presentations, and pathophysiology.

Line diagrams accompany 90 percent of the cases in this text to help provide the reader with visualization of the pathology being discussed. I hope the diagrams will serve as a refresher and supportive element when the interpreter encounters a similar case in his or her practice.

The intent of this author is to provide a foundation for the late beginner to early intermediate orthopedic MR reader in a concise structure with excellent image quality and diagrammatic representation of the disease.

I have chosen to omit the study of the spine from this text because I prefer not to duplicate the abundance of information already available on this subject. In addition, I have not examined the temporomandibular joint because this subject seems more relevant in a text on neural disease, a study of the head and neck, or in a dental text.

Orthopedic MR is in its infancy, and it can be reasonably predicted that it will account for 50–60 percent of MR volume at most sites. My own MR experience has now exceeded 50,000 cases, and at The Christ Hospital we have performed over 5,000 knee examinations. Orthopedic MR now accounts for 60 percent of our volume.

Stephen J. Pomeranz, MD

ACKNOWLEDGMENTS

I would like to thank my dedicated secretary Diana Vester. Without her help and organizational skills, this text could not have been completed. I would also like to extend my appreciation to my fellow in magnetic resonance, L. Eugene Arrington, now a staff radiologist specializing in MR at University Hospital in Augusta, Georgia, for his patience, dedication, and extraordinary computer skills. I would like to thank my staff in magnetic resonance at The Christ Hospital in Cincinnati, Ohio, for their diligence in filming cases and helping me to oversee photographic aspects of this text, and my colleagues and members of the Radiology Department at The Christ Hospital, especially its chairman, Owen L. Brown, for assisting me in locating interesting cases. I would like to thank the administration of The Christ Hospital and its president, Jack Cook, who gave me their generous support; my friends and colleagues from around the world who have sent me case material and allowed me to include it in this teaching file text; and, finally, the patients themselves, including professional athletes, who have given me permission to use their examinations in this textbook anonymously.

SPECIAL ACKNOWLEDGMENT

I would like to express my appreciation to my parents, Harriet and Paul, for their tremendous support in my former life as a child and adolescent. They are joined by my in-laws, Helen and Jim Kereiakes, who have provided a sounding board and their support in my academic endeavors.

Stephen J. Pomeranz, MD

CONTENTS

PART I

Knee

CASE 1

Differential Diagnosis of Normal Anatomy

HISTORY: Identify the structures indicated by the arrows in these images. (Figs. 1-1 and 1-2: sagittal volumetric acquisition fast scan contiguous 1.5-mm sections.)

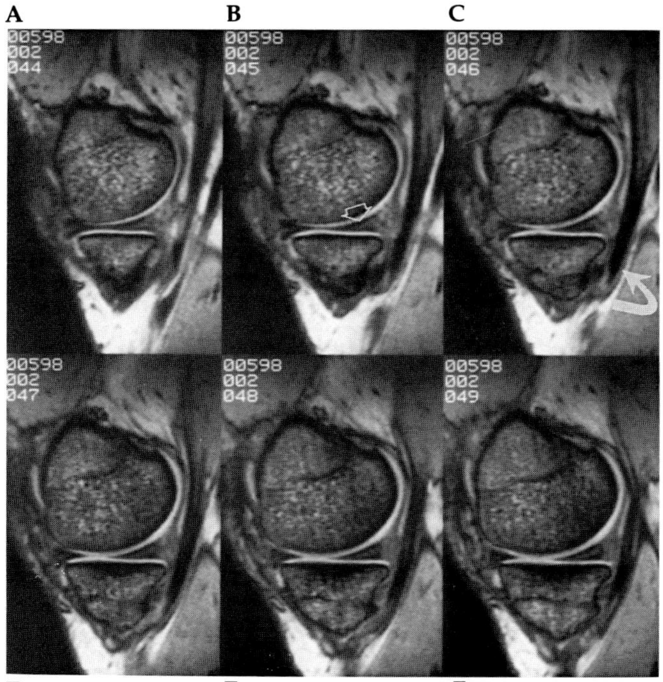

FIGURE 1-1

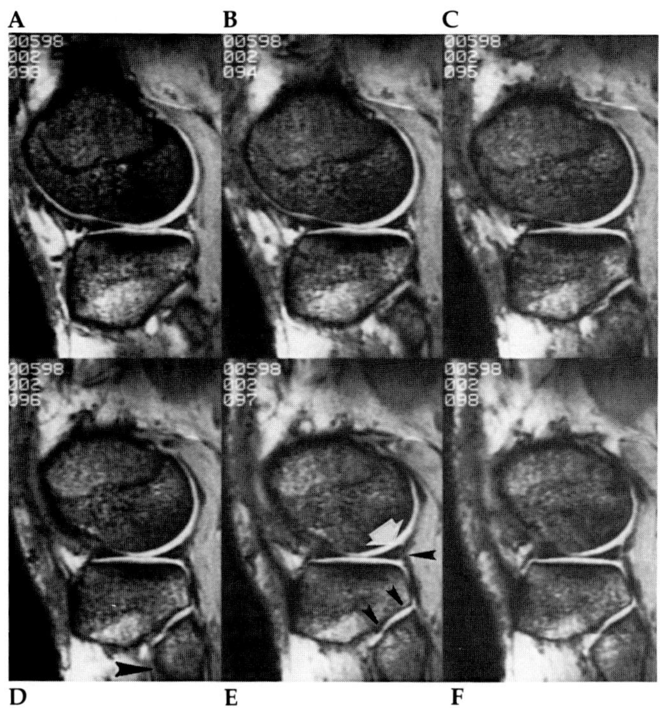

FIGURE 1-2

DISCUSSION: The thin sagittal sections shown in Figures 1-1 and 1-2 are obtained through the lateral and medial menisci. The medial meniscus (Fig. 1-1) is banana shaped when viewed in the axial projection and relatively consistent in length. Its posterior aspect (open arrow in Fig. 1-1*B*) is taller, longer, and wider than its anterior aspect. This asymmetry of the medial meniscus distinguishes medial from lateral in the sagittal plane. The medial meniscus has very tight attachments to the medial collateral ligament via capsular fibers and the coronary ligaments. The intercondylar tibial attachments just deep to the anterior and posterior meniscal horns are known as the ligamentous meniscal roots. The pes anserine tendon complex (curved arrow, Fig. 1-1*C*) inserts on the tibia and consists of the semitendinosus, gracilis, and sartorius tendons. It also identifies the medial side of the knee. Posterior cysts of the gastrocnemius semimembranosus bursa wrap about and dissect superior and inferior to this complex. The first sagittal sections through the medial meniscus transect the anterior and posterior meniscal bodies. Only deeper sections into the imaging volume (6–9.0 mm deep) in the sagittal plane image the true anterior and posterior medial meniscal horns.

The lateral meniscus (Fig. 1-2) is relatively symmetric anterior to posterior, and this relationship identifies the lateral side of the knee in the sagittal projection (two symmetric triangles). In the axial plane the lateral meniscus is C-shaped with a narrower radius of curvature than the medial meniscus. The length of the anterior horn of the lateral meniscus is extremely variable and can be congenitally foreshortened. Therefore, it may normally appear small or hypoplastic on sagittal sections. The attachments of this meniscus to the ligamentous anatomy are looser than the attachments of the medial meniscus. Initially, sagittal sections through the lateral meniscus show a bow tie shape. Deeper sections show the meniscus separating into two symmetric hypointense triangles anteriorly and posteriorly (horizontal arrowhead in *E*). The hyaline cartilage (white arrow in *E*) of the lateral femoral condyle is hyperintense on gradient-echo (fast scan) imaging. The tibiofibular cartilaginous interface (paired arrowheads in *E*) is a site of potential tibiofibular bursitis. The bursal space in this location is collapsed and not visible unless distended by fluid.

DIAGNOSIS: The MR images show normal medial and lateral meniscal anatomy.

CASE 2

Anatomy and Knee Variants

HISTORY: A 36-year-old woman reported acute anterior "knee strain" while jogging. The patient had fallen but experienced minimal symptoms until the following day. What is the MRI diagnosis? (Figs. 2-1 and 2-2: sagittal, magnified, T1-weighted images of the anterior and posterior lateral meniscal horns, obtained with a surface coil.)

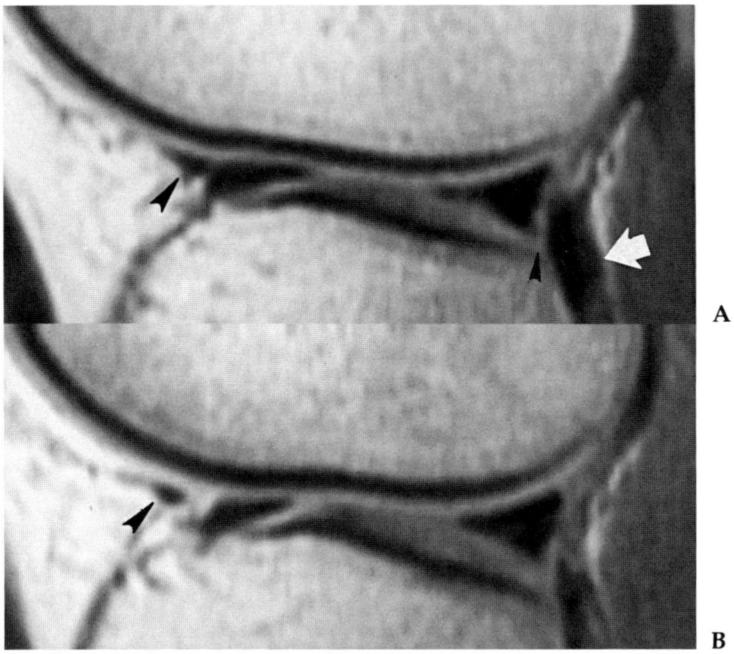

FIGURE 2-1

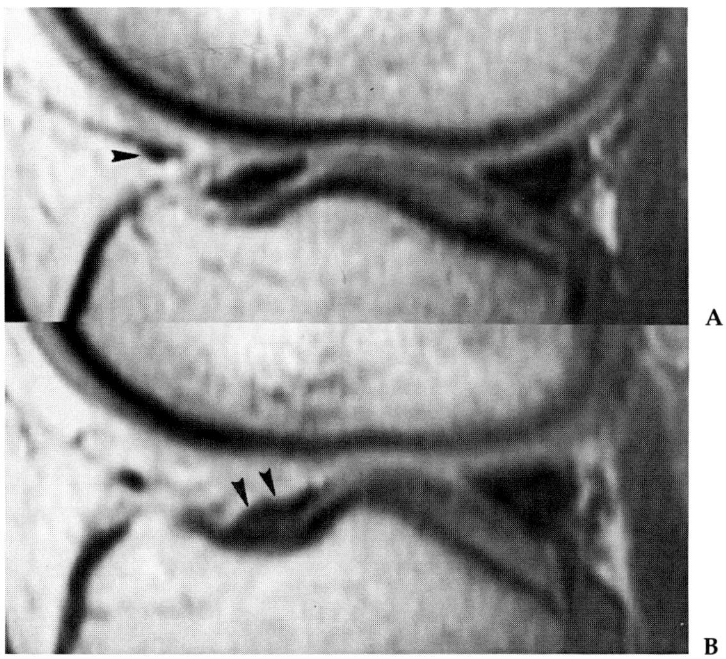

FIGURE 2-2

DISCUSSION: This case illustrates two points. First, the area of hypointense signal located in front of the anterior horn of lateral meniscus (large arrowheads in Fig. 2-1) is not an avulsed meniscal fragment but the normal transverse meniscal ligament and accompanying punctate hypointense inferolateral geniculate artery branches. This is a normal finding that may migrate anteriorly on progressive adjacent sagittal sections. It follows a transverse mediolateral anatomic course, from anterior meniscus to anterior meniscus. The transverse meniscal ligament averages 6.0 to 8.0 mm in diameter. The lateral anterior meniscal root (paired arrowheads in Fig. 2-2*B*) attaches to a notch in the tibia. Knowledge of this anatomy precludes misdiagnosis of avulsion anterolateral meniscus tear.

The second point has to do with the popliteus tendon (white arrow in Fig. 2-1*A*) and its bursal reflection (small black arrowhead). The tendon penetrates the meniscocapsular junction of the lateral meniscus. The tendon itself is hypointense. It arises from the proximal fibula and courses medially and caudally, merging with its parent muscle along the posterior aspect of the knee. The popliteus tendon is analogous to the pronator teres in the arm in that it unlocks the screw-home mechanism in the knee joint following extension. The popliteus reflection may fill with fluid or blood after knee injury, resembling a posterior tear on MRI; however, the vertical orientation and posterior migration on serial sagittal sections prevent this error. The anterolateral meniscal root is indicated by the paired arrowheads in Figure 2-2*B*.

DIAGNOSIS: The MR images show the normal transverse meniscal ligament, popliteus tendon and reflection, and the lateral meniscal root.

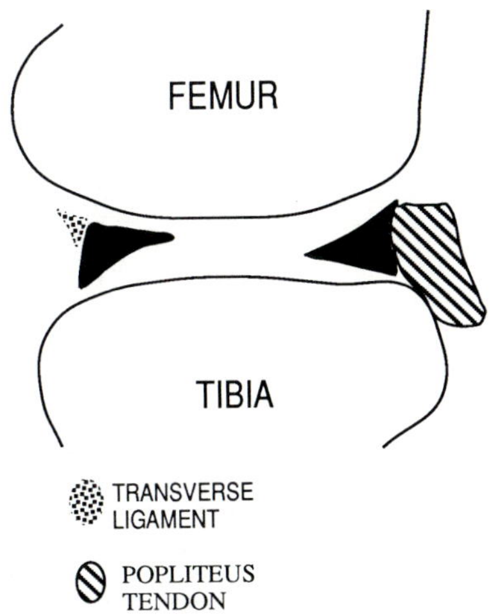

FIGURE 2-3

CASE 3

Differential Diagnosis of Postoperative Knee Pain

HISTORY: A 31-year-old woman who had previously undergone knee surgery reported chronic knee pain of 8 months' duration. From the imaging findings, what was the earlier surgical procedure? (Figs. 3-1 and 3-2: coronal and sagittal proton-density MR images, TR/TE 1,400/20 msec, 14.0-cm FOV, 56 × 128 pixel matrix, 3.0-mm sections, 2 excitations.)

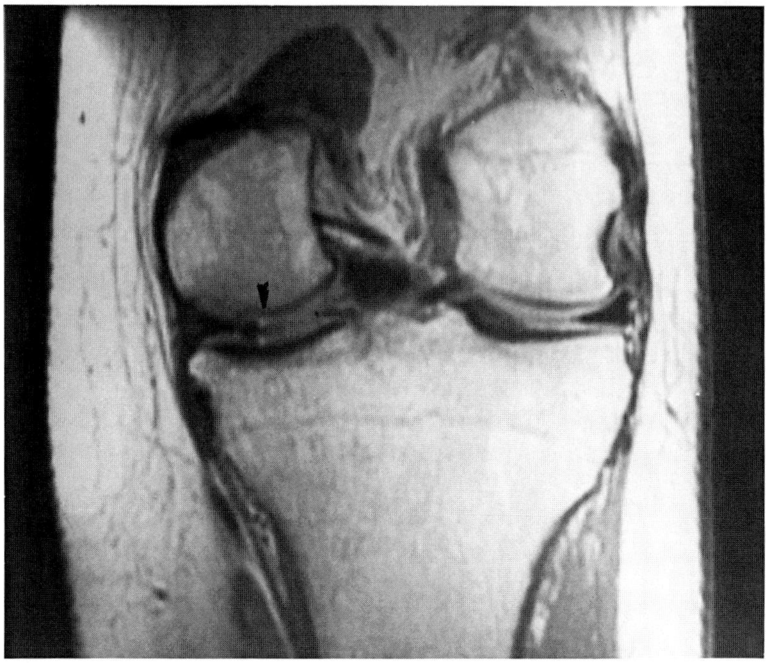

FIGURE 3-1

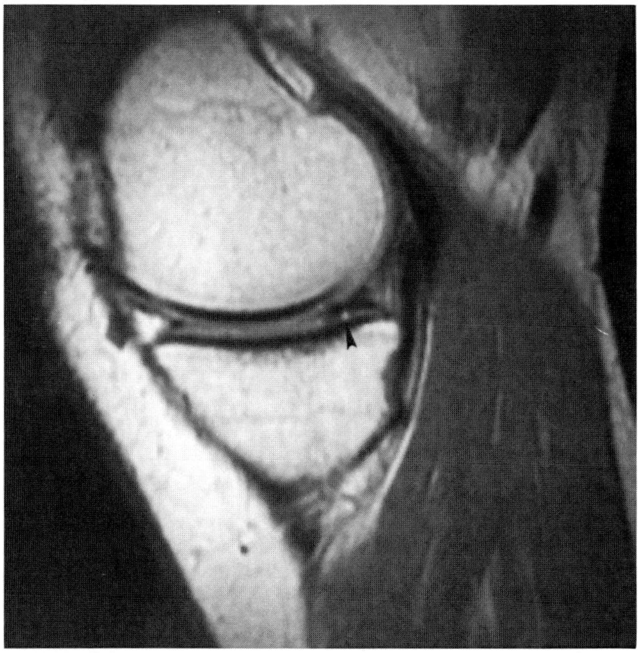

FIGURE 3-2

DISCUSSION: The anterior horn of the medial meniscus is extremely small and has been partially resected. This confirms that the patient has had a meniscectomy. In addition, evidence of a meniscal repair with oversewing of the tear is provided by the focal punctate hyperintense areas seen in the femoral and tibial cartilages in both the coronal and sagittal projections (arrowheads), and in the posterior meniscal body and posterior meniscal horn. These areas of higher signal intensity represent metallic nonferromagnetic suture lines. Suture lines may be seen with oversewn meniscal tissue or after meniscal transplantation. The partially resected meniscus appears truncated and amputated and is smaller than normal. Bizarre triangular meniscal shapes may be seen; however, tear may only be diagnosed when true oblique intrameniscal signal alteration is present. More extensive meniscal resection produces a homogeneous fluid signal intensity, and the MRI appearance may be indistinguishable from that of meniscal agenesis.

DIAGNOSIS: An anterior medial meniscectomy has been performed, with posterior medial meniscal repair.

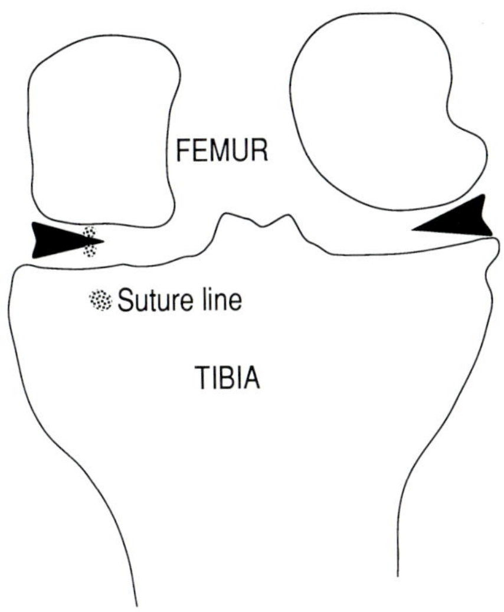

FIGURE 3-3

CASE 4

Differential Diagnosis of Normal Anatomy

HISTORY: Identify the structure creating the linear oblique band of low signal intensity projecting between the femoral condyles and the hypointense bands demarcated by arrowheads. (Fig. 4-1: coronal T1-weighted image.)

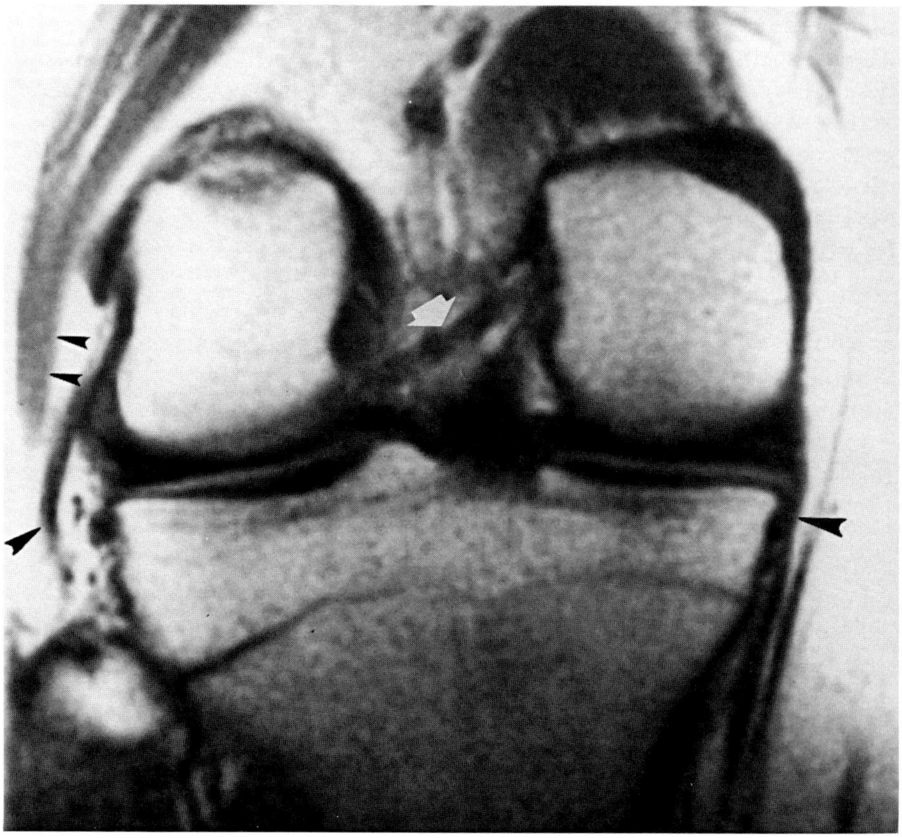

FIGURE 4-1

DISCUSSION: The hypointense oblique band (white arrow) represents the ligament of Wrisberg, also known as the meniscofemoral ligament. It extends from the posterior horn of the lateral meniscus to the lateral surface of the medial femoral condyle superiorly. This ligament lies directly behind the posterior cruciate ligament; therefore, if one follows the posterior cruciate ligament on serial coronal sections, one may find the ligament of Wrisberg.

Just anterior to the posterior cruciate ligament is a thin structure (not shown), the Humphrey ligament, a branch of the Wrisberg ligament. The posterior cruciate ligament is sandwiched between the Humphrey ligament and the ligament of Wrisberg. The Humphrey ligament fuses with the posterior cruciate ligament in 80% of anatomic specimens. These structures control posterior displacement of the tibia on the femur and add additional stabilization against excessive varus and valgus angulation.

The lateral collateral complex is composed of three main elements: the iliotibial band, the fibular collateral ligament (single arrowheads), and the biceps femoris tendon. The biceps muscle (paired arrowheads) and its tendon, along with the fibular collateral ligament, join to form the conjoined tendon. The iliotibial band attaches to the tibial Gerdy tubercle. The fibular collateral ligament arises from the lateral femoral epicondyle just below the origin of the popliteus tendon and inserts on the fibula.

DIAGNOSIS: The band of low signal intensity between the femoral condyles is the ligament of Wrisberg. Also identified is the fibular collateral ligament.

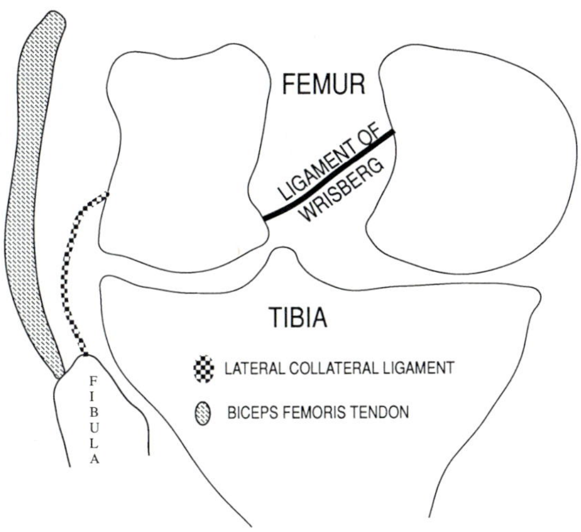

FIGURE 4-2

CASE 5

Differential Diagnosis of Normal Anatomy

HISTORY: Identify the structures indicated by the small arrowhead, the medium-sized arrowhead, the large arrowhead, and the group of three arrowheads. (Figs. 5-1 and 5-2: sagittal multiecho proton-density (5-1) and T2-weighted (5-2) MR images, TR/TE 1,200/20, 80 msec.)

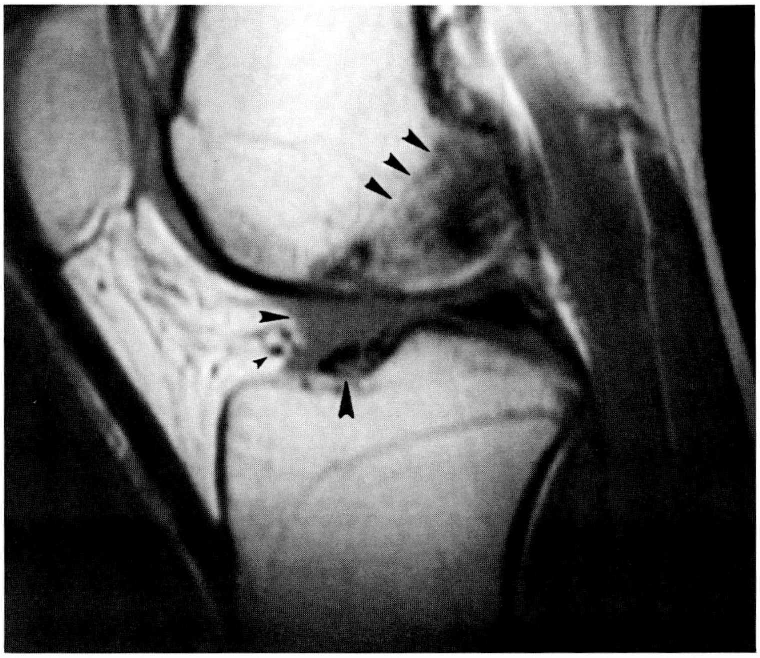

FIGURE 5-1

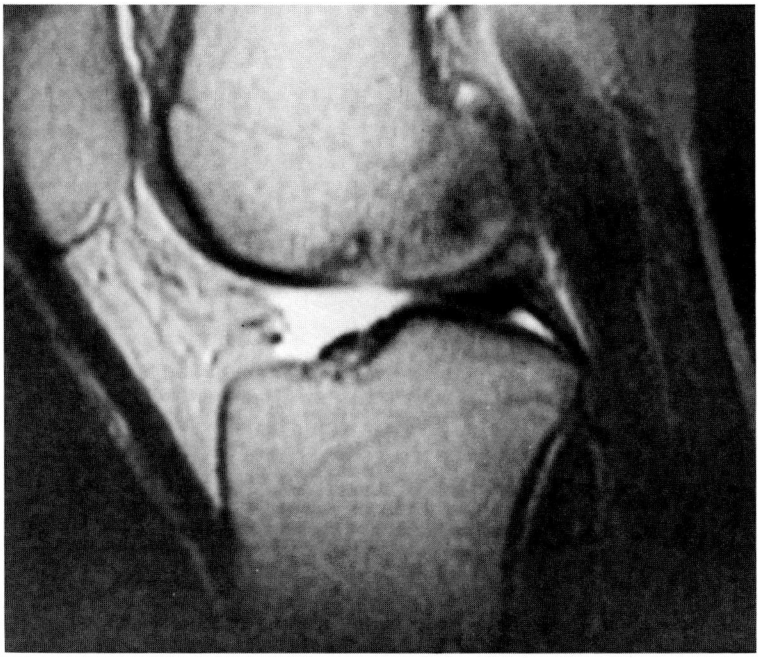

FIGURE 5-2

DISCUSSION: These sagittal sections, obtained through the notch of the knee just lateral to the insertion of the anterior cruciate ligament (not shown), show several normal anatomic structures or variations. The transverse meniscal ligament (small arrowhead in Fig. 5-1) is discussed in case 2. The anterior meniscosynovial recess (medium-sized arrowhead) may be quite redundant, particularly along the lateral side of the knee, and may wrap around the anterolateral meniscal root (large arrowhead). With large effusions, it may obscure visualization of the lateral meniscal horn altogether, but this is a rare site for a true tear (<2% of all tears).

The three arrowheads grouped together demarcate a volume averaging artifact that arises from the cortical interface of the lateral femoral condyle. Occasionally this straight hypointense interface will simulate the appearance of an intact anterior cruciate ligament.

DIAGNOSIS: Shown is a normal transverse meniscal ligament with a normal lateral anterior meniscal root and a fluid-filled anterolateral meniscosynovial recess. A volume averaging artifact is discernible along the medial aspect of the lateral femoral condyle.

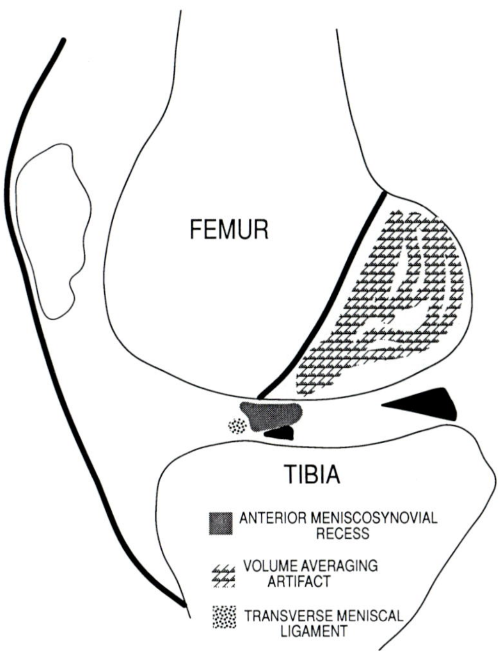

FIGURE 5-3

C A S E 6

Differential Diagnosis of Meniscal Tear

HISTORY: A 31-year-old woman presented with posterior knee pain. Is a true tear present? (Fig. 6-1: sagittal proton-density MR images, TR/TE 1,000/20 msec, 14.0-cm FOV, 4.0-mm sections, 192 × 256 pixel matrix, 2 excitations. Multiformat (four-on-one) contiguous sections.)

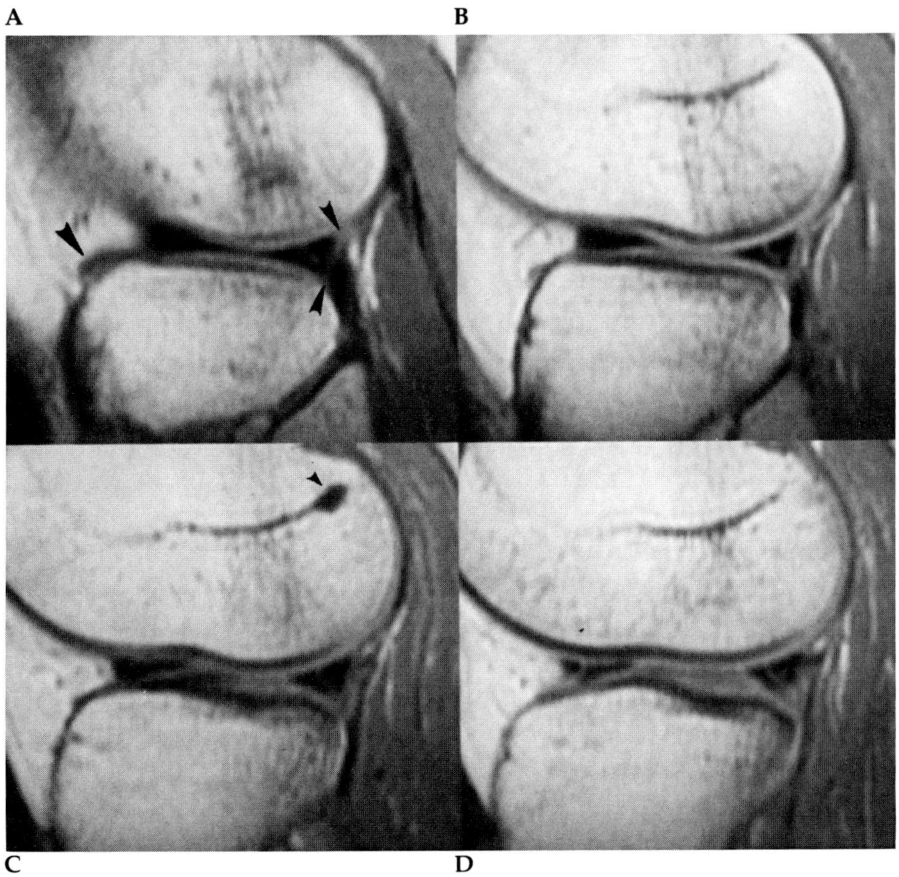

FIGURE 6-1

DISCUSSION: The longer length of the posterior meniscal body relative to the anterior meniscal body identifies the medial compartment of the knee. The capsular interface is seen as a thick gray band posteriorly. A subtle area of punctate intermediate signal intensity (arrowhead) is seen at the junction of the anterior and posterior meniscal bodies. Edge tears of this type are often small and may exist only on one section. They may have a rolled edge or parrot beak shape when viewed in the axial projection. Since sagittal views are obtained tangentially to the abnormality, confirmation of this peripheral lesion is made with orthogonal coronal sections. Gradient-echo, free induction decay imaging (fast scan) can be used to confirm the presence of true tear in either plane. Volume imaging (three-dimensional Fourier transform) with fast scan 1.5-mm sections is an alternative method of confirming very small meniscal tears.

DIAGNOSIS: The patient had a peripheral medial meniscal body tear.

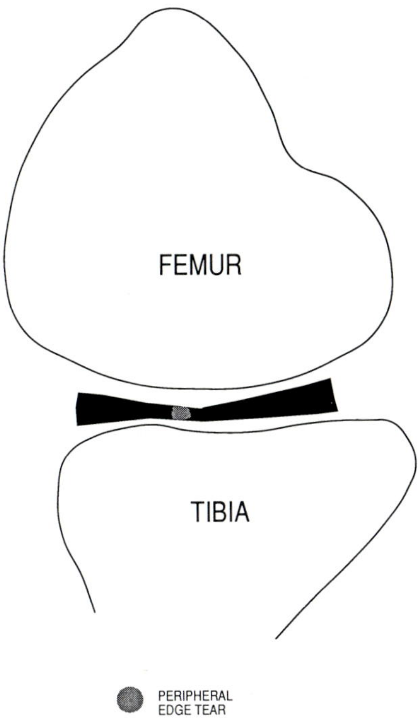

FIGURE 8-2

CASE 9

Differential Diagnosis of Meniscal Tear

HISTORY: A 43-year-old man reported medial knee pain for one month after sustaining a twisting injury during a tennis match. What is the MRI diagnosis? Is a meniscal body tear or myxoid signal change present? Identify the structures indicated by the arrows in Fig. 9-1. (Figs. 9-1 and 9-2: sagittal and coronal proton-density images, TR/TE 1,200/20 msec.)

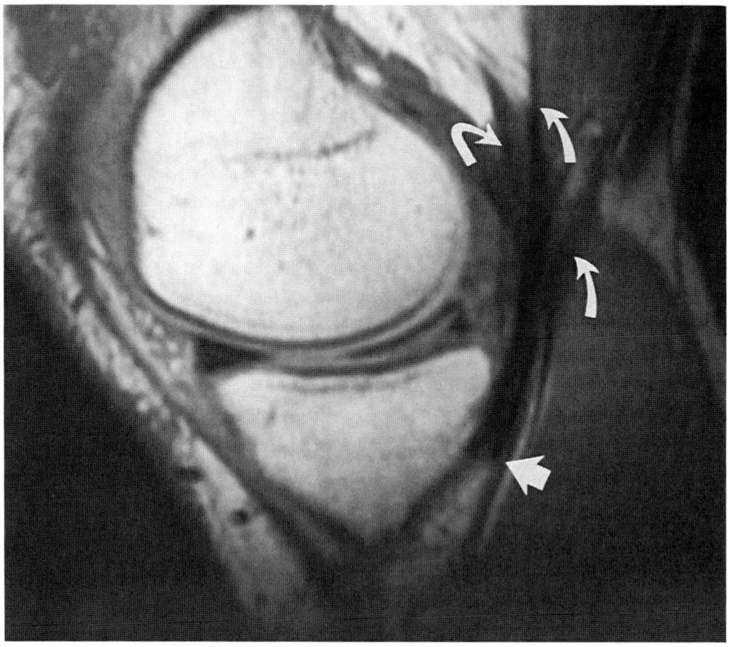

FIGURE 9-1

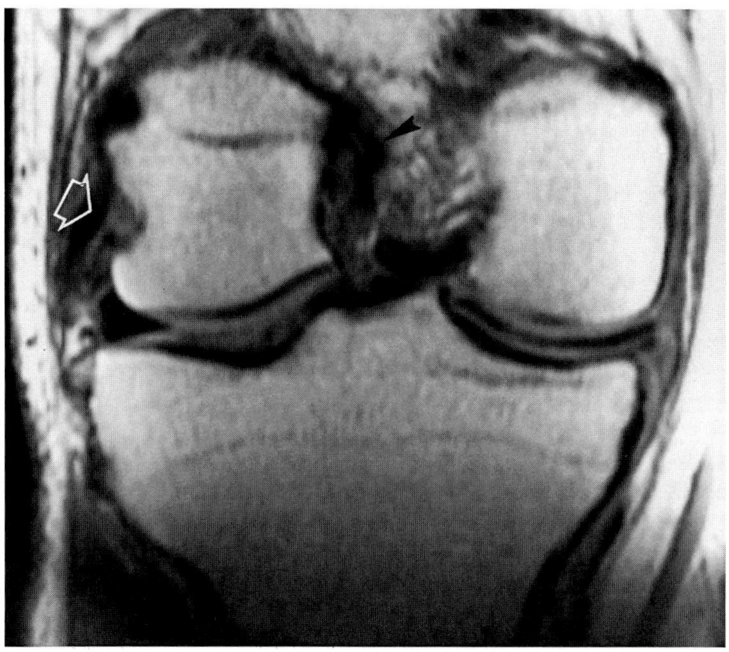

FIGURE 9-2

DISCUSSION: The posterior body of the medial meniscus has an oblique area of intermediate signal intensity with several features inconsistent with simple myxoid intrameniscal signal change: (1) the signal is too bright, (2) it does not have a horizontal Y or fork shape associated with it (see Case 7), (3) it is oblique rather than horizontal, and (4) it is contiguous with the tibial articular surface in the sagittal and coronal planes. Localization of this true peripheral tear to the medial meniscus can be inferred by identifying the components of the pes anserinus complex (arrows in Fig. 9-1): the combined insertions of the tendinous expansions of the semitendinosus, gracilis, and sartorius muscles. The medial location is also confirmed by visualization of the fibular collateral ligament (open arrow in Fig. 9-2) arising from the lateral femoral condylar protuberance, and the linear (arrowhead in Fig. 9-2) and laterally positioned anterior cruciate ligament. The anterior cruciate ligament has a more globular and gray signal in this patient due to hematoma and edema in its sheath from recent injury.

DIAGNOSIS: The patient has an oblique medial meniscal body and posterior horn edge tear with anterior cruciate ligament injury.

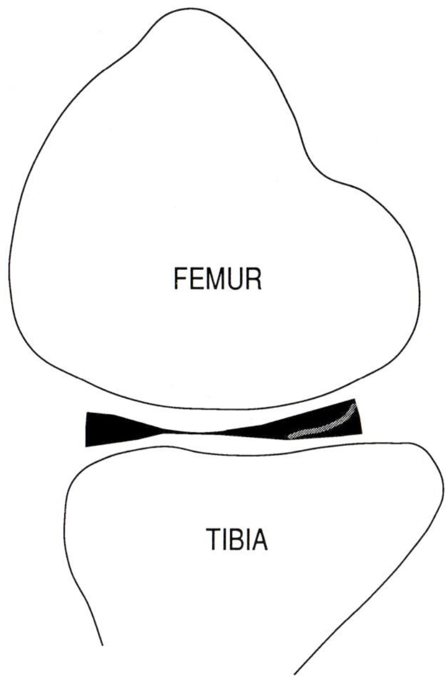

FIGURE 9-3

CASE 10

Differential Diagnosis of Anterior Knee Pain

HISTORY: A 17-year-old patient sustained acute anterior knee pain after a fall while playing basketball. Does MRI show a true tear or pseudotear? (Fig. 10-1: sagittal proton-density image, TR/TE 1,400/20 msec, 14.0-cm FOV, 128 × 256 pixel matrix, 3.0-mm sections, 2 excitations.)

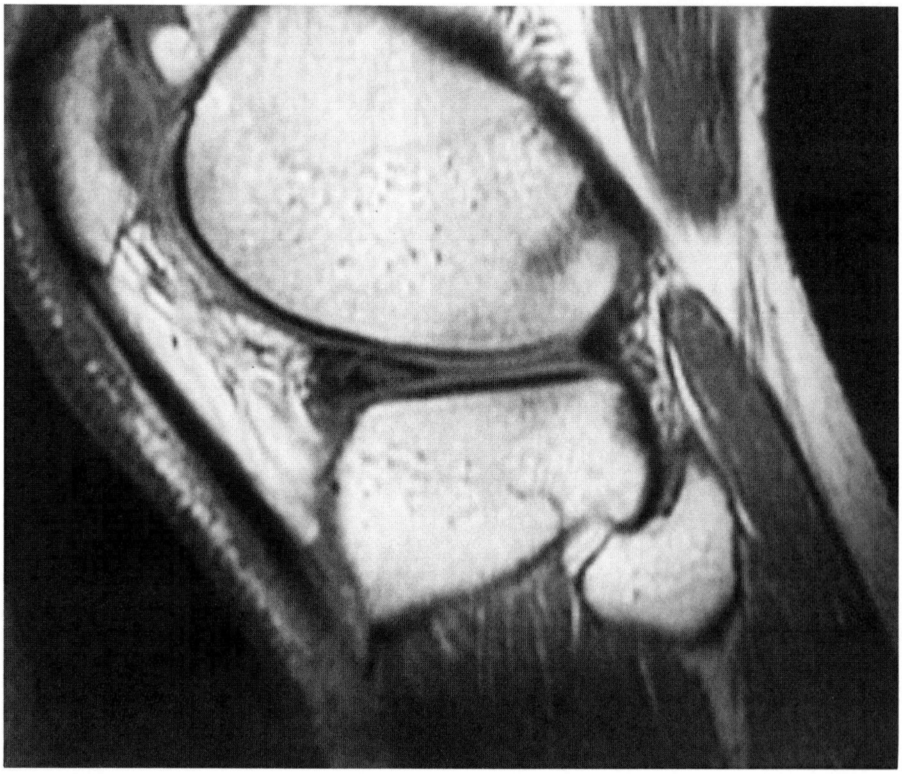

FIGURE 10-1

DISCUSSION: This case illustrates both a real and a false finding. The real finding consists of the confluent signal in the anterior body of the lateral meniscus (see drawing, Fig. 10-2) that represents lateral meniscal body tear. True tears of the anterior horn of the lateral meniscus occur in fewer than 1 in 150 tears. Also, note that the posterior aspect of the meniscus is truncated along its anterior margin.

Anterior to the meniscal complex and in front of the tear is the transverse meniscal ligament, separated from the true meniscus by an oblique line. This interface represents areas of potential bursal reflection that can accumulate fluid, giving the appearance of a tear.

In summary, both a pseudotear and a true tear exist.

DIAGNOSIS: MRI shows a lateral meniscal body tear with anterior body extension adjacent to a pitfall of the transverse ligament.

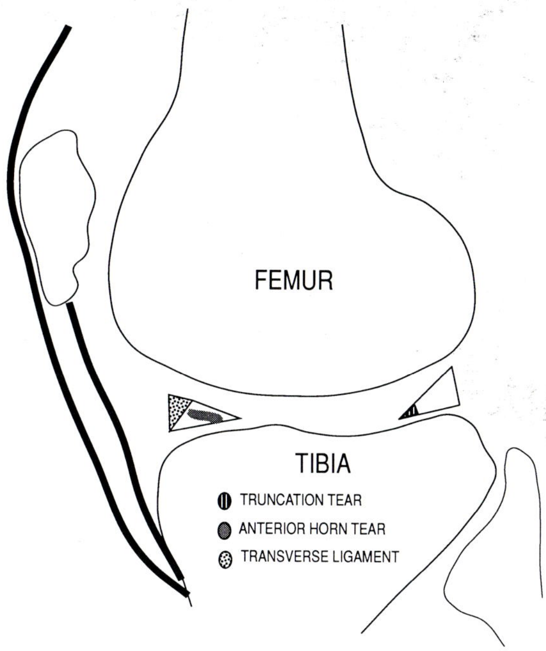

FIGURE 10-2

CASE 11

Differential Diagnosis of Chronic Anterior Knee Pain

HISTORY: A 31-year-old ballet dancer reported chronic anterior knee pain. What is the MRI diagnosis? (Fig. 11-1: Sagittal proton-density MRI, TR/TE 1,400/20 msec, 14.0-cm FOV, 256 × 126 pixel matrix, 3.0-mm sections, 2 excitations.)

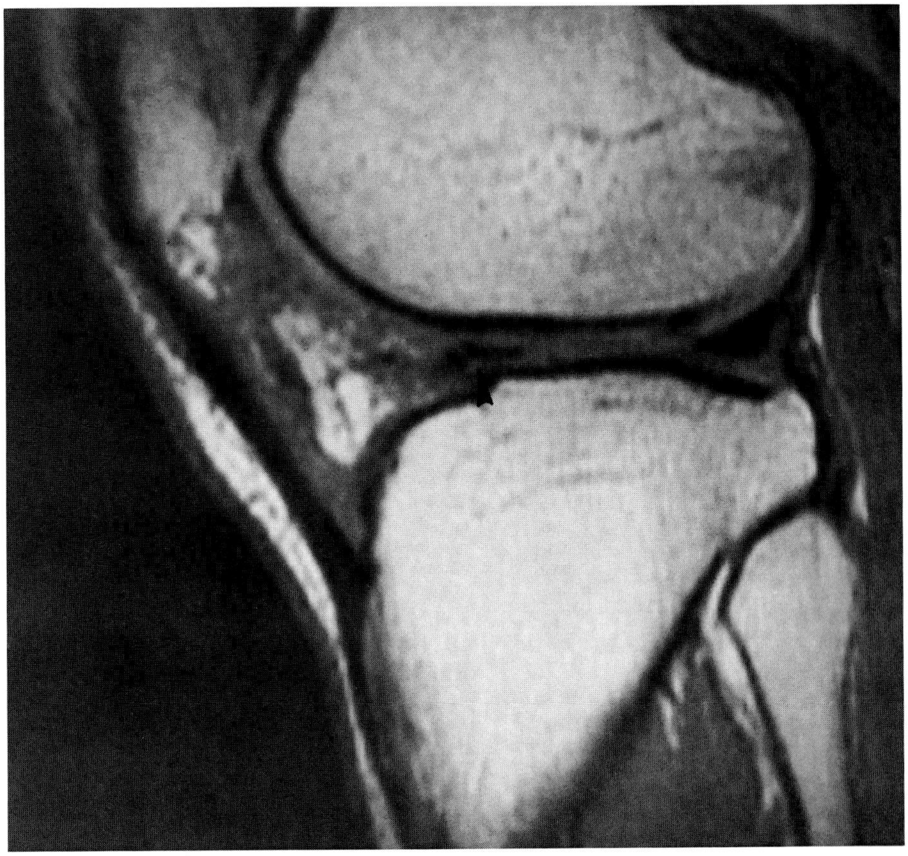

FIGURE 11-1

DISCUSSION: The anterior horn and anterior body of the lateral meniscus are barely visible and have been previously resected. A faint oblique linear area of intermediate signal intensity courses through the residual meniscal tissue (arrowhead), compatible with tear in the meniscal remnant. The signal of the intrapatellar fat has been completely replaced by intermediate signal intensity, and no Hoffa fat is visible in this section. The patient has undergone a partial Hoffa fat pad resection; subsequent fibrosis and fat necrosis in this region produced the current appearance.

DIAGNOSIS: The patient has previously undergone anterior meniscal body and anterior lateral horn resection with partial resection of the Hoffa fat pad. A tear is present in the residual remnant of the anterolateral meniscus. Fibrosis is present in the area of the Hoffa fat pad resection.

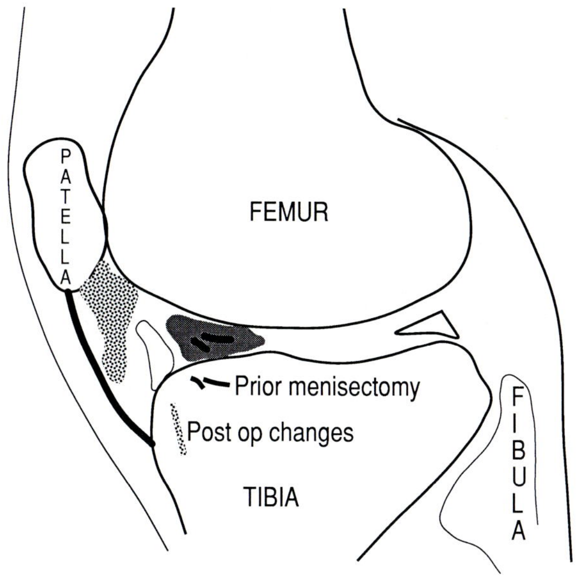

FIGURE 11-2

CASE 12

Differential Diagnosis of Chronic Knee Pain

HISTORY: A 36-year-old woman with known rheumatoid arthritis reported chronic knee pain. What is the MRI diagnosis? (Figs. 12-1*A* and *B*: sagittal multiformat contiguous fast scan images, TR/TE 1,000/15 msec, 18.0-cm FOV, 192 × 256 pixel matrix, 4.0-mm sections, 2 excitations. Fig. 12-2: coronal proton-density image, TR/TE 1,000/20 msec, 14.0-cm FOV, 128 × 256 pixel matrix, 4.0-mm sections, 2 excitations.)

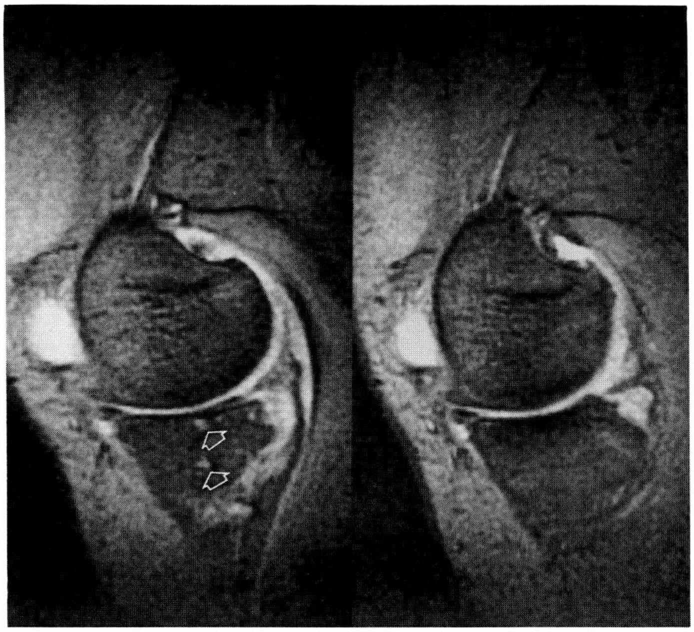

A **B**

FIGURE 12-1

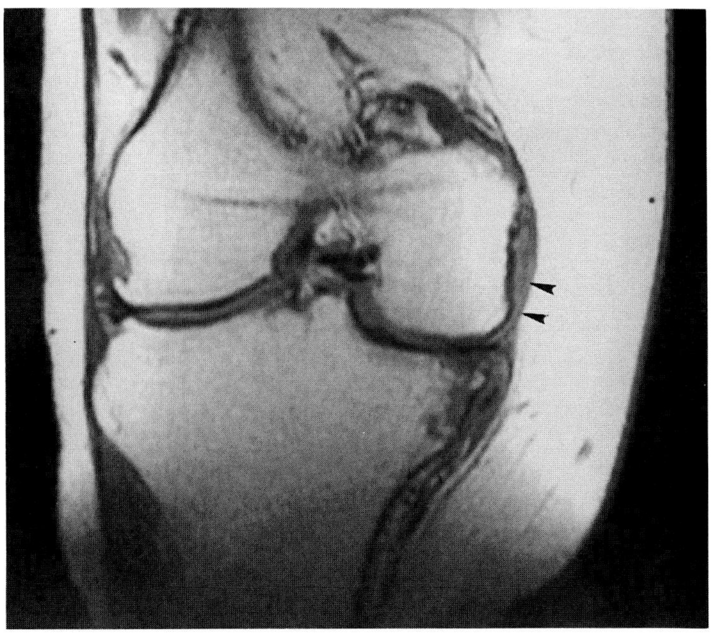

FIGURE 12-2

DISCUSSION: Extremely small menisci are present in the sagittal views, which raises the possibility of meniscectomy or bucket-handle tear. The patient has known systemic arthropathy. The cartilage pads and synovium appear redundant, with joint effusion and synovial thickening, especially posteriorly in the sagittal views. Pannus formation has involved the subchondral bone, seen as hyperintense intramedullary signal (arrows in Fig. 12-1*B*) in the tibia in the sagittal plane and as hypointense signal in the coronal view medially. The capsule is markedly thickened in the coronal projection (arrowheads in Fig. 12-2). Capsular thickening is diagnosed when the hyperintense fat pad just medial to the joint line is replaced by intermediate signal intensity. In addition to meniscectomy and a bucket-handle tear, other causes of small menisci include osteoarthritis, rheumatoid arthritis, juvenile rheumatoid arthritis, relapsing polychondritis, and mixed connective tissue disease.

DIAGNOSIS: The patient has rheumatoid arthritis with small menisci.

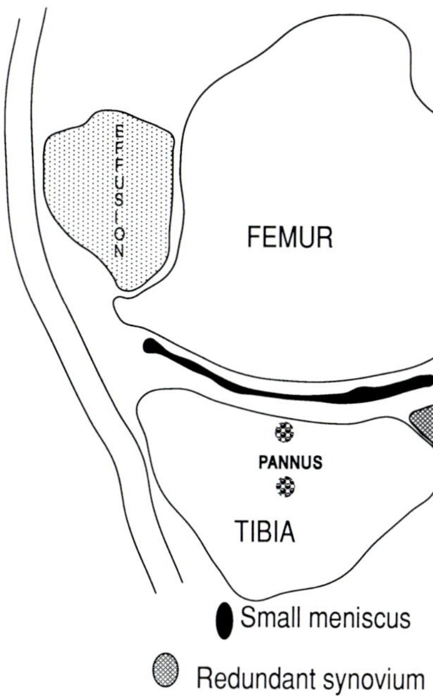

FIGURE 12-3

CASE 13

Differential Diagnosis of Meniscal Tear and Anterior Knee Pain

HISTORY: A 19-year-old soccer player who sustained a varus hyperextension injury during play complained of intermittent locking of the knee and pain for 3 months. Without the aid of arrows, identify four findings in this case. (Fig. 13-1: sagittal proton-density image, TR/TE 1,200/20 msec.)

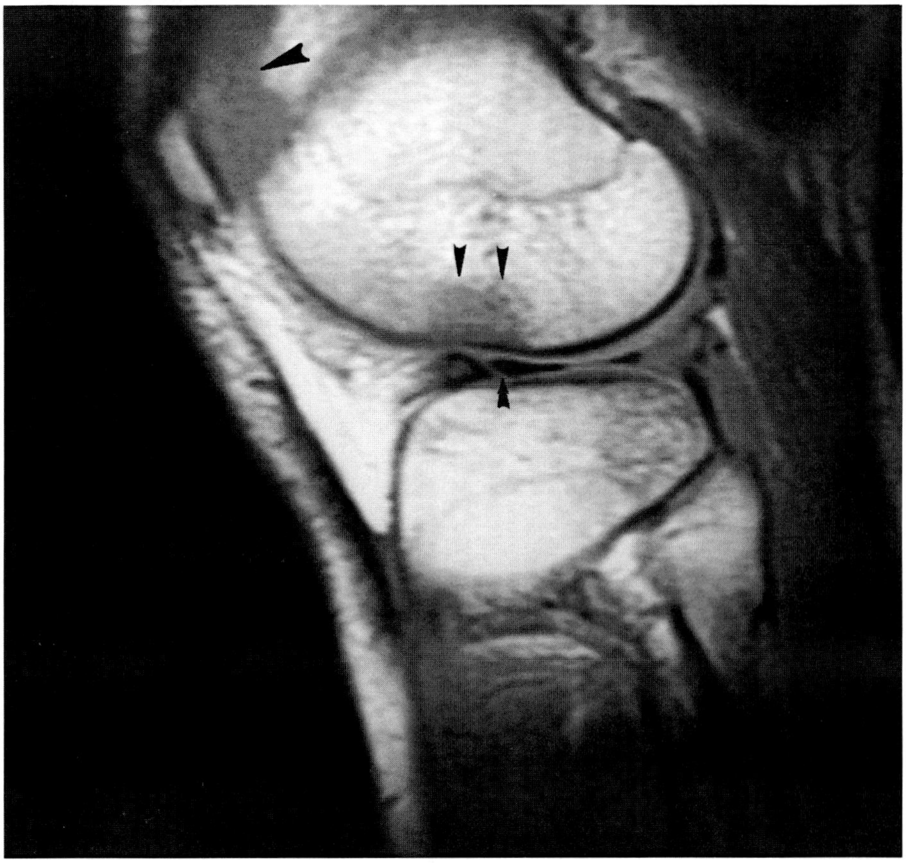

FIGURE 13-1

DISCUSSION

1. The retropatellar bursa is filled with intermediate signal intensity blood-tinged fluid (large arrowhead).
2. A moderately marginated area of decreased signal intensity is apparent along the subchondral surface of the lateral femoral condyle (arrowheads). This is the most common site of bone bruise in the knee following sports-related knee trauma. There is normally a small notch or dip in the anterolateral femoral condyle in this location that may predispose to bone contusion. Normally this area exhibits barely perceptible signal hypointensity on T1-weighted or proton-density images; however, the signal change is too pronounced in this case to be normal.
3. Similarly, the posterosuperior aspect of the tibial plateau exhibits diminished signal intensity due to direct contusion from an axial loading force of the femur against its surface during varus stress. Directly craniad to the posterior tibial plateau, the popliteus reflection is filled with intermediate signal intensity blood-tinged fluid. The posterolateral meniscus appears extremely small.
4. The most significant finding is the diminutive posterior body of the lateral meniscus and a sequestered area of hypointense signal containing a gray spot in its center. This area is separated from the anterior meniscal body by a thin vertical line (small arrowhead) and lies directly beneath the femoral bone injury. Although the appearance resembles that of the transverse meniscal ligament complex, the hypointense area is too large, and, coupled with the small posterior segment, is compatible with a sequestered meniscal fragment. This variant of the bucket-handle tear is actually a rip in the posterior meniscus that has folded over on itself anteriorly, a free fragment. The terms "folded-fragment sign" or "folded meniscal tear" describe its appearance in the sagittal projection.

DIAGNOSIS: The patient has joint hemarthrosis with femoral and tibial bone contusions and a folded-fragment lateral meniscal tear.

CASE 14

Differential Diagnosis of Meniscal Tear

HISTORY: A 47-year-old woman who had sustained a skiing injury presented with intermittent locking of the knee. (Figs. 14-1*A* and *B*: sagittal proton-density images; Figs. 14-2*A* and *B*: coronal proton-density images; TR/TE 1,200/20 msec.)

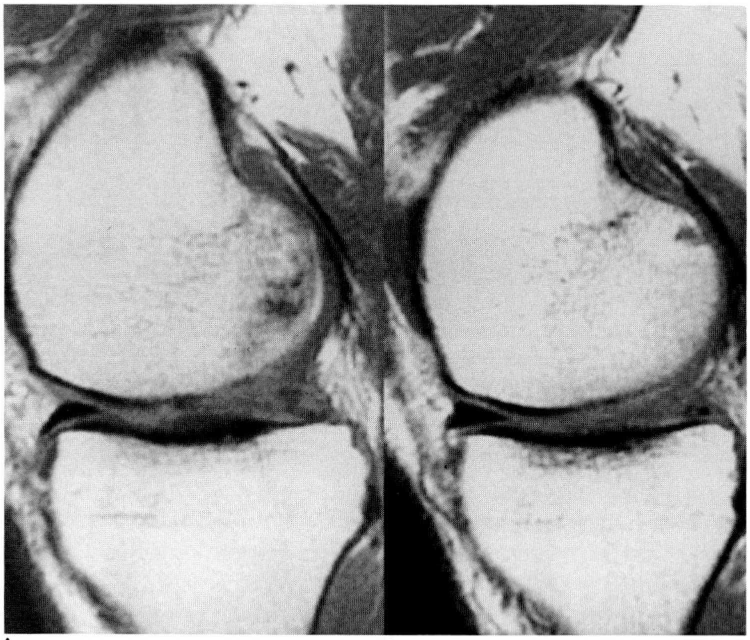

A **B**

FIGURE 14-1

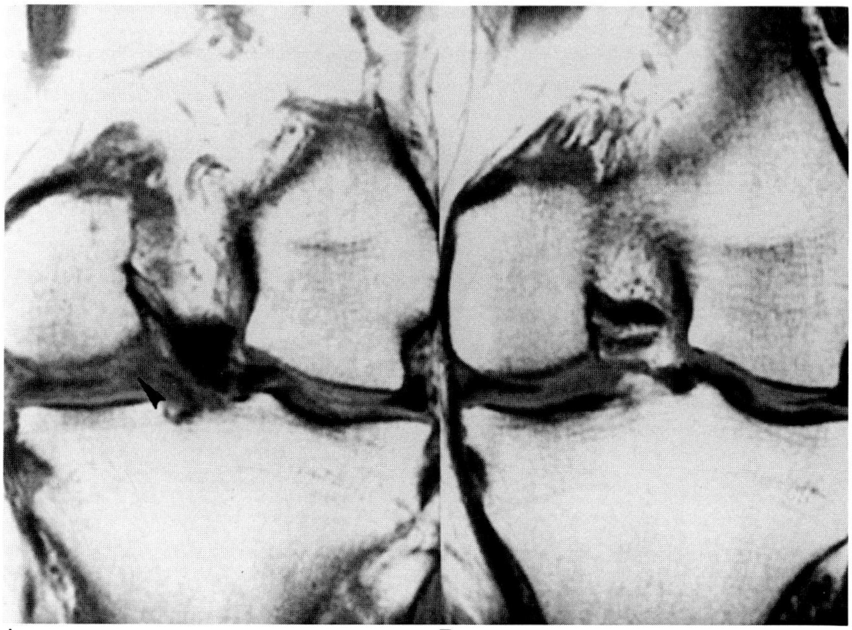

A **B**

FIGURE 14-2

DISCUSSION: A bucket-handle tear in the meniscus (see Fig. 14-3) leaves a gaping hole in the meniscus that is filled with fluid or blood. The inner edge of the meniscus may migrate deeper into the knee and may be identified on MRI if it is of reasonable size. Sagittal sections through the portion of the meniscus that is not torn may show meniscal truncation, small size, and bizarre shape, but might not demonstrate signal alteration. A sagittal section obtained directly through the gap or tear will show only the signal of proteinaceous or hemorrhagic fluid and not the hypointense meniscal triangle. This is true of the posteromedial horn in this case (Fig. 14-1). The site of truncation is identified in the coronal plane (arrowhead in Fig. 14-2*A*), and it is through this location that the sagittal projection was obtained. A free, hypointense meniscal piece in the notch of the knee is not visible.

DIAGNOSIS: The patient has a bucket-handle tear of the inner edge of the posterior horn of the medial meniscus.

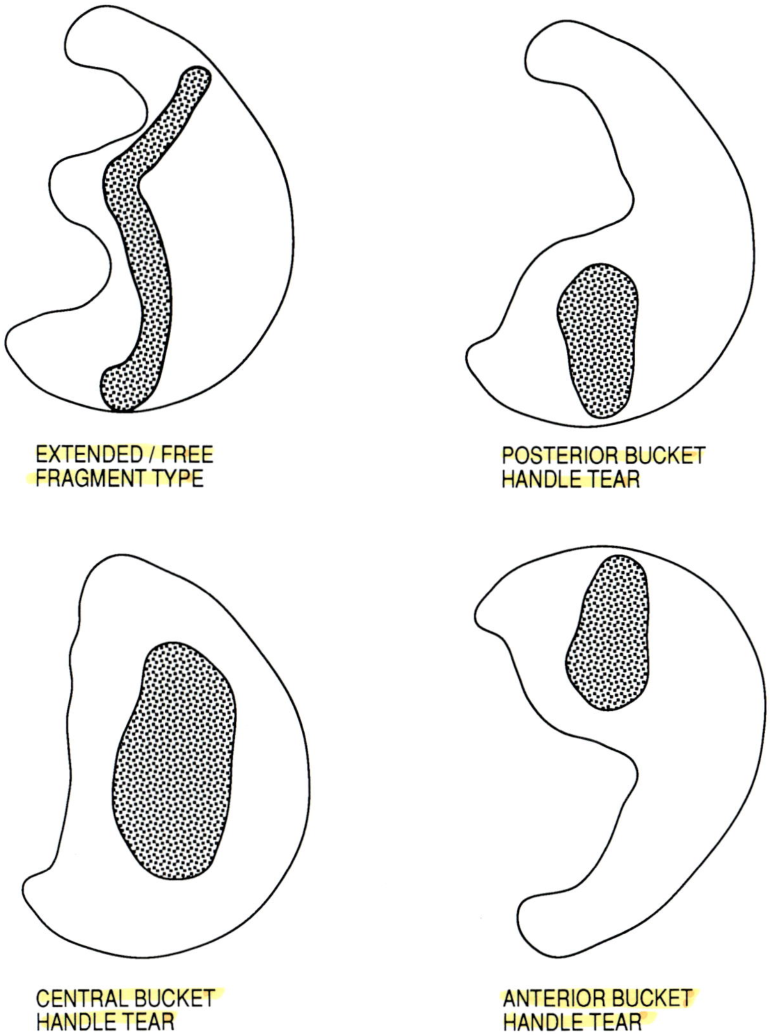

FIGURE 14-3

CASE 15

Differential Diagnosis of Acute Knee Pain

HISTORY: A 25-year-old man sustained left knee trauma in a motorcycle accident. MRI shows a bucket-handle medial meniscus tear, a partial anterior cruciate ligament tear, and a large joint effusion. What is the underlying condition? (Fig. 15-1: sagittal multiecho proton-density (*A*) and T2-weighted (*B*) images, TR/TE 1,400/20, 80 msec. Fig. 15-2: coronal, and Fig. 15-3: sagittal proton-density images, TR/TE 1,100/20 msec. FOV = 14.0 cm, 192 × 256 pixel matrix, 4.0-mm section thickness.)

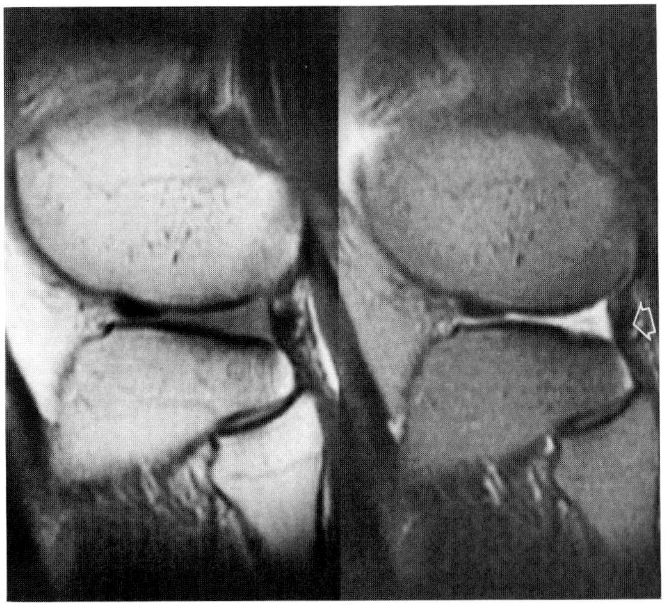

A B

FIGURE 15-1

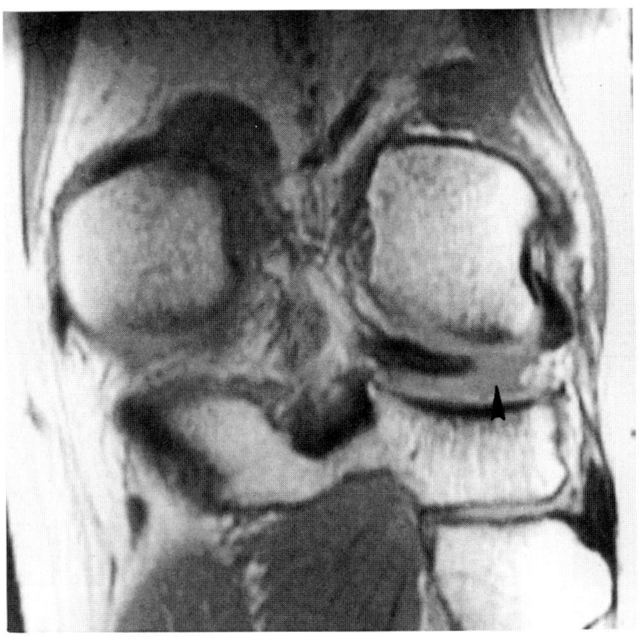

FIGURE 15-2

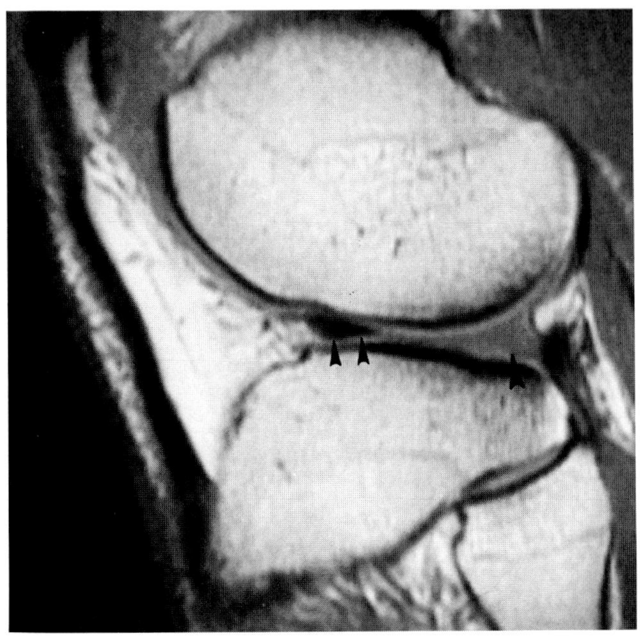

FIGURE 15-3

DISCUSSION: The sagittal images are obtained through the lateral meniscus posterior and anterior body/horn junction. The entire posteromid- and posterior horn is replaced by water-intensity signal. One possibility is complete avulsion of the meniscus and its replacement by fluid or edema. An alternative consideration is prior meniscectomy; however, this patient has definitely not had meniscectomy. The final and least common possibility is congenital hypoplasia or absence of the posterior horn and body of the lateral meniscus. This is an unusual condition, occurring in fewer than one in 1,600 cases, and this is the only case we have observed in over 10,000 MRI studies of the knee. Suspicion that this is not a meniscal tear is raised by the fact that there is no accompanying bone injury, cartilaginous injury, meniscal fragmentation, or loose body. In fact, the surrounding tissues are normal. Bone or cartilage injuries, including bruises, accompany as many as 60% of meniscal tears.

The intrameniscal signal is homogeneous, a finding militating against trauma. The remaining popliteus tendon is identified (clear arrow in Fig. 15-1*B*). The area of incomplete hypoplasia is demonstrated in the coronal and sagittal views (arrowhead in Fig. 15-2). The sagittal view confirms the presence of a hypointense intact triangular lateral anterior meniscal horn and body (arrowheads in Fig. 15-3).

DIAGNOSIS: The patient has congenital absence of the posterolateral meniscus.

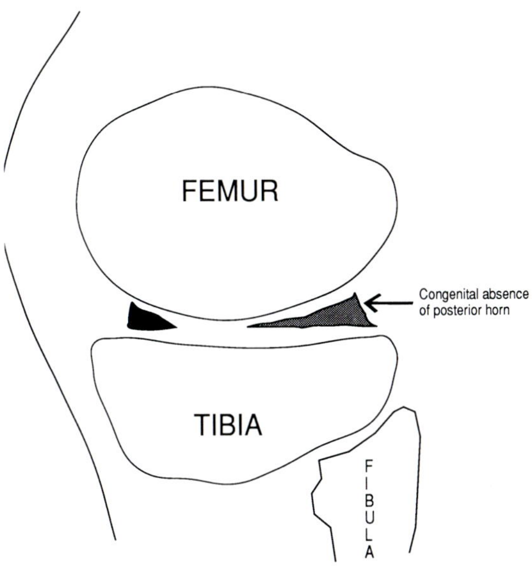

FIGURE 15-4

CASE 16

Differential Diagnosis of Meniscal Tear

HISTORY: A 28-year-old man presented with lateral knee pain 1 year after knee surgery. What are the MRI findings? (Fig. 16-1: sagittal multiecho proton-density MRI. Fig. 16-2: sagittal multiecho T2-weighted MRI.)

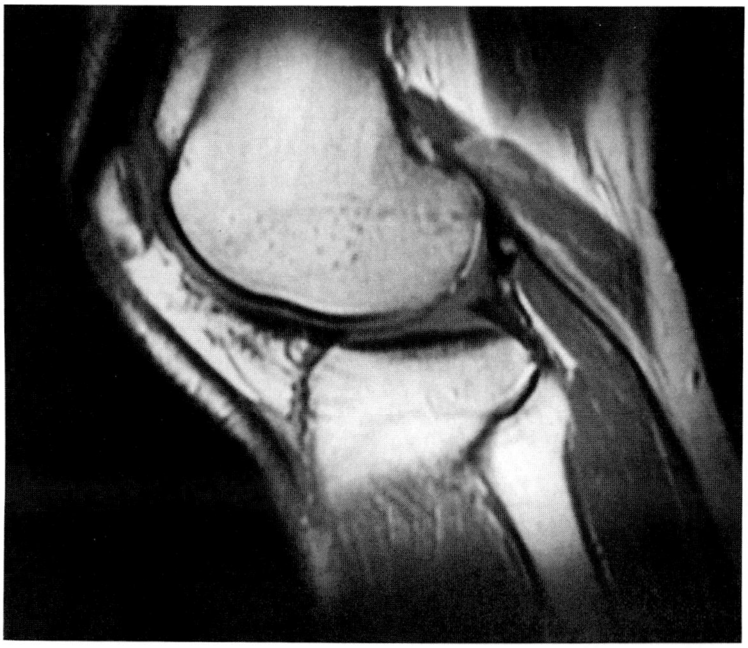

FIGURE 16-1

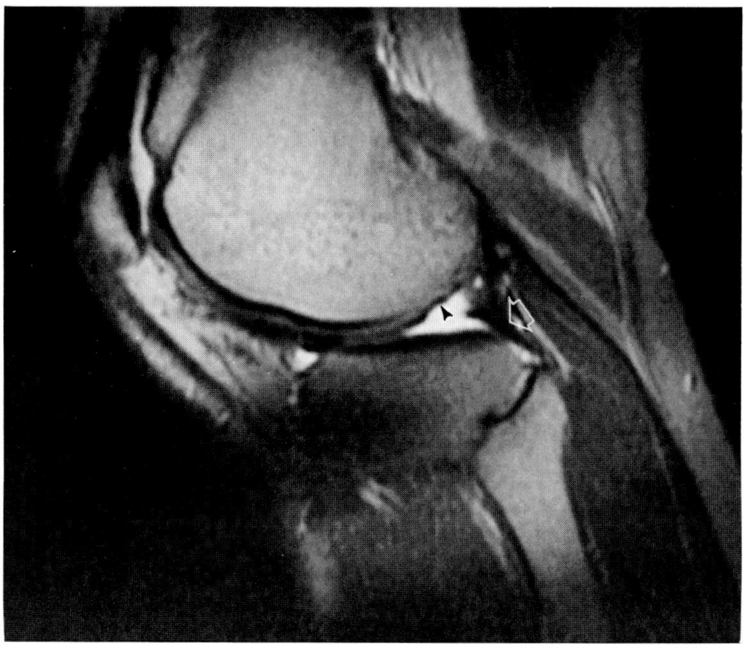

FIGURE 16-2

DISCUSSION: The homogeneous intermediate signal on the proton-density image and the hyperintense signal on the T2-weighted image replace the posterior aspect of the lateral meniscal body and posterior horn in these sagittal images. Such homogeneous bright signal can only be produced by meniscectomy or congenital absence of the posterior meniscal body and posterior horn. Bucket-handle tears are inhomogeneous and are often associated with bone (>50%) or ligamentous (>30%) injury. The hypointense popliteus tendon is demonstrable (open arrow in Fig. 16-2) and should not be mistaken for residual meniscal tissue. The posterior femoral condylar hyaline cartilage appears attenuated (arrowhead in Fig. 16-2). This finding accounts for the patient's symptoms. Because this ulcer is broad and deep but spares the underlying bone, it pathologically corresponds to a grade III ulcer, according to the classification of Outerbridge. A small joint effusion is present.

DIAGNOSIS: The patient has undergone prior meniscectomy of the posteromedial meniscus. MRI shows a current joint effusion and a hyaline cartilage ulcer or chondromalacia, grade III.

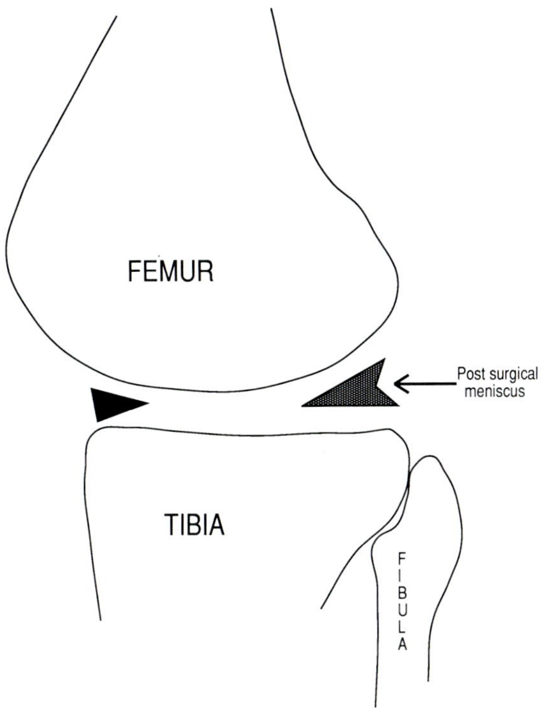

FIGURE 16-3

CASE 17

Differential Diagnosis of Acute Knee Pain

HISTORY: A 35-year-old woman sought medical attention after twisting her knee during a tennis match. What is the MRI diagnosis? (Figs. 17-1*A–D*: coronal (four-on-one) proton-density images, TR/TE 1,000/20 msec, 14.0-cm FOV, 128 × 256 pixel matrix, 3.0-mm sections, 2 excitations.)

A B

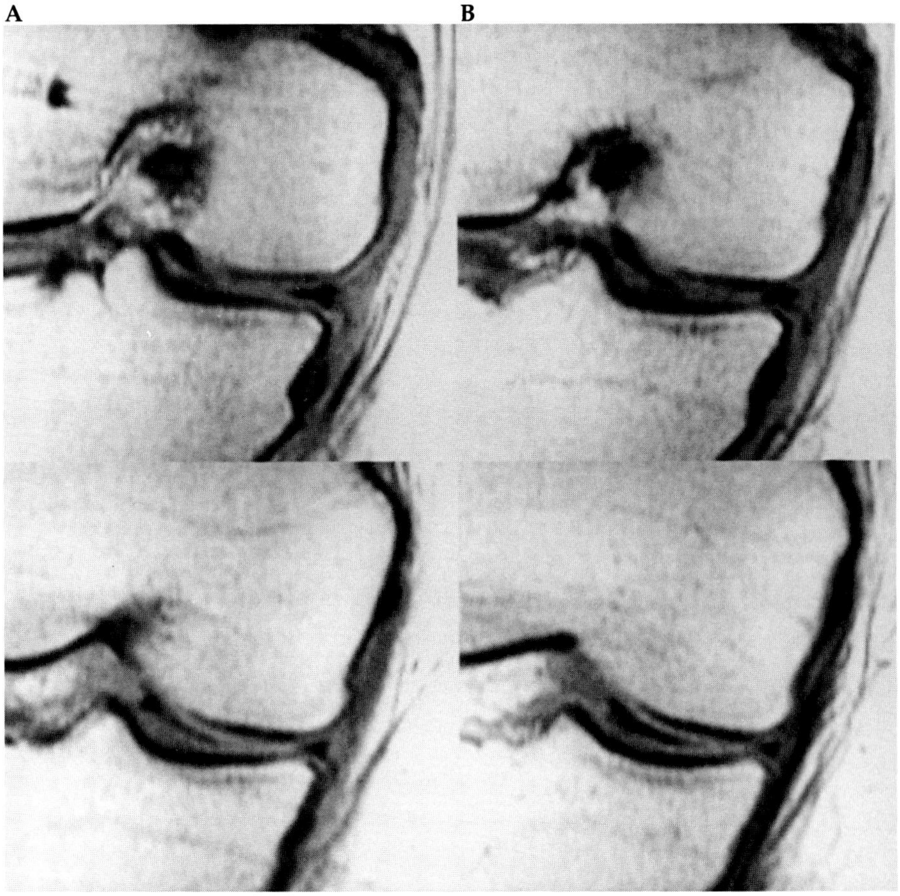

C D

FIGURE 17-1

DISCUSSION: The contiguous coronal images show separation of the medial meniscus, with a peripheral hypointense triangular fragment separated from a deeper and more lateral hypointense triangular fragment. The separation is diagramed in Figure 17-2. The more peripheral of the fragments is quite small, which suggests a bucket-handle tear. Signs of bucket-handle tear and the views that best show these signs are as follows:

1. small size (sagittal or coronal),
2. bizarre shape (sagittal),
3. truncation (sagittal),
4. persistent separation of fragments (coronal),
5. hypointense free fragment (coronal),
6. total absence of normal hypointense meniscal signal (sagittal).

DIAGNOSIS: The patient has a bucket-handle tear of the medial meniscus.

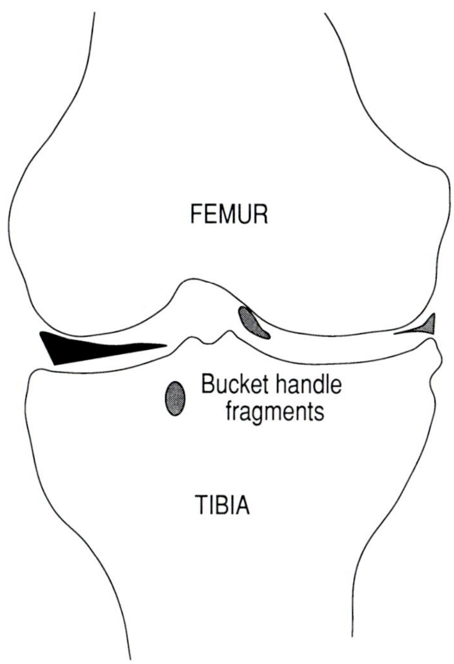

FIGURE 17-2

CASE 18

Differential Diagnosis of Meniscal Tear

HISTORY: A 41-year-old woman described a sensation of fullness along the lateral joint line. What is the MRI diagnosis? (Figs. 18-1*A* and *B*: coronal multiformat radial fast scan images (gradient recalled free induction decay), TR/TE 400/12 msec, 15° flip angle, 4.0-mm, 18.0-cm FOV, 256 × 192 pixel matrix, 2 excitations.)

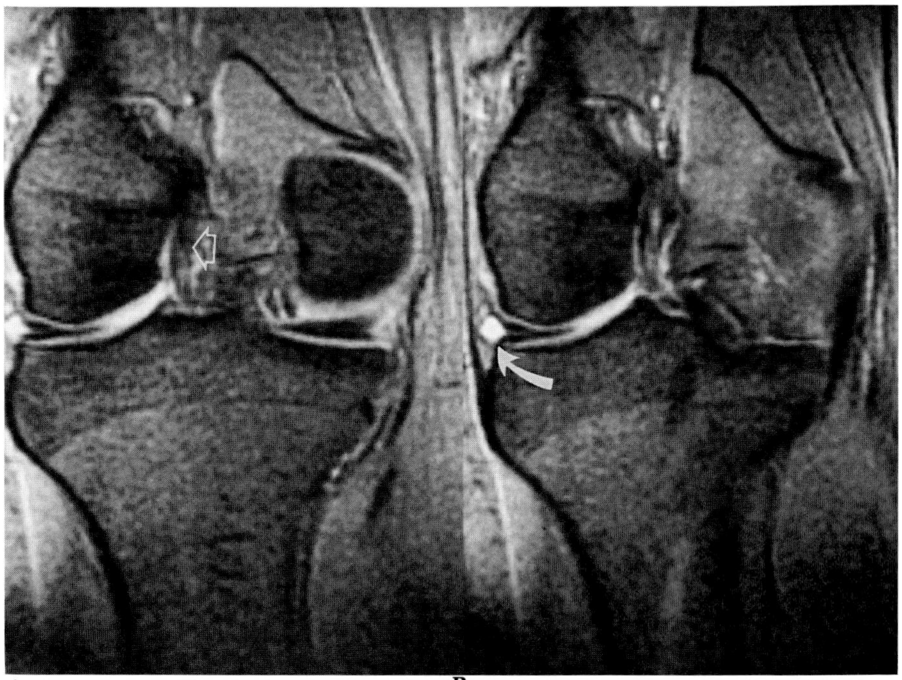

FIGURE 18-1

DISCUSSION: Fast scan images are used to display the relationship of subtle meniscal pathology to the meniscal surface and to highlight the hyperintense signal of masses, particularly cystic masses, about the knee. These images are obtained in the orthogonal projection with contiguous sections. They can also be obtained in radial fashion, like the spokes of a wheel plotted around and perpendicular to the meniscus, which theoretically makes identification of articular surface communication of meniscal signal easier. We use radial sections only in selected difficult cases.

In this case, a section tangent to the hyperintense 1.0-cm mass clarifies the relationship of the area of homogeneous bright signal intensity to the lateral meniscal body. A thin, hyperintense line that is barely perceptible traverses the lateral meniscus, terminating as a small homogenous signal alteration (curved arrow in *B*). This view shows the typical appearance, size, and location of a lateral meniscal cyst, commonly associated with a horizontal degenerative split tear. Meniscal cysts tend to be smaller on the lateral side of the knee and more often symptomatic. The lateral compartment of the knee is identified by the anterior cruciate ligament (clear arrow in *A*).

DIAGNOSIS: The patient has a lateral meniscal cyst with horizontal meniscal tear.

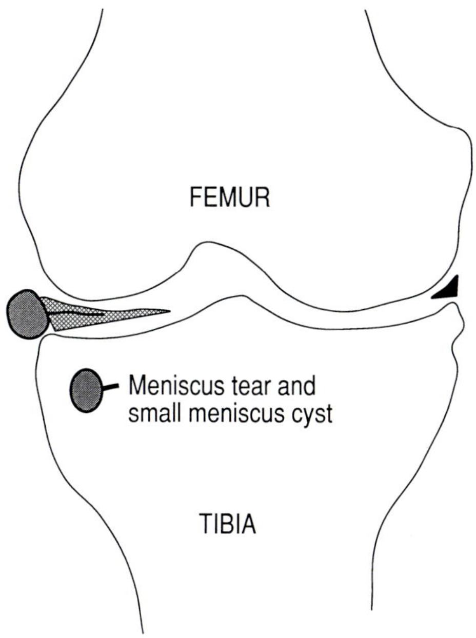

FIGURE 18-2

CASE 19

Differential Diagnosis of Meniscal Tear

HISTORY: A 41-year-old woman described a sensation of fullness along the lateral joint line. What is the MRI diagnosis? (Figs. 19-1*A* and *B*: coronal multiformat (two-on-one) radial fast scan images (gradient recalled free induction decay), TR/TE 400/12 msec 15° flip angle, 4.0-mm sections, 18.0-cm FOV, 256 × 192 pixel matrix, 2 excitations.)

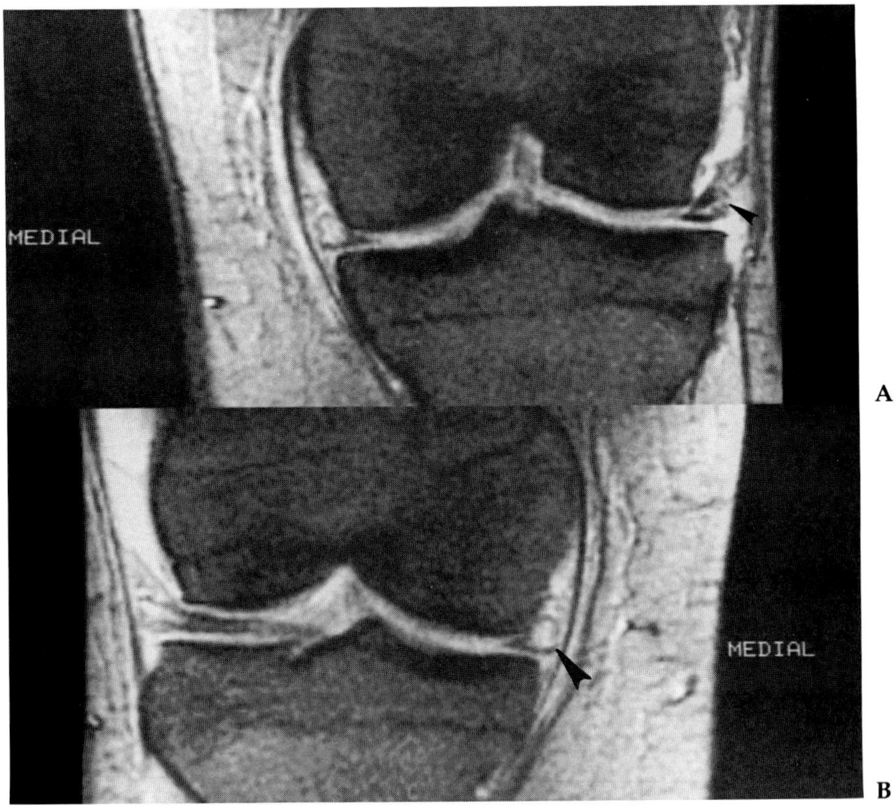

FIGURE 19-1

DISCUSSION: These two fast scan images were obtained in the radial mode, then flipped horizontally with respect to each other. The angle of the coronal slice is slightly different between *A* and *B*. *A* is an orthogonal coronal section; *B* is a paracoronal or 7° oblique coronal section. The lateral side of the knee is identified by the straight iliotibial hypointense band. The medial side is labeled, and the curved, hypointense tibial collateral complex is apparent. In *A*, a linear hyperintense line communicates with the peripheral capsular surface (arrowhead) as well as the deeper articular surface. In the paracoronal section (*B*) the signal from the lateral meniscus has an entirely different shape. This is the rationale for employing radial sections in the evaluation of meniscal tears: the appearance varies with the section angle. Imaging a meniscus at multiple angles ensures that an accurate pictorial view of the intrameniscal signal shape and its relationship to the articular surface will be obtained.

The bright signal in the medial meniscus (arrowhead in *B*) is rounded, globular, and too pronounced to represent normal myxoid signal change. However, it does not clearly communicate with an articular surface in the images shown. Inspection of adjacent sections and planes in such a case is critical. At surgery the lesion was found to be an intrameniscal cyst.

DIAGNOSIS: The patient has a horizontal tear through the lateral meniscus and a medial intrameniscal cyst.

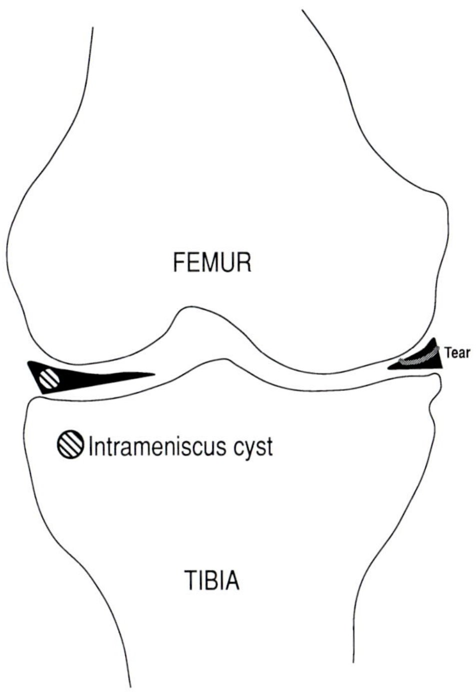

FIGURE 19-2

CASE 20

Differential Diagnosis of Meniscal Tear

HISTORY: A 57-year-old man presented with medial knee pain and crepitus. What is indicated by the arrowheads? (Fig. 20-1: sagittal T1-weighted MRI. Fig. 20-2: lateral radiograph.)

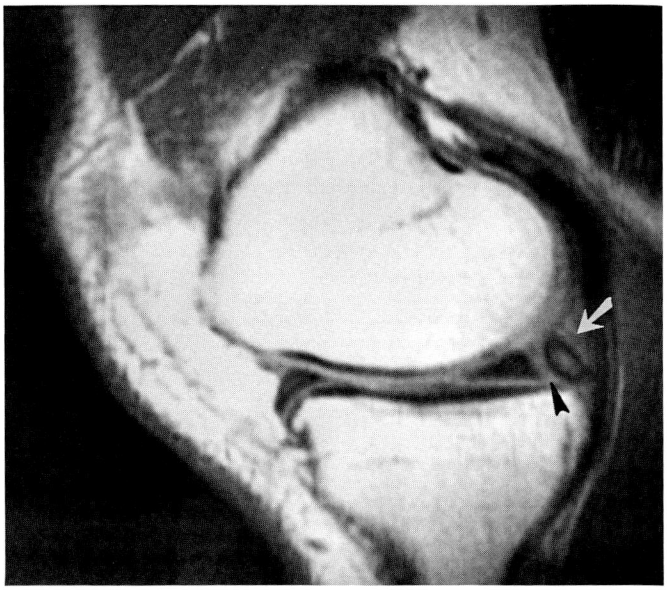

FIGURE 20-1

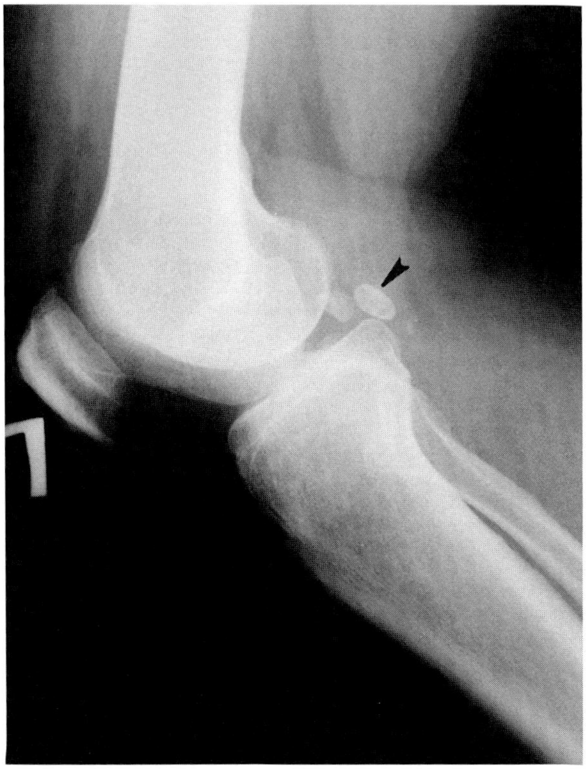

FIGURE 20-2

DISCUSSION: A sagittal section taken from the medial side of the knee shows a separation of intermediate signal intensity (arrowhead in Fig. 20-1) between the posterior meniscal horn and a hypointense area posterior to it. The hypointense area represents a calcific intracapsular loose body (arrowhead in Fig. 20-2) but contains a central nidus of brighter signal intensity than its rim on MRI. Calcification may produce different signal intensities, depending on its origin or content. Cortical bone alone is hypointense on T1 and T2 sequences. Posthemorrhagic calcifications often have hyperintense centers and hypointense rims on both T1- and T2-weighted images. Some calcific fragments may contain medullary bone or yellow marrow and therefore may also have bright signal in their center on T1-weighted images that decreases in intensity on T2-weighted images. This accounts for the signal seen in this loose calcific body, visible with the fabella on the lateral radiograph. Calcification is most easily seen on true T2-weighted images or fast scan images, where it is more hypointense and often surrounded by hyperintense joint fluid. The arrowhead in Figure 20-1 demarcates the posterior joint capsule (its anterior component), which is split by the calcific mass. Another vertical area of intermediate signal intensity represents the remainder (arrow) of the split posterior joint capsule (its posterior component). The importance of obtaining conventional radiographs in interpreting musculoskeletal MR images cannot be overemphasized. Without the conventional radiograph in this case, a misdiagnosis of vertical meniscal tear might have been made.

DIAGNOSIS: The patient has an intraarticular (intracapsular) calcific loose body.

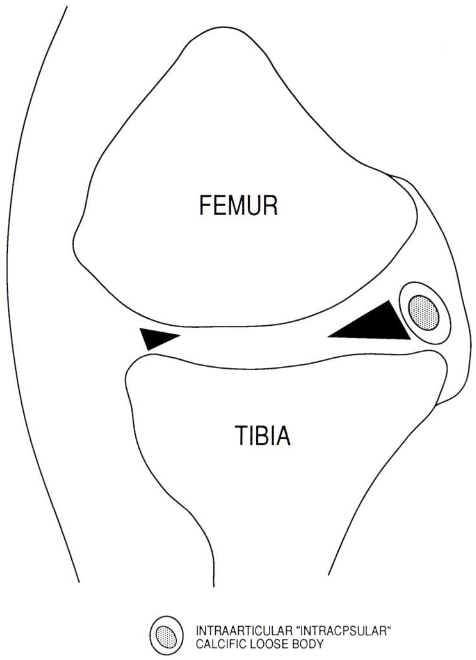

FIGURE 20-3

CASE 21

Differential Diagnosis of Meniscal Disease

HISTORY: A 29-year-old woman described medial knee pain for 7 months after sustaining a varus stress injury. (Figs. 21-1*A* and *B*: contiguous sagittal proton-density images, TR/TE 1,200/20 msec, 3.0-mm sections.)

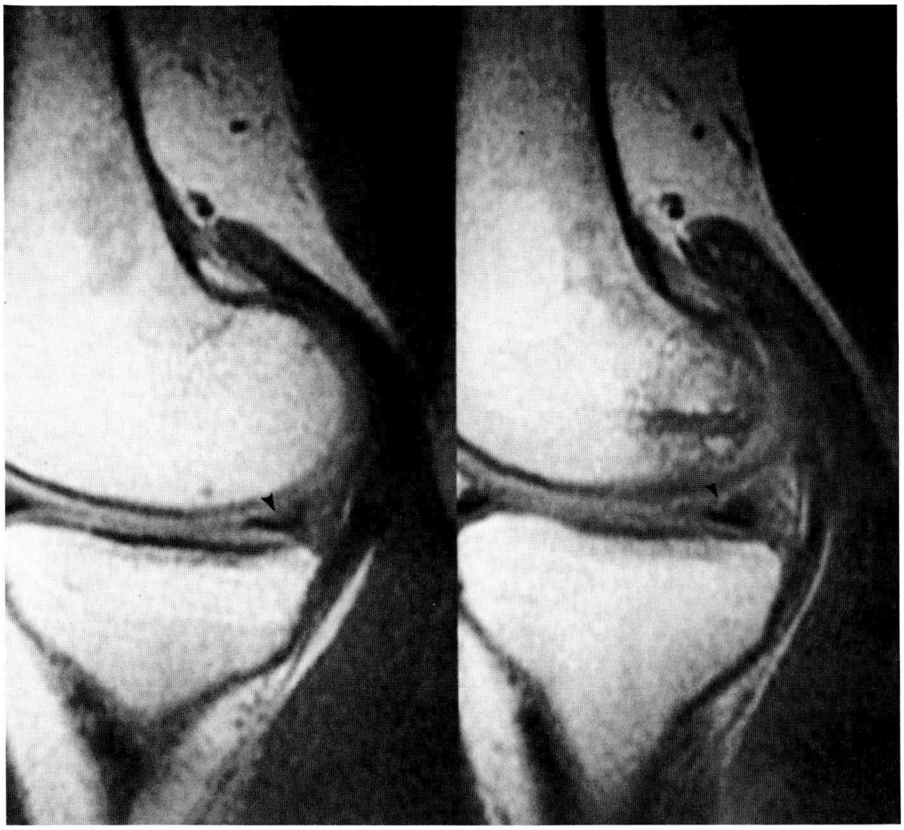

A **B**

FIGURE 21-1

DISCUSSION: The posterior aspect of the body and posterior horn of the medial meniscus demonstrates a short, thick, curved or hook-shaped area of increased signal intensity (arrowhead in *A* and *B*) along its superior articular surface margin on at least two contiguous sagittal sections. This type of tear is more commonly seen in the lateral meniscus at the junction of the posterior horn and meniscal body. These tears are so small that they may be seen on only one sagittal section, but with an FOV of less than 18.0 cm and with 4.0-mm sections or smaller, visualization is unlikely. Most commonly these lesions occur on the inner free edge, as in this case, and have oblique vertical and lateral components. Fast scan gradient-echo/low flip angle imaging may be extremely useful in confirming these tears and differentiating them from volume averaging artifacts. The arthroscopic appearance in the axial projection is reminiscent of a parrot's beak.

DIAGNOSIS: The patient has a parrot beak medial meniscal tear.

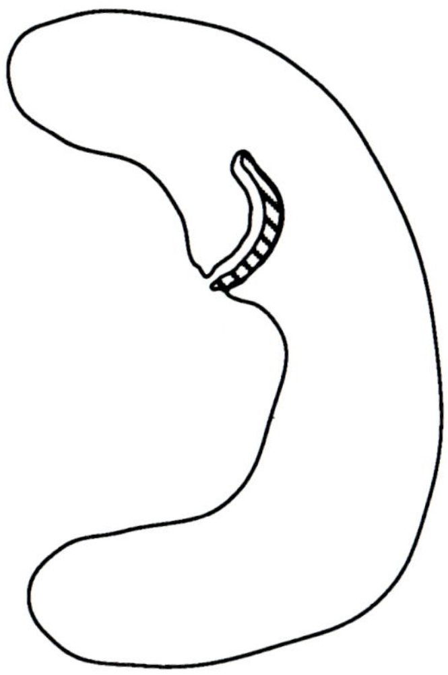

FIGURE 21-2

CASE 22

Differential Diagnosis of Meniscal Disease

HISTORY: A 33-year-old man described medial knee pain following a skiing injury. What is the MRI diagnosis? (Fig. 22-1: sagittal, and Fig. 22-2: coronal multiformat adjacent contiguous 4.0-mm sections, 192 × 256 pixel matrix.)

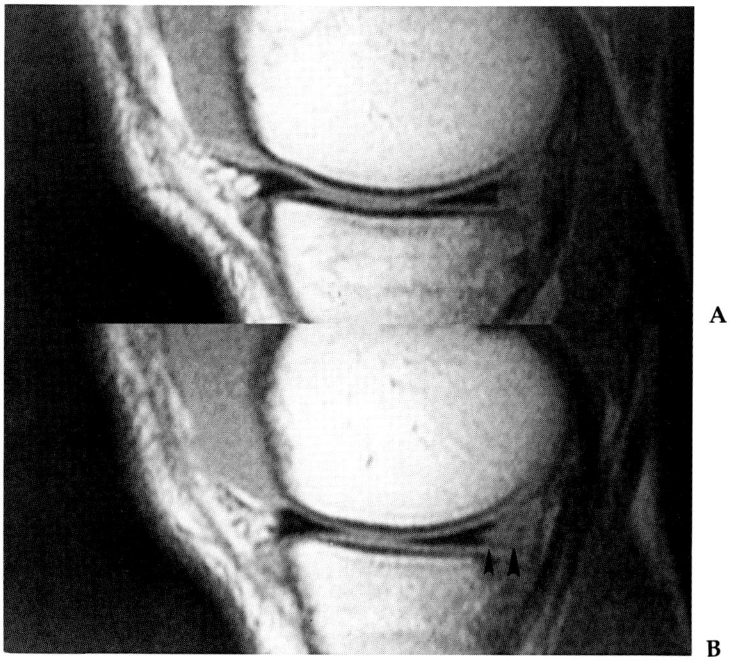

FIGURE 22-1

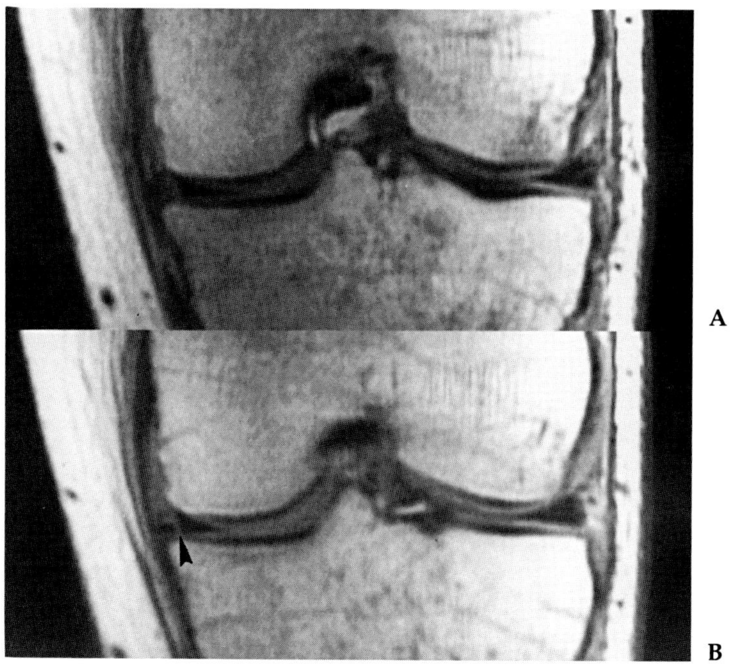

FIGURE 22-2

DISCUSSION: MRI criteria for diagnosing meniscal tears are primarily based on intrameniscal signal alterations or abnormalities in meniscal shape or size, or truncation. Occasionally the meniscus itself remains intact following trauma but separates from its peripheral capsular attachments (arrowheads in Fig. 22-1*B*). Because the medial meniscal capsular attachments are quite tight, detachment along this medial interface may be accompanied by collateral ligamentous injury and frank capsular tear. With capsular tear, arthroscopy may be contraindicated, since the fluid used for joint irrigation may leak from the joint space into soft tissues, producing a compartment syndrome.

Posteriorly, meniscal attachments are somewhat looser than midmedial or meniscal body attachments. When these detach (a form of meniscal tear), as in this case, the posterior meniscal margin becomes malaligned relative to the posterior tibial margin, creating an offset (see Fig. 22-3) of >1.0 cm on serial sections. The posterior and superior medullary signal of the tibial surface, normally bright, is decreased on proton-density or T1-weighted images, owing to intraskeletal edema. This edema appears hyperintense on T2-weighted images. In the coronal projection, a peripheral intrameniscal component to the tear is visible (arrowhead in Fig. 22-2*B*).

DIAGNOSIS: The patient has a medial meniscocapsular separation, with a peripheral midbody meniscal tear and bone contusion.

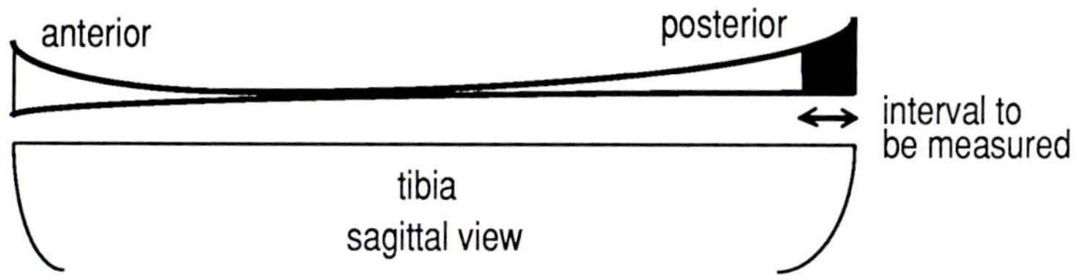

FIGURE 22-3

CASE 23

Differential Diagnosis of Acute Knee Pain

HISTORY: A 17-year-old professional tennis player reported inability to extend her leg and anterior knee pain after sustaining a twisting injury in a match 1 week earlier. Identify the areas or abnormalities designated by arrows and arrowheads in Figures 23-1 and 23-2. (Fig. 23-1: sagittal, and Fig. 23-2: coronal spin-density MR images, TR/TE 1,000/20 msec, 4.0-mm sections, 14.0-cm FOV, 256 × 128 pixel matrix, 2 excitations.

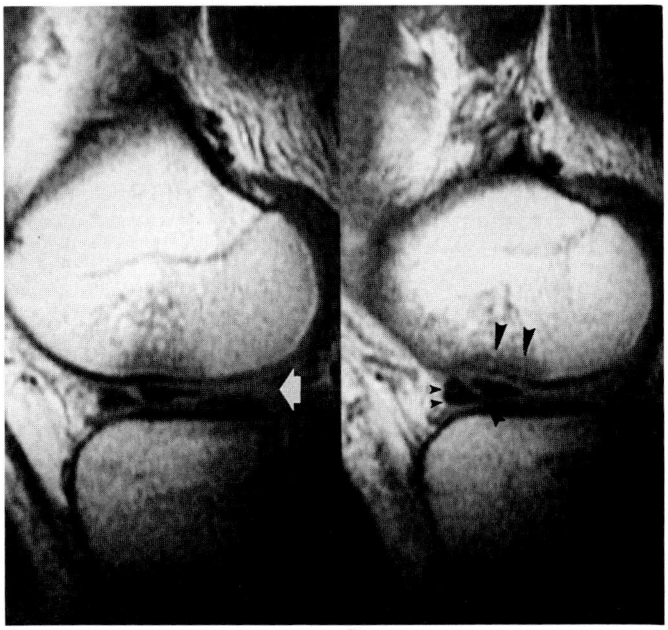

A B

FIGURE 23-1

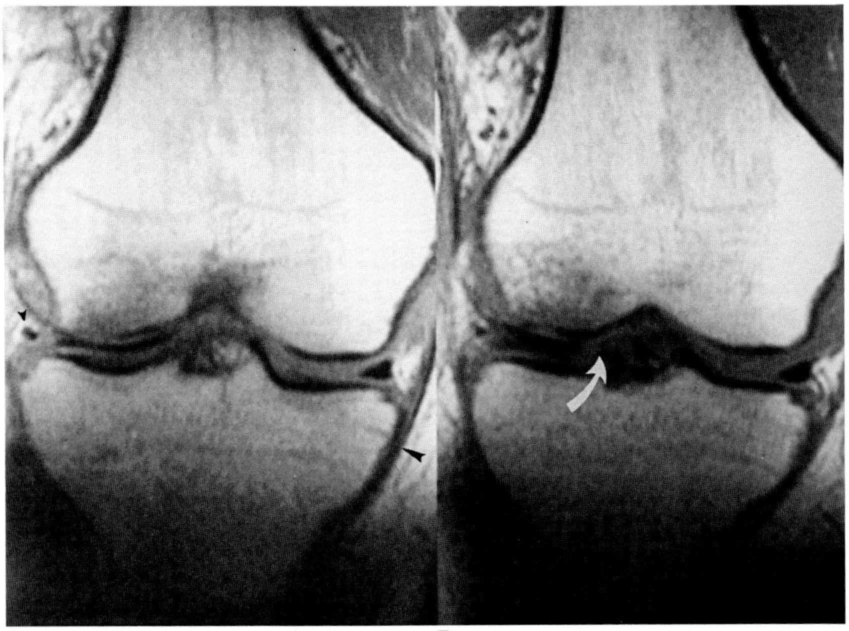

A B

FIGURE 23-2

DISCUSSION: In the sagittal views, angled through the lateral meniscal body, no posterior horn or body is visible (white arrow in Fig. 23-1*A*); it can also be ascertained from these views that the patient has not had a prior meniscectomy. Meniscal hypoplasia is a rare condition that is characterized by intermediate homogeneous T1 signal and is not associated with other signs of injury. Instead, the posterior meniscal body and posterior horn have flipped over on themselves. A cleft (large arrowhead in Fig. 23-1*B*) now separates fragments of the folded posterior meniscal elements (more anteriorly positioned) from the anterior meniscal horn (more posteriorly located). This configuration simulates that of the transverse meniscal ligamentous (TMJ) configuration as it separates from the anterior meniscal horn. However, the anterior triangle-shaped hypointense abnormal folded meniscus (paired small arrowheads in Fig. 23-1*A*) is too large and is not round like the TMJ. An overlying femoral medial condylar bone contusion is present (paired large arrowheads in Fig. 23-1*B*).

Abnormalities in the meniscus periphery consisting of a free lateral meniscal fragment (small arrowhead in Fig. 23-2*A*) are demarcated in the coronal projection. This also is a bucket-handle tear (see Fig. 23-3). A free meniscal fragment deep in the notch of the knee is visible in Figure 23-2*B* (white arrow). The diagnosis of bucket-handle tear is also strongly suggested by the small lateral meniscal height in Figure 23-2*A*. The hypointense lateral femoral condylar bruise is also apparent in the coronal projection. The medial side of the knee is identified by the tibial collateral component of the medial collateral complex (large arrowhead in Fig. 23-2*A*).

DIAGNOSIS: The patient has a bone contusion, a bucket-handle tear with folding of the posterior horn and posterior body anteriorly, a free meniscal fragment medially, and an avulsed meniscal fragment laterally.

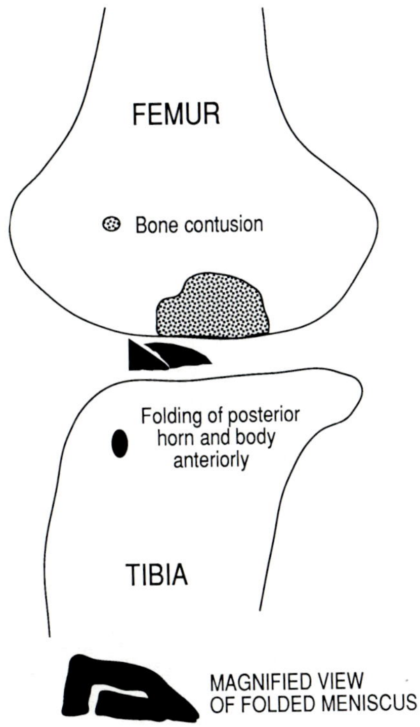

FIGURE 23-3

CASE 24

Differential Diagnosis of Meniscal Tear

HISTORY: A 45-year-old man sustained a valgus stress injury to the knee and hyperextension while skiing. What is the MRI diagnosis? (Fig. 24-1: sagittal contiguous 3.0-mm proton-density MR images. Fig. 24-2: fast scan gradient-echo MR images.)

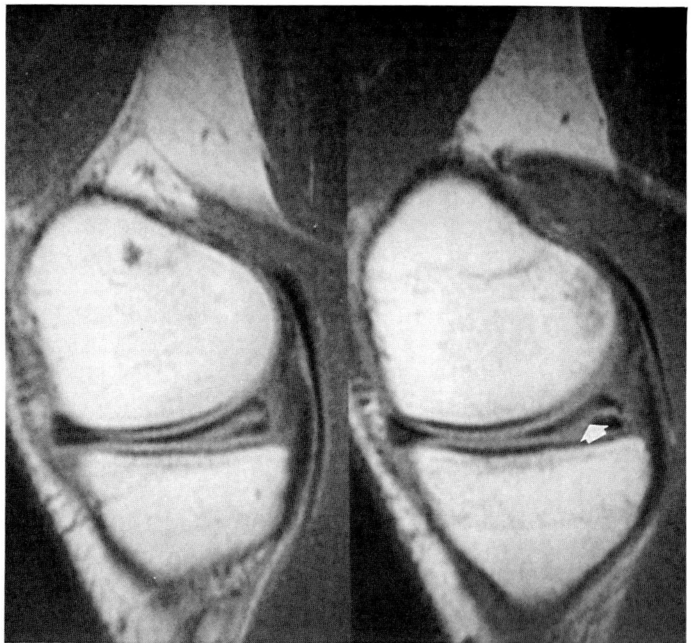

A B

FIGURE 24-1

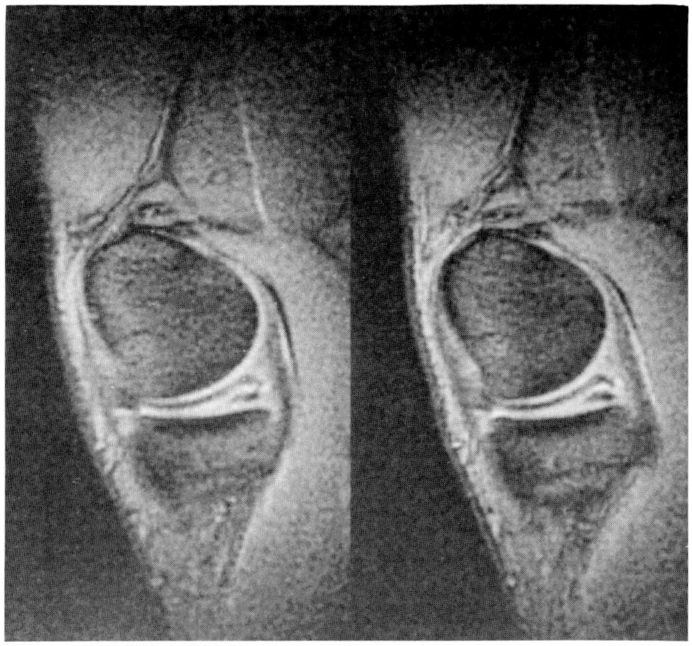

A B

FIGURE 24-2

DISCUSSION: A horizontal and slightly obliquely oriented intrameniscal signal (white arrow in Fig. 24-1*B*) is present in the posteromid portion of the medial meniscus. This is identified as the medial side in the sagittal view from the absence of the fibula and the presence of pes anserinus tendons. Note also that the posterior aspect of the medial meniscus is taller than the anterior aspect on the normal medial side. The menisci on the lateral side of the knee are symmetric in height.

The intrameniscal signal extends to the tibial surface, permitting a comparison of different imaging techniques: on fast scans the meniscal tear appears bright, on T1-weighted or spin-density scans it appears gray. Fast scan can be most helpful in confirming tear, as it is sensitive to the hyperintense water signal. Because water has an extremely long T2 relaxation time, repeated application of rapid low flip angle pulses without a 180° pulse allows a steady state to build up in the x-y or horizontal plane.

Finally, although the signal seen is somewhat horizontal in orientation, it cannot be simple intrameniscal myxoid signal, since (1) the signal is too pronounced, (2) it communicates with the tibial articular surface, and (3) the signal changes are pronounced on at least two sections and are seen in two projections.

Although it is tempting to regard this tear as arising from the true posterior meniscal horn, the lesion is too peripheral and not deep enough into the imaging volume to be in this location. True posterior horn tears arise 3.0 to 6.0 mm from the posterior meniscal root (see Fig. 24-3).

DIAGNOSIS: The patient has a posterior midbody medial meniscal tear.

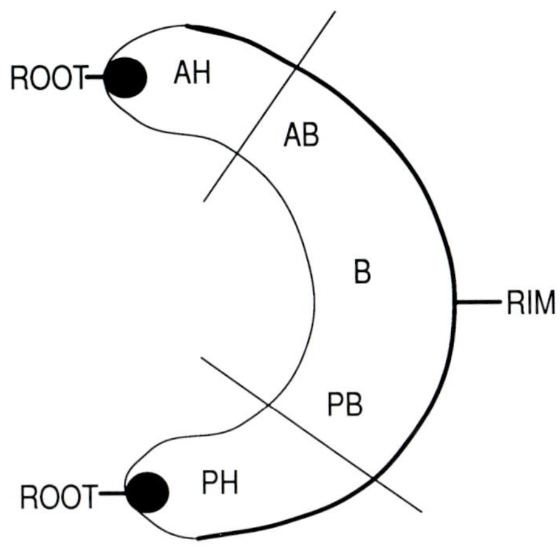

AH = ANTERIOR HORN
AB = ANTERIOR BODY
B = BODY
PB = POSTERIOR BODY
PH = POSTERIOR HORN

FIGURE 24-3

CASE 25

Differential Diagnosis of Postsurgical Knee Pain

HISTORY: A 31-year-old man who had undergone medial meniscal transplantation 4 months earlier reported persistent medial knee pain. (Fig. 25-1: sagittal, and Fig. 25-2: coronal multiformat (four-on-one) multisection, single-echo, proton-density images, TR/TE 1,000/20 msec, 4.0-mm sections, 14.0-cm FOV, 256 × 128 pixel matrix, 2 excitations.)

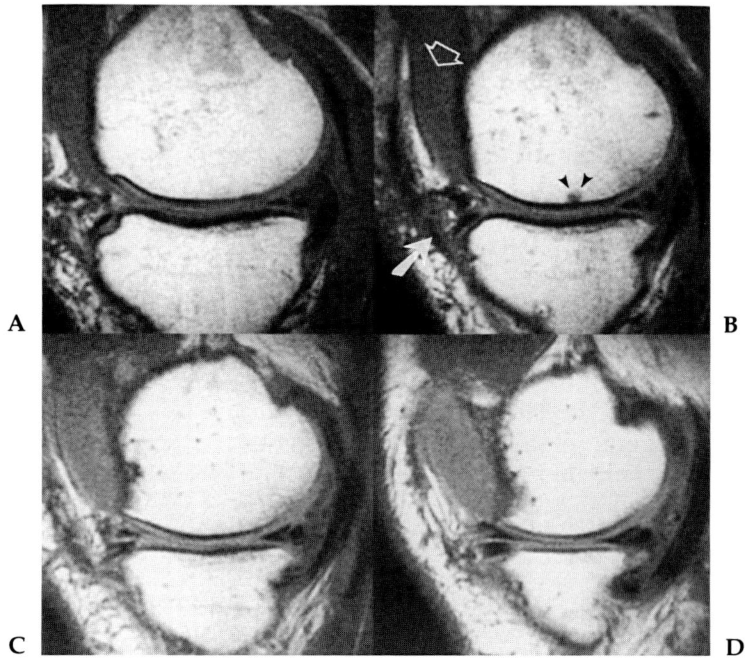

FIGURE 25-1

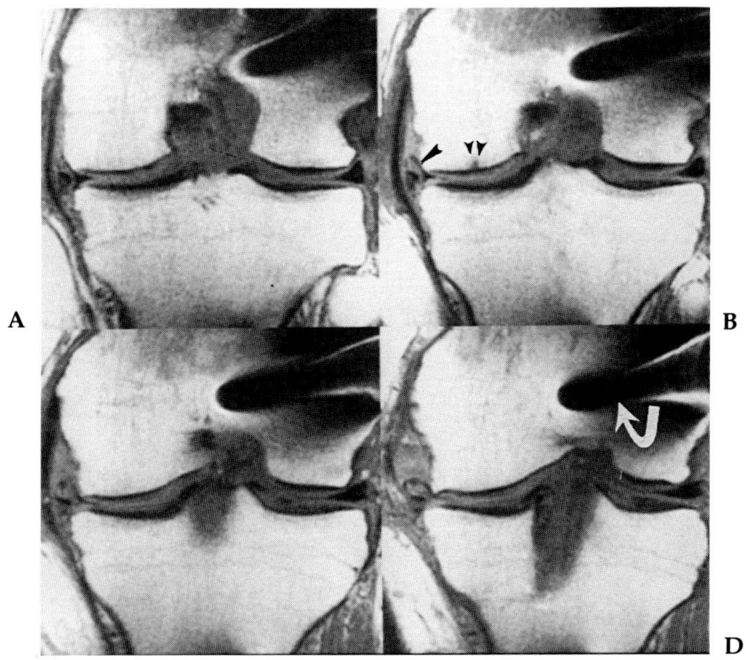

FIGURE 25-2

DISCUSSION: Meniscal transplantation is a new procedure in which cadaveric meniscal allograft is used. The allograft is irradiated with a minimum of 1 million rad to achieve both viral and bacterial sterilization. Most often, meniscal transplantation is performed on patients who have had near-total meniscectomy at an early age. The meniscus transplant is sewed to a thin residual peripheral rim or ridge of the native meniscus, and the inner tips of the menisci are anchored to meniscal roots with sutures or bone plugs (see Fig. 24-3). A major problem with meniscal transplantation is the axial loading forces on the transplant, which may produce meniscal peripheralization as the meniscus rips away from its anchored peripheral margin and deep meniscal roots.

On coronal sections, if one draws a line from the medial femoral condylar eminence to the tibial plateau, the meniscus appears peripheral (extends off the tibial plateau) and contains abnormal intrameniscal signal with adjacent capsular thickening. The sagittal images confirm the presence of knee effusion (open arrow in Fig. 25-1*B*) but also show vertical posterior and horizontal anterior foci of abnormal intrameniscal signal compatible with a tear in the transplanted meniscus. Normally, a globular area of intermediate signal intensity fills the transplanted meniscus secondary to radiation-related effect, but when focal linear or horizontal signal extends through the meniscus in all projections and extends to the articular surface, a diagnosis of tear is likely. The tear appears hook-shaped in Figure 25-2*B* (single arrowhead).

Incidentally noted is an area of intermediate signal intensity in the adjacent infrapatellar fat pad secondary to prior surgery (arrow in Fig. 25-1*A*), as well as a hypointense subchondral ulceration in the underlying bone (paired arrowheads in Fig. 25-2*B*). A ferromagnetic artifact (curved white arrow in Fig. 25-2*D*) in the coronal images is created by a surgically placed lateral femoral condylar staple.

DIAGNOSIS: The patient has a medial tear in the meniscal transplant, with transplant avulsion and peripheralization.

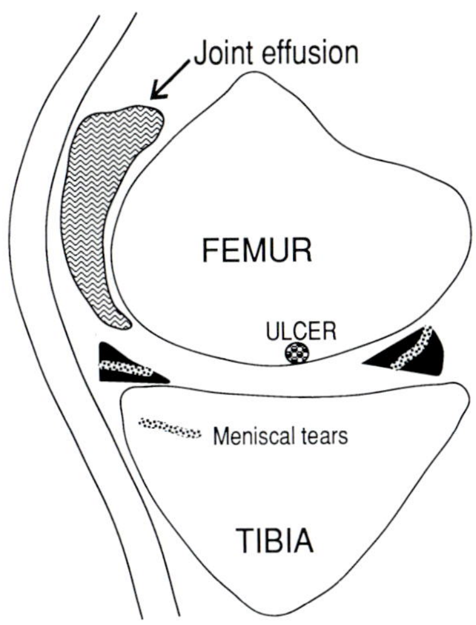

FIGURE 25-3

CASE 26

Differential Diagnosis of Chronic Knee Pain

HISTORY: A 36-year-old man presented with chronic knee pain and clicking or joint crepitus. What is the MRI diagnosis? (Fig. 26-1: coronal, and Fig. 26-2: sagittal multiformat contiguous 3.0-mm proton-density MR images obtained through the lateral meniscus (in Fig. 26-1).

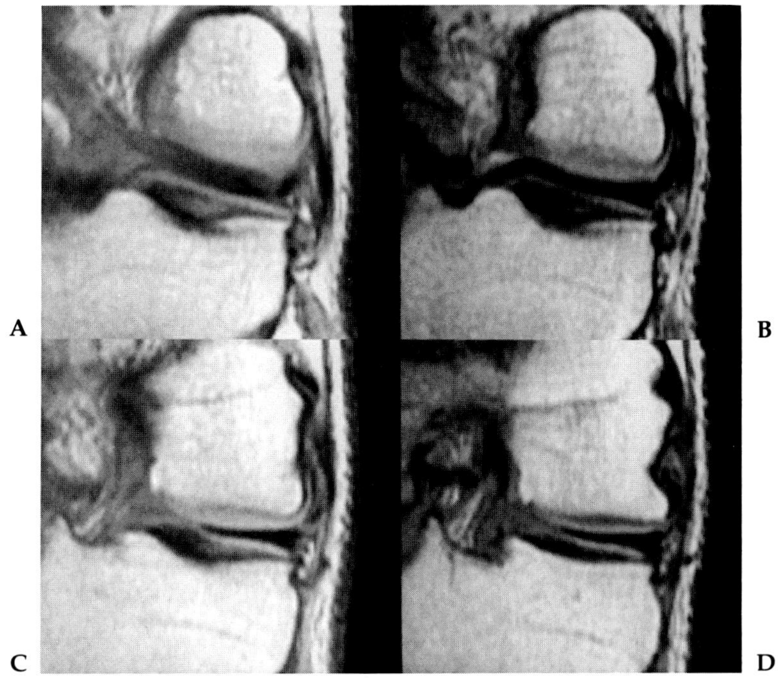

FIGURE 26-1

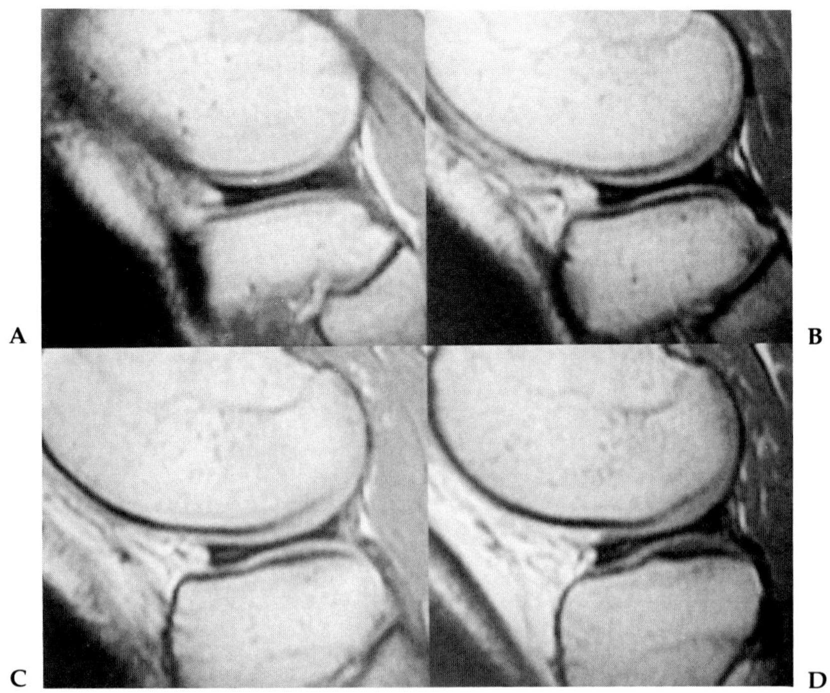

FIGURE 26-2

DISCUSSION: In the sagittal plane, the meniscus has an hourglass shape on multiple sections rather than appearing as two separate triangles. The hourglass shape may be seen on one section or on two 3.0-mm sections, but should never be seen on more than two sections. Also, the meniscus extends deeply toward the femoral notch in the coronal projection. It never tapers to its normal triangular configuration.

These are typical findings of discoid meniscus. Discoid meniscus is most common on the lateral side, occurring in 2% of the population, and is rare on the medial side (0.3%). It is a congenital condition with associated musculoskeletal deformities that include hypoplasia of the lateral femoral condyle, fibular muscular defects, hypoplasia of the fibular head, ectasia or aneurysm of the inferior lateral geniculate artery, and hypoplasia of the lateral tibial spine.

The typical clinical presentation includes clicking or snapping of the knee with pain or tenderness during joint flexion and extension. The clicking is most commonly due to the femoral condyle rocking and overriding the anterior horn of the discoid meniscus. The majority of discoid menisci are asymptomatic; however, this anomaly is said to predispose to internal derangement. The appearance of the hourglass or "bow-tie" shape of the meniscus on more than two 5.0-mm sagittal sections (or three 3.0-mm sections) is known as the "two-cut" rule and is a reliable sign of discoid meniscus.

DIAGNOSIS: The patient has a discoid meniscus.

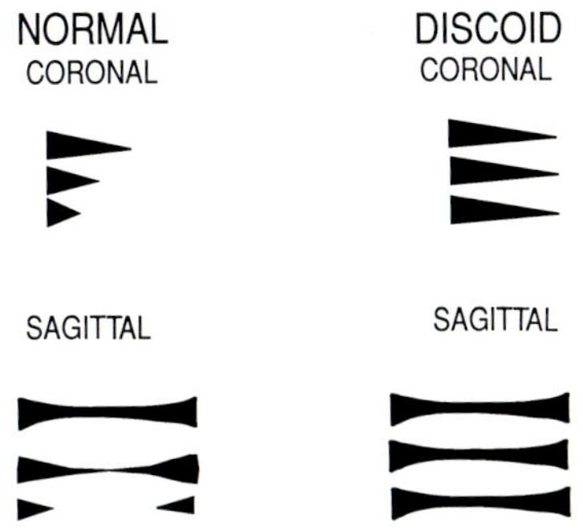

FIGURE 26-3

CASE 27

Differential Diagnosis of Chronic Knee Pain

HISTORY: Three different anatomic test cases are presented. What is the MRI diagnosis in each case? Identify the anatomy designated by arrows and arrowheads. (Fig. 27-1: Case 1. Coronal T1-weighted MR image, 5-mm section thickness. Fig. 27-2: Case 2. Sagittal T1-weighted MR images, 5-mm section thickness. Fig. 27-3: Case 3. Sagittal T1-weighted MR images, 5-mm section thickness.)

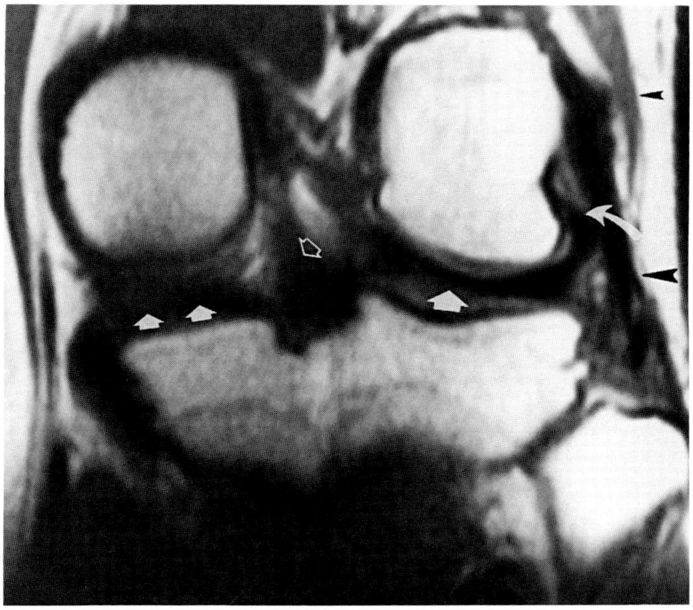

FIGURE 27-1

A B C D

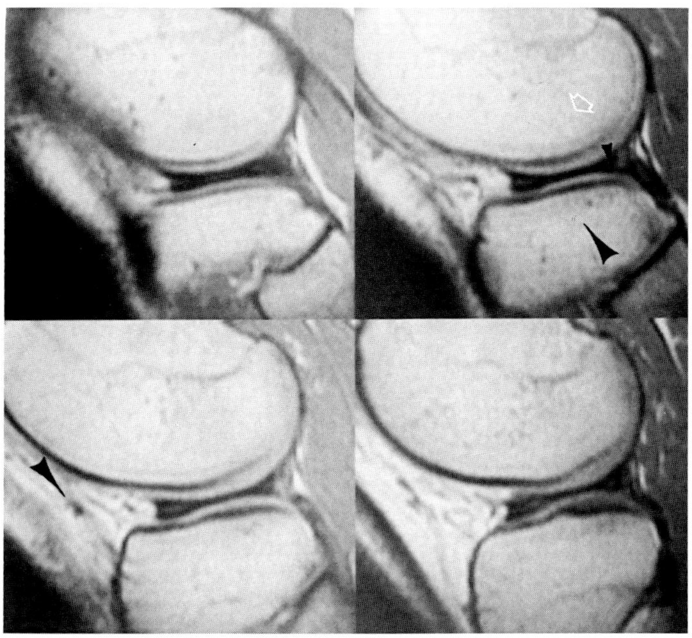

FIGURE 27-2

A B C

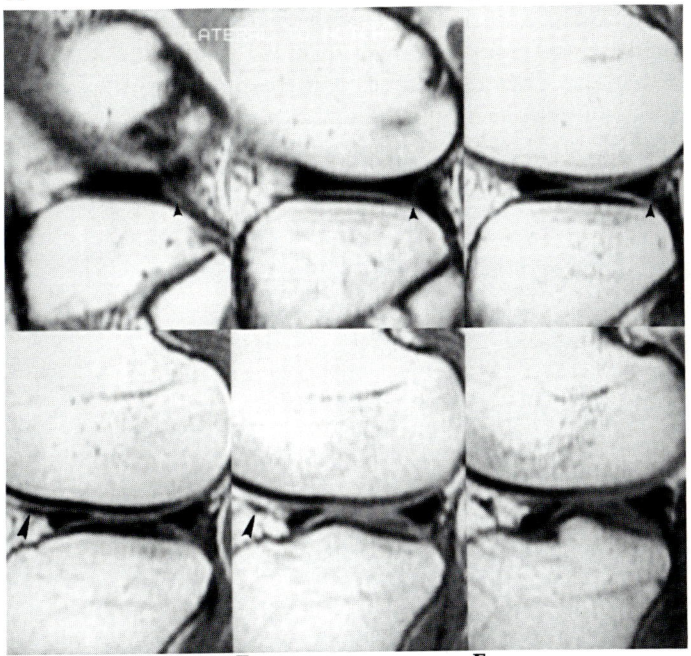

D E F

FIGURE 27-3

DISCUSSION: The following structures are identified on the coronal T1-weighted image in Figure 27-1: biceps femoris distal muscle (small black arrowhead), popliteus tendon in its hiatus (curved white arrow), conjoined tendon with contributions from the fibular collateral and biceps femoris (large black arrowhead), posterior cruciate ligament (open arrow), and the posteromedial joint capsule (paired white arrows).

Identified in Figure 27-2*B* are the transverse meniscal ligament (large arrowhead) and the popliteus reflection (small arrowhead). The configuration of the lateral meniscus on this section is normal. The true posterior lateral meniscus horn has an hourglass or rectangular shape in the coronal plane when sectioned at a tangent to its horizontal axis. If this configuration persists for more than two contiguous 5.0-mm sections, the diagnosis of discoid meniscus is certain. In the normal subject, the lateral meniscus has a deep center convex downward or concave upward like the center of a soup bowl. Therefore, coronal sections may also give the impression that the meniscus is separated into two parts, as in a true bucket-handle tear (compare case 17).

The diagnosis of discoid meniscus is discussed in detail in case 26. The sagittal configuration of a discoid meniscus is shown again for comparison with the normal sagittal meniscus (Fig. 27-3). The normal meniscus begins to separate into two symmetric triangles anteriorly and posteriorly after the second sagittal section. In contrast, the anterior and posterior menisci remain connected in discoid menisci.

DIAGNOSIS: Case 1: Normal anatomy. Case 2: Discoid meniscus. Case 3: Normal anatomy.

CASE 28

Differential Diagnosis of Ligamentous Disorders of the Knee

HISTORY: A 46-year-old man sustained an acute hyperextension injury following a blow to the anterior knee while playing soccer. What is the MRI diagnosis? (Fig. 28-1: sagittal multiformat two-on-one multiecho proton-density (*A*) and T2-weighted (*B*) MR images, 14.0-cm FOV, 192 × 256 pixel matrix, 4.0-mm sections, 2 excitations. Fig. 28-2: sagittal T1-weighted image.)

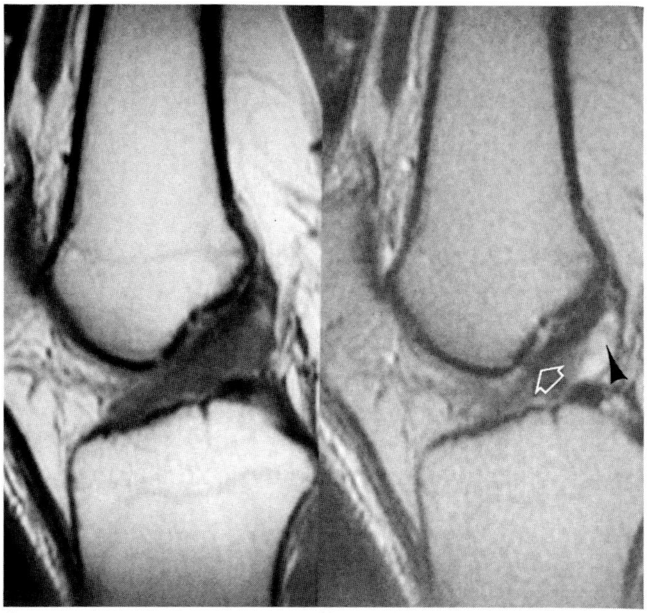

A **B**

FIGURE 28-1

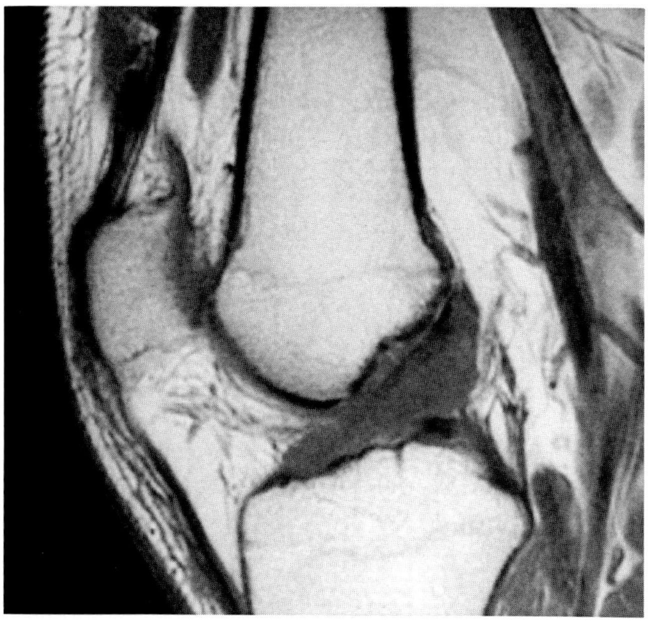

FIGURE 28-2

DISCUSSION: The anterior cruciate ligament (ACL) courses posterosuperolaterally, originating in the medial aspect of the lateral femoral condyle and inserting on the tibial plateau approximately 1.0 cm posterior to its anterior border. The ACL is grayer, straighter, thinner in caliber, and more difficult to visualize than the posterior cruciate ligament (PCL). The ACL is extrasynovial but is invested by a sheath of intermediate signal intensity that is often volume averaged in the sagittal plane. The ligament is seen as a dark hypointense band surrounded by poorly defined areas of gray signal that do *not* become hyperintense on T2-weighted images.

Visualization of the ACL should be attempted in both coronal and axial planes; there is a tendency to look only at the sagittal images. If the ACL is not seen in the sagittal plane, even with thin sections (4.0 mm or less), there is insufficient basis for diagnosing complete ACL transection. However, inability to visualize the ACL in two planes (sagittal and coronal or paracoronal) is sufficient basis for diagnosing complete ACL transection, provided the sections were obtained correctly. A common cause of poor visualization of the ACL is hyperflexion, hyperextension, or external overrotation.

In this case, the straight hypointense band of the ACL is seen on proton-density images but is better visualized on T2-weighted images (arrow in Fig. 28-1*B*). Multiecho sagittal T-2 weighted imaging with a 4.0- or 5.0-mm section is currently our method of choice for ACL visualization when standard single-echo imaging fails. The intermediate signal intensity of the sheath is barely visible on long echo time images, and therefore the hypointense ACL stands out. When this sheath fills with fluid or blood, it will usually become more hyperintense, further highlighting the hypointense ligament. In normal subjects, a small amount of fluid will collect along the medial portion of the lateral anterior meniscosynovial recess adjacent to the ACL tibial insertion site. Hyperintense signal posterior to the ACL is not normally seen on T2-weighted images. When it occurs (arrowhead in Fig. 28-1*B*), and some persistent hypointense linear ligamentous fibers are still present, a diagnosis of partial ACL injury can be made.

DIAGNOSIS: The patient has a partial ACL tear.

CASE 29

Differential Diagnosis of Ligamentous Disorders of the Knee

HISTORY: A 23-year-old football player presented with a 3-year history of poorly defined "knee injury" that had been treated with 4 months of rest and inactivity. What is the MRI diagnosis? (Fig. 29-1: sagittal multiecho proton-density MR image; Fig. 29-2: T2-weighted MR image; 16.0-cm FOV, 128 × 256 pixel matrix, 4.0-mm sections, 2 excitations.)

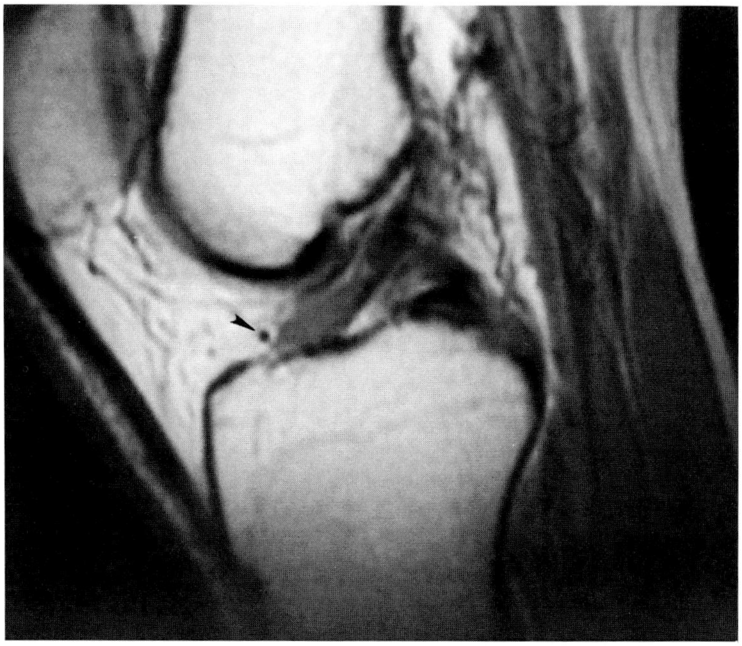

FIGURE 29-1

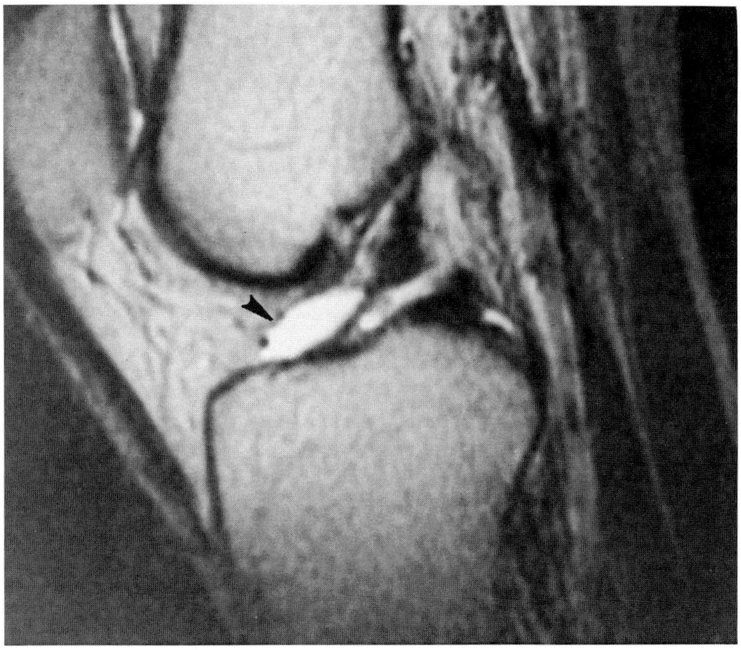

FIGURE 29-2

DISCUSSION: Because the surrounding structures become more hyperintense relative to ligamentous tissue on T2-weighted images, the anterior cruciate ligament (ACL) is more easily seen in this sequence (Fig. 29-2). While T2* free induction decay fast-scan imaging gives the appearance of a T2 effect, the ligament is not as well seen as on true T2-weighted spin-echo sequences. Oblique paracoronal images or three-dimensional volumetric acquisitions with 1.0 to 2.0-mm sections in the sagittal plane may be used to define the boundaries and course of the ACL. However, such techniques are time-consuming and too cumbersome to use with spin-echo multiecho sequences.

A fluid collection (arrowhead in Fig. 29-2) adjacent to the tibial insertion of the ACL lies in the medial portion of the lateral meniscosynovial recess just behind the transverse meniscal ligament (arrowhead in Fig. 29-1). Fluid is seen in this location in 3% of normal subjects in our series of over 6,000 MRI studies of the knee.

The lobulated, hypointense "lumpy–bumpy" appearance of the ACL on T2-weighted images is compatible with fibrosis around a previously repaired or healed partial ACL tear. Since the Hoffa fat pad is homogeneous and the patient has never had surgery, a healed partial tear is the correct diagnosis.

DIAGNOSIS: The patient has a chronic, healed tear of the ACL.

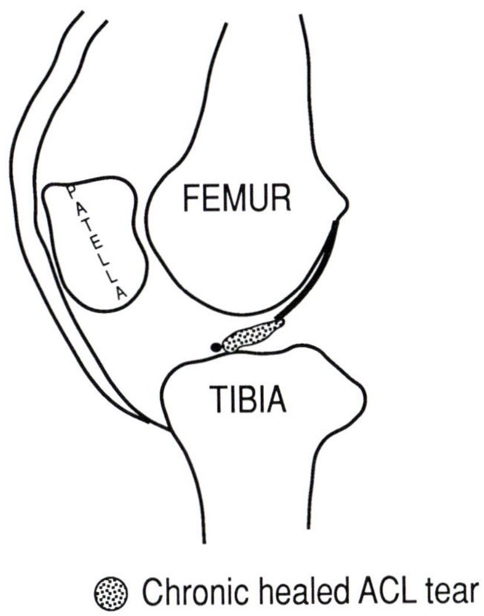

FIGURE 29-3

CASE 30

Differential Diagnosis of Acute Knee Pain

HISTORY: A 36-year-old woman sustained acute "knee strain" in a fall while jogging, with minimal symptoms until the following day. What is the MRI diagnosis? (Fig. 30-1: sagittal multiecho, multiformat proton-density image (*A*) and T2-weighted image (*B*).)

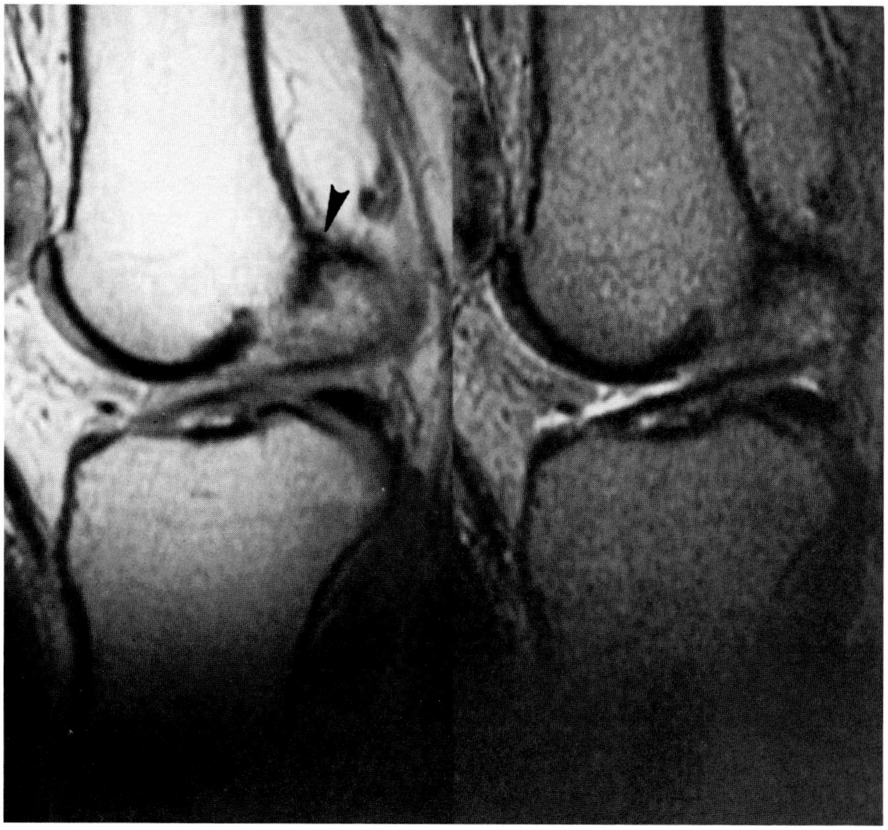

FIGURE 30-1

DISCUSSION: A small amount of hyperintense fluid bathes the tibial insertion of the anterior cruciate ligament (ACL) or lies just anterior to it. However, the course of the ACL in this case is inappropriate. Normally it should extend more craniad or proximally toward the posteromedial surface of the lateral femoral condyle (arrowhead in *A*). In this case it courses in an almost straight posterior direction. Therefore, the femoral attachment of the ACL has been avulsed.

It is critical to identify any bone fragment that has been avulsed with proximal-end ACL injuries, as the surgical procedure often must change to accommodate the fragment. In this case, no bone fragment is present.

DIAGNOSIS: The femoral end of the ACL is avulsed.

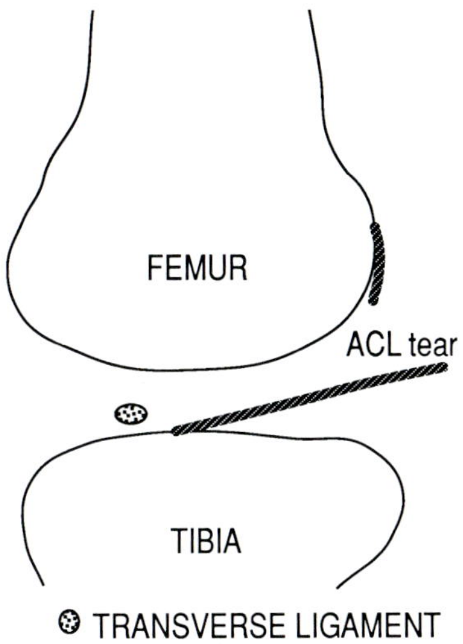

FIGURE 30-2

CASE 31

Differential Diagnosis of Anterior Knee Pain

HISTORY: A 26-year-old athlete presented with distal anterior thigh and suprapatellar pain, particularly on extension. What is the MRI diagnosis? (Fig. 31-1: sagittal proton-density image, TR/TE 1,000/20 msec.)

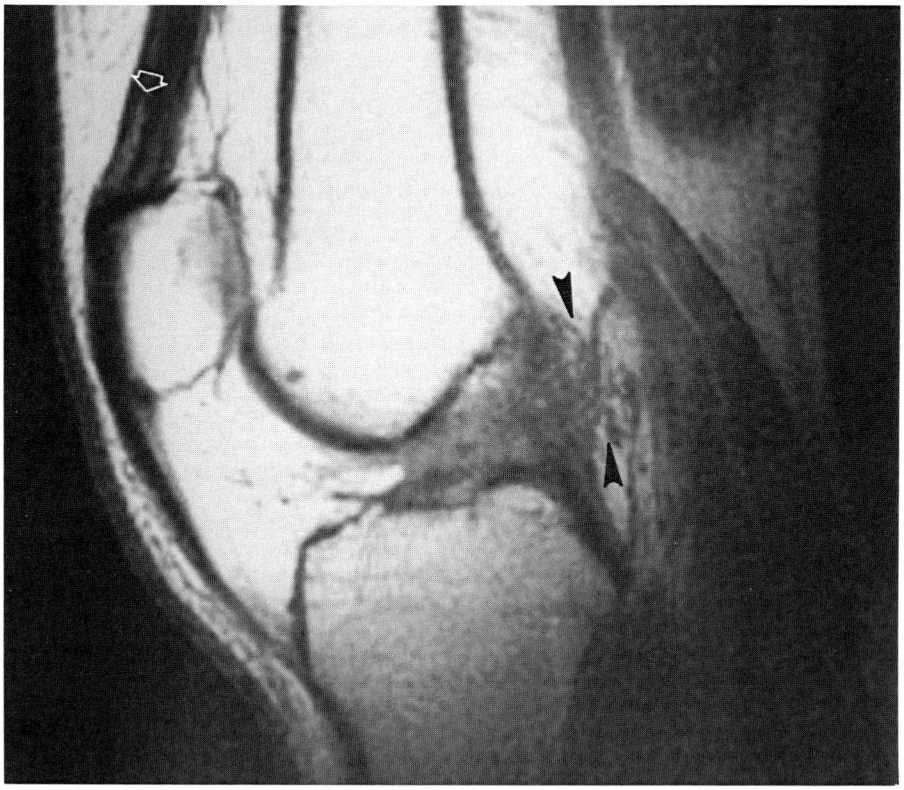

FIGURE 31-1

DISCUSSION: Quadriceps avulsion injuries and tendinitis are not common diagnoses in athletes. Avulsion injury of the proximal patellar epiphysis is more common than quadriceps tendinitis. The pain experienced with tendinitis is aching, with point tenderness over the quadriceps, discomfort on hypoflexion, and a sense of fullness around the quadriceps tendon. With acute onset, the major differential diagnosis is quadriceps tendon rupture.

MRI of tendon rupture shows the normal hypointense tendon as noncontiguous and replaced by intermediate signal intensity blood or fluid on T1-weighted or spin-density imaging. Poorly defined foci of increased signal intensity replace the normal tendinous linear anatomy (open arrow). Tendinitis presents as an intratendinous linear band of increased signal intensity, with or without a circumferential peritendinous signal increase; however, the linear contour and the internal constituents of the tendon can be traced longitudinally. Complete rupture is accompanied by a mass of intermediate or high signal intensity at the rupture site.

This patient has also experienced a complete anterior cruciate ligament (ACL) tear (see Fig. 31-2). The midsubstance of the ACL cannot be traced and is replaced by foci of intermediate signal intensity. Another useful sign of ACL injury is the "spider sign." The wavy foci of intermediate signal intensity (arrowheads), best seen on T1-weighted or proton-density images, represent fragments of frayed ACL fibers.

DIAGNOSIS: The patient has quadriceps tendinitis with an anterior cruciate ligament tear.

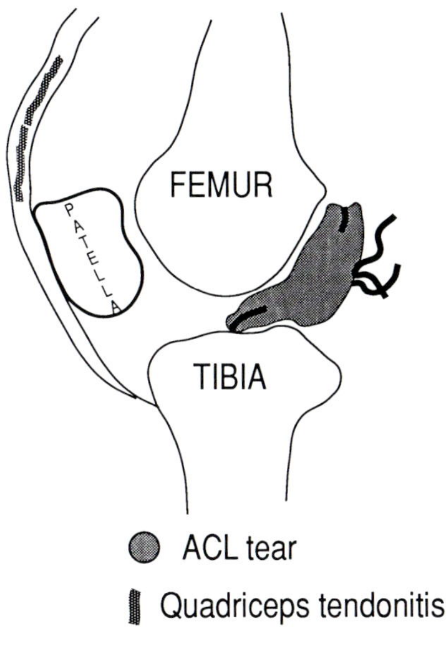

FIGURE 31-2

CASE 32

Differential Diagnosis of Knee Mass

HISTORY: A 27-year-old man sustained an injury during a tennis match. The pain is exacerbated by running. Is the ACL tear partial or complete? (Fig. 32-1: sagittal spin-density MRI, TR/TE 1,000/20 msec, 4.0-mm sections, 14.0-cm FOV, 2 excitations, 256 × 128 pixel matrix.)

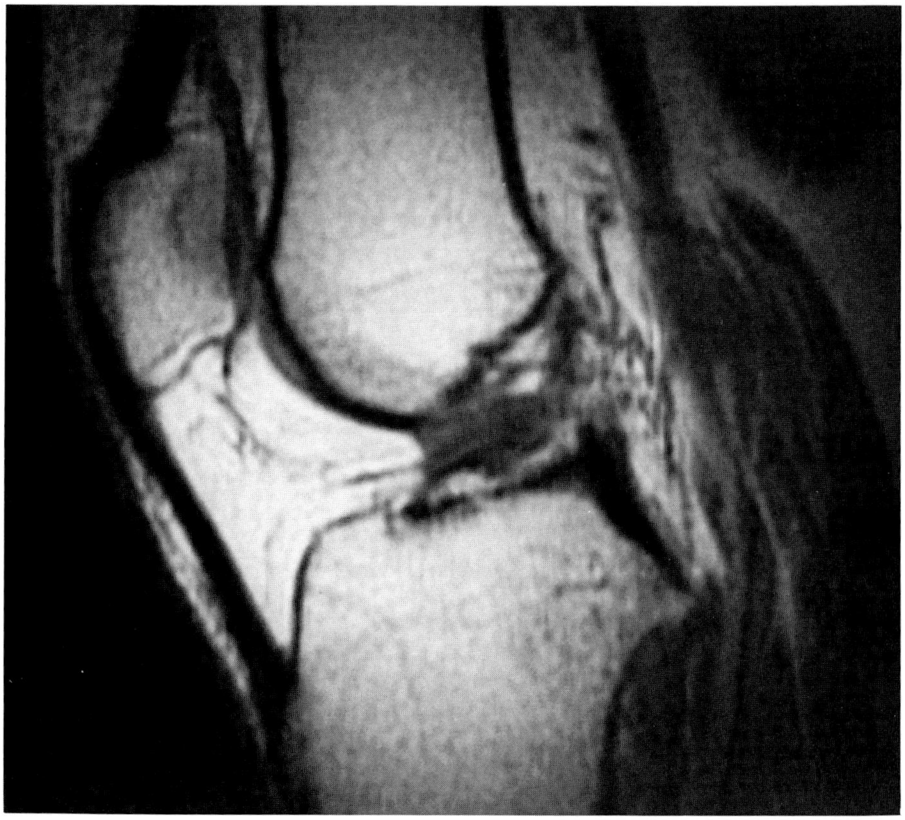

FIGURE 32-1

DISCUSSION: Sagittal images at the level of the anterior cruciate ligament (ACL) reveal an elliptical mass of intermediate signal intensity that replaces the linear hypointense signal of the ACL midsubstance. The ACL is best visualized with 10° of external rotation, thin sections, multi-echo T2-weighted and spin-density images, or high resolution 1.0- to 2.0-mm three-dimensional volumetric images. When the ACL ruptures, acute hemorrhage and edema at the rupture site, while extrasynovial, are invested by a thin sheath that delimits this acute phenomenon. The appearance of a pseudomass is created on spin-density or T1-weighted images. The presence of this pseudomass without any demonstrable hypointense linear oblique fibers running through it on proton-density or T2-weighted imaging is highly suggestive of complete ligamentous rupture.

Clinically, ACL injury may be suspected by the drawer test: anterior displacement of the tibia on the femur at 90° of flexion. The result is reported in maximal displacement of the involved knee minus displacement of the normal knee, in millimeters. Since the ACL is multibanded, the Lachman test (similar to the drawer test) is performed in 20° to 30° of flexion. A side-to-side difference of 2.5 mm is abnormal.

DIAGNOSIS: A pseudomass of the ACL is present, secondary to midsubstance rupture.

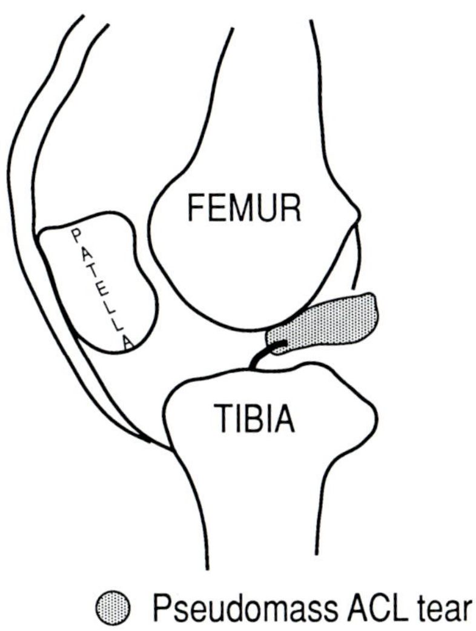

FIGURE 32-2

CASE 33

Differential Diagnosis of Knee Mass

HISTORY: A 66-year-old man sustained a hyperextension injury after a fall from a ladder. The patient had extreme pain on hyperflexion. Is the ACL tear partial or complete? (Fig. 33-1: sagittal, and Fig. 33-2: coronal spin-density MR images, TR/TE 1,000/20 msec, 4.0-mm sections, 14.0-cm FOV, 2 excitations, 192 × 256 pixel matrix.)

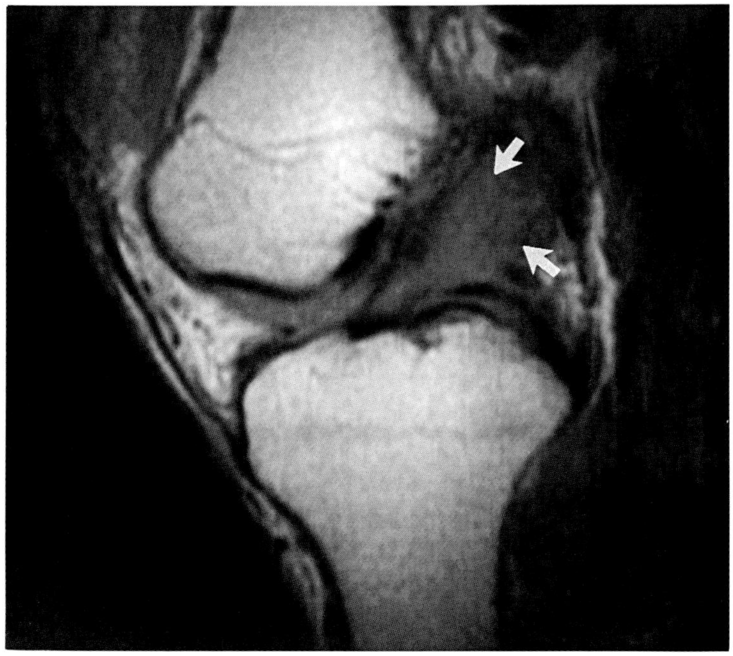

FIGURE 33-1

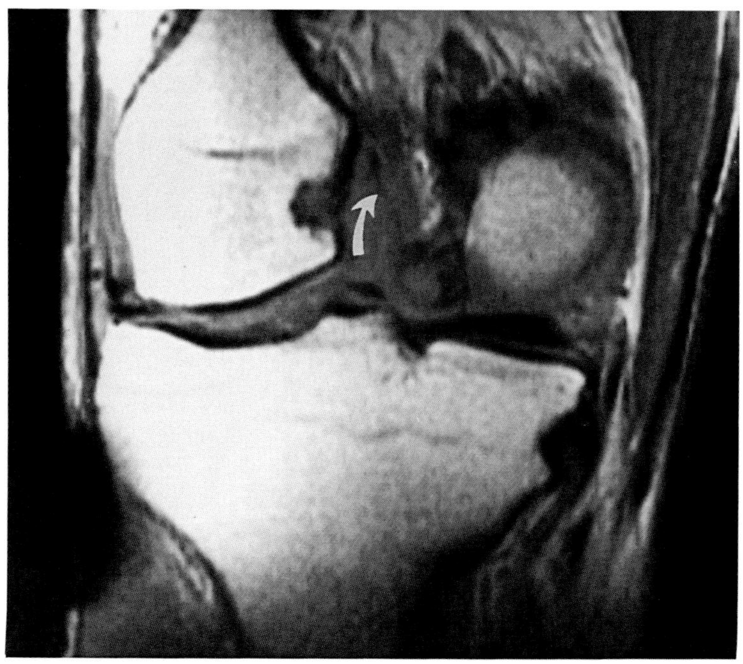

FIGURE 33-2

DISCUSSION: A large homogeneous area of intermediate signal intensity circumscribes the anterior cruciate ligament (ACL). Intact fibers of the ACL appear as thin, linear, hypointense foci in both sagittal and coronal projections (curved arrows). The gray area (straight arrow in Fig. 33-1) represents a large hematoma or proteinaceous fluid collection that is demarcated by the joint capsule and the sheath that invests the ACL. In this case, the coronal view was obtained to confirm that several ligamentous fibers remain intact. The ACL is at least 11.0 to 13.0 mm in size in the normal adult; therefore, this ligament is too small. The differential diagnosis of such a small ACL includes hypoplasia, atrophy of a native graft ACL, partial tear, and the ACL of a normal child. In normal young children, less than 10 years old, the diameter of the ACL is in the range of 6.0 to 10.0 mm.

As described in case 32, the clinical signs of an ACL tear include a positive Lachman test and the anterior drawer sign.

DIAGNOSIS: A pseudomass of the ACL is present, secondary to midsubstance rupture.

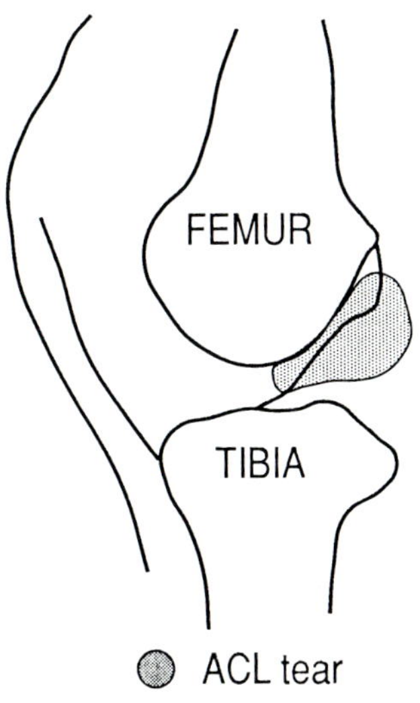

FIGURE 33-3

CASE 34

Differential Diagnosis of Ligamentous Disease of the Knee

HISTORY: A 27-year-old man received an anterior cruciate ligament allograft. The images shown are sagittal proton-density sections obtained 1 week (Fig. 34-1), 3 months (Fig. 34-2), and 5 months (Fig. 34-3) after surgery. What is the MRI diagnosis? (Figs. 34-1 through 34-3: sagittal T1-weighted MR images, TR/TE 700/20 msec.)

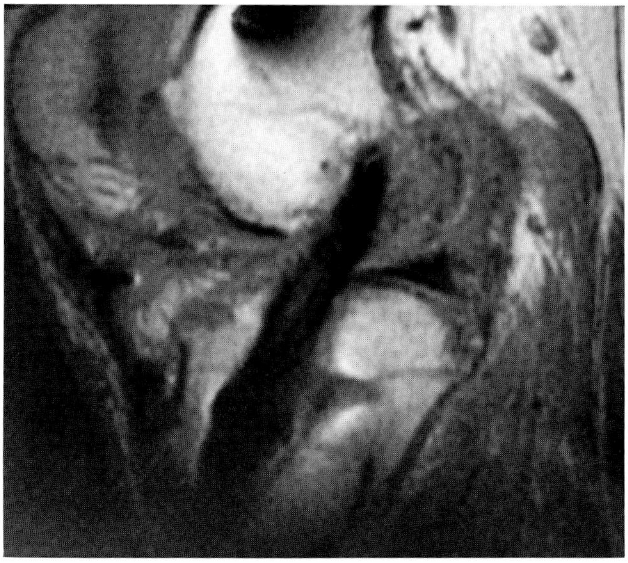

FIGURE 34-1

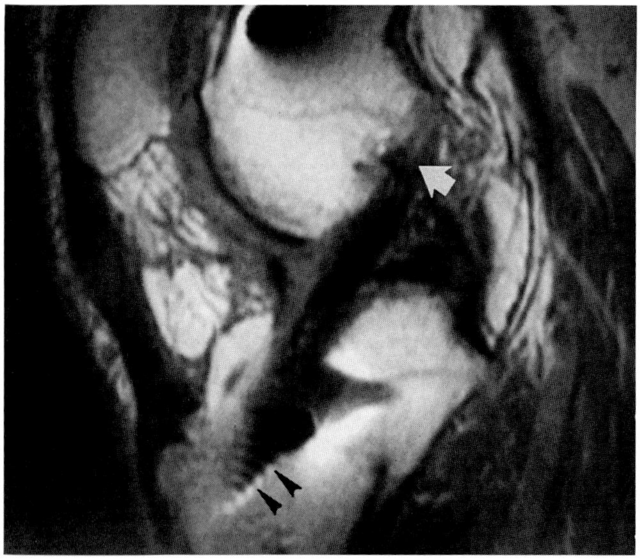

FIGURE 34-2

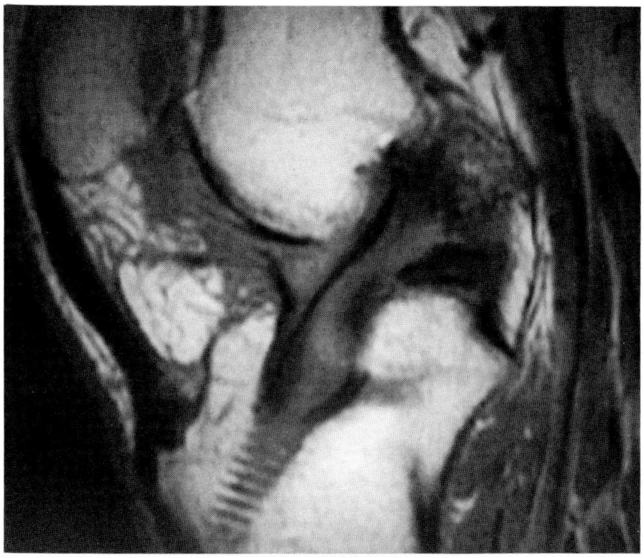

FIGURE 34-3

DISCUSSION: Anterior cruciate ligament (ACL) allografts are commonly taken from cadaveric infrapatellar tendon. These grafts are usually 11.0 to 12.0 mm thick. Smaller sizes are due to undersizing (uncommon) or atrophy (common). Because the tendon requires tensile forces to maintain its integrity, lack of weight-bearing or inability to ambulate may contribute significantly to atrophy. The graft at 1 week after surgery exhibits normal integrity or thickness. Progressive atrophy due to diminishing tensile forces occurred (arrow in Fig. 34-2) subsequently.

The graft is usually buried in a tibial tunnel (paired arrowheads in Fig. 34-2) that is drilled posterosuperiorly to anteroinferiorly through the tibia. The tunnel should exit the tibia anteriorly at the tibial tubercle and exit the tibial plateau just behind the anterior tibial spine in the sagittal view. It should attach to the posterosuperior lateral femoral condyle in the coronal view. The tendon is then pulled through this tunnel and anchored at its femoral and tibial ends by bone plugs, usually harvested with the graft. The caudal graft end may be stapled to the anterior tibial surface. Interference screws, used to press the bone plugs against the tunnel walls, may produce nonferromagnetic artifacts, particularly severe on fast scan and T2-weighted images. If such metallic hardware is present, these sequences should be avoided.

At 3 to 6 weeks, the tunnel usually fills with small to moderate amounts of fluid. However, if T2-weighted rather than spin-density sequences can be used, the hypointense tendon is easily contrasted with hyperintense fluid. More fluid is seen in a tunnel housing atrophic tendons.

Besides T2-weighted sagittal images, oblique coronal images perpendicular to the tendon course offer a simple way of assessing ACL graft diameter, radius, or area. Oblique images parallel or tangent to the course of the graft are a further option that we (rarely) employ to improve graft visualization.

DIAGNOSIS: The ACL allograft has atrophied.

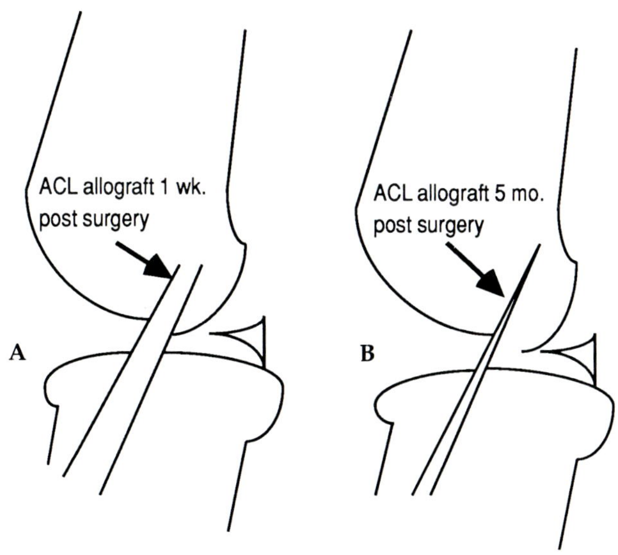

FIGURE 34-4

CASE 35

Differential Diagnosis of Acute Knee Pain

HISTORY: A 17-year-old girl presented with severe knee pain, tenderness, and a sensation of instability after a field hockey–related injury. At least four abnormalities are associated with this case. What are the MRI diagnoses? (Figs. 35-1 and 35-2: sagittal multiformat (four-on-one contiguous proton-density (Fig. 35-1, Fig. 35-2*A*, *C*) and T2-weighted (Fig. 35-2*B*, *D*) MR images, 14.0-cm FOV, 192 × 256 pixel matrix, 4.0-mm sections, 2 excitations. Fig. 35-3: coronal multiformat (four-on-one) contiguous proton-density MR images.)

A B C D

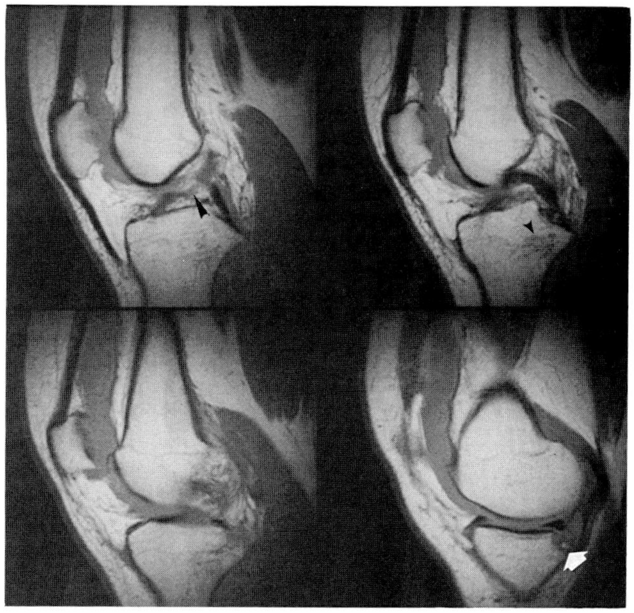

FIGURE 35-1

A B C D

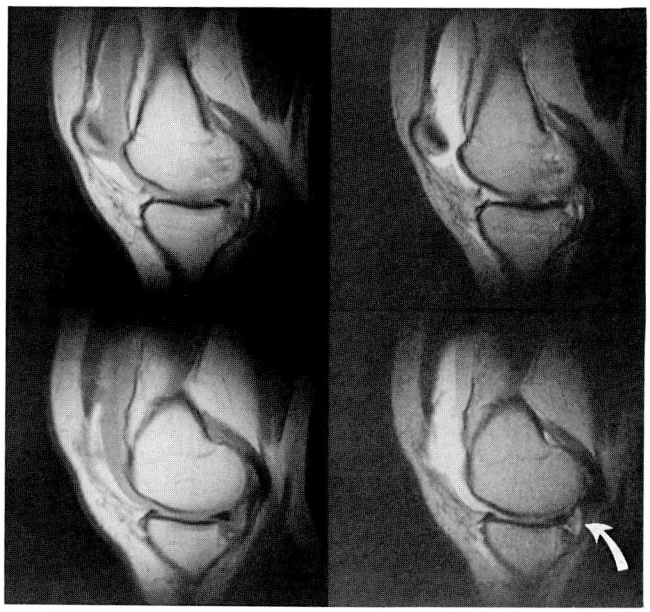

FIGURE 35-2

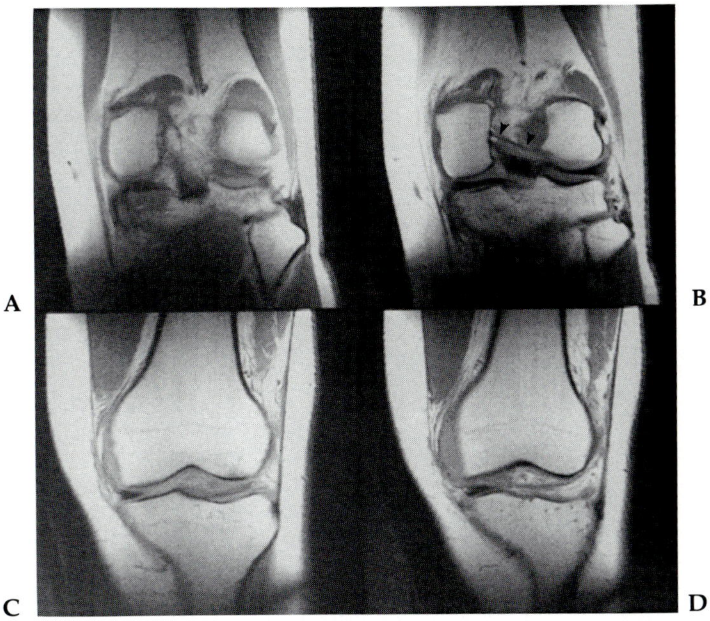

FIGURE 35-3

DISCUSSION: The major findings in this case can be extracted from the images shown. The midsubstance of the anterior cruciate ligament is interrupted (arrowhead in Fig. 35-1*A*). However, the cause of the patient's knee pain is related to a chip fracture of the posteromedial aspect of the tibial plateau, best seen in Figure 35-1*D* (white arrow). Associated hemorrhage lies just above this fracture fragment (curved arrow in Fig. 35-2*D*), within the capsular reflection. The resulting hypointensity in and around the posterior tibia is also easily seen in the coronal projection.

A fluid–fluid–fat interface is visible in the suprapatellar bursa (Fig. 35-2).

Irregular linear hypointense foci of signal alteration in the posterior tibia (arrowhead in Fig. 35-1*B*) represent stress fracture lines.

The normal ligament of Wrisberg is outlined (paired arrowheads in Fig. 35-3*B*).

DIAGNOSIS: The patient has a posteromedial tibial plateau chip fracture, joint effusion, a torn anterior cruciate ligament, and a tibial plateau stress fracture.

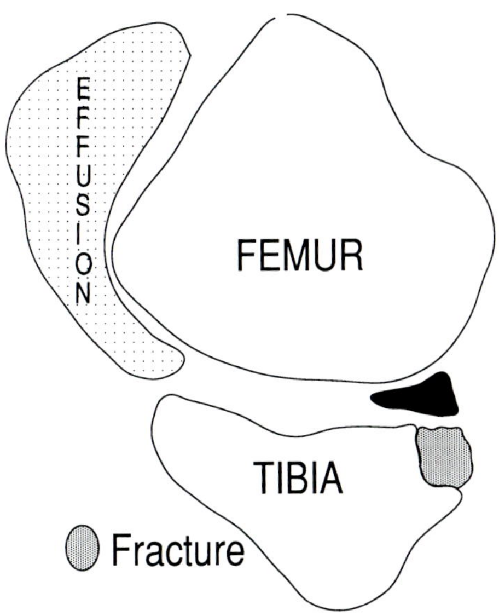

FIGURE 35-4

CASE 36

Differential Diagnosis of Acute Trauma

HISTORY: A 17-year-old boy sustained an acute blow to the medial aspect of the knee during a football game. What is the MRI diagnosis? (Fig. 36-1: coronal multiformat (four-on-one) proton-density MR images, TR/TE 1,400/20 msec, 14.0-cm FOV, 128 × 256 pixel matrix, 3.0-mm sections, 2 excitations. Fig. 36-2: proton-density, coronal magnification views of the lateral side of the knee in the same patient.)

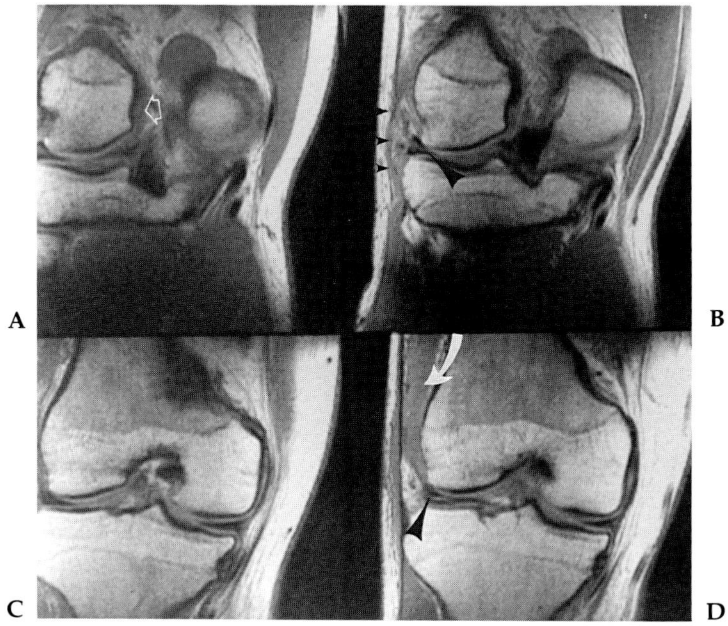

FIGURE 36-1

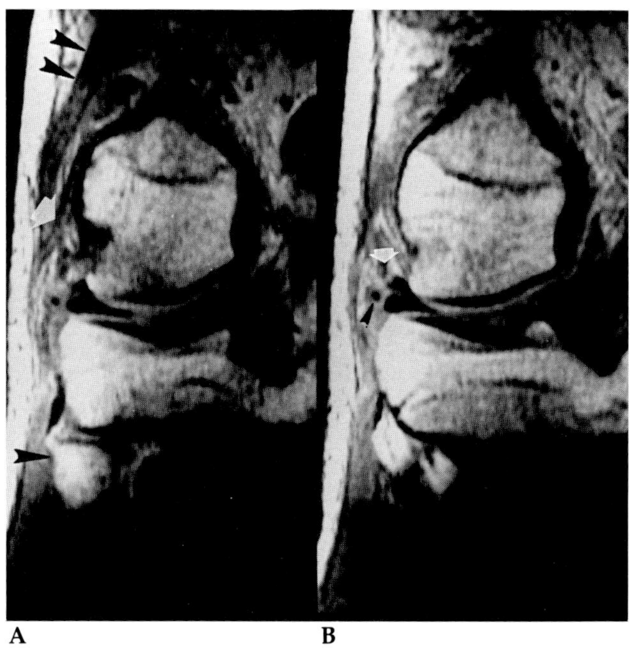

FIGURE 36-2

DISCUSSION: The signal communicating with the articular surface and the capsular surface is apparent in the lateral meniscal body (arrowhead in Fig. 36-1*B*) and anterior horn (arrowhead in Fig. 36-1*D*). Anterior horn tears are rare, occurring in less than one in 100 to 200 cases of meniscal injury.

The lateral collateral complex in this patient is abnormal. The iliotibial band is the most anterior and superficial component, with its distal attachment on the lateral Gerdy tubercle. Edema and hemorrhage are present around the iliotibial band as it attaches (triple arrowheads in Fig. 36-1*B*). The biceps femoris muscle (paired arrowheads in Fig. 36-2*A*) and tendon will join with the fibular collateral ligament to form the conjoined tendon that inserts on the fibular head. The intermediate signal intensity joint capsule lies deep to these structures and provides less pronounced knee support than its medial counterpart.

Hypointense fragments of the fibular collateral ligament can be seen just lateral to the lateral meniscus (single arrowhead in Fig. 36-2*B*). The linear hypointense fibers of the fibular collateral ligament cannot be seen on the coronal sections, although its remnant (normally a curvilinear black band) is seen as subtle intermediate signal (white arrow in Fig. 36-2*B*). The fibular head is identified in Figure 36-2*A* by a horizontal black arrowhead. We use the following MR grading system to quantify the severity of lateral collateral complex (LCC) injuries:

Grade I: Capsular edema (intermediate signal intensity).

Grade II: Capsular edema with one of the LCC structures injured or interrupted: the biceps femoris tendon, fibular collateral ligament, or iliotibial band.

Grade III: Capsular edema with complete interruption of the conjoined tendon, with or without rupture of the iliotibial band.

The hypointense band of the linear ACL is replaced by intermediate signal intensity just medial to the lateral femoral condyle (open arrow in Fig. 36-1*A*). Also present is a joint effusion in the lateral retinacular space (curved arrow in Fig. 36-1*D*).

DIAGNOSIS: MRI disclosed conjoint tendon rupture, injury of the iliotibial band without complete tear, lateral meniscal body and anterior horn tear, joint effusion, and ACL injury.

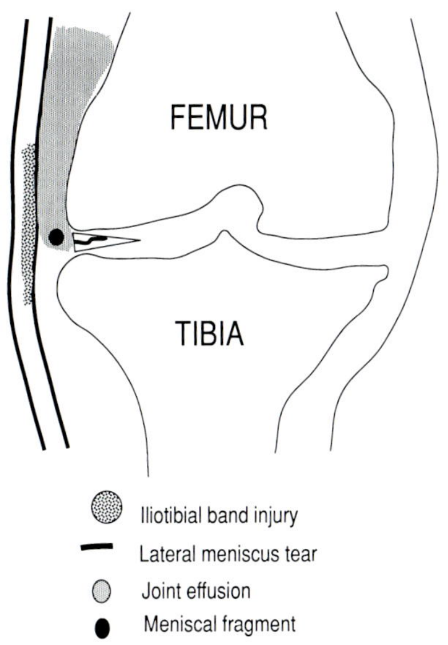

FIGURE 36-3

CASE 37

Differential Diagnosis of Acute Trauma and Ligamentous Disease

HISTORY: A 30-year-old professional running back in the National Football League presented with medial knee pain and tenderness but no clinical evidence of instability. He was at the bottom of a pile of tacklers when several larger players fell on his leg, which was held in extension. What is the MRI diagnosis? (Fig. 37-1: multiformat (two-on-one) coronal proton-density (*A*) and T2-weighted (*B*) MR images, TR/TE 1,400/20, 80 msec, 14.0-cm FOV, 128 × 256 pixel matrix, 3.0-mm sections, 2 excitations.)

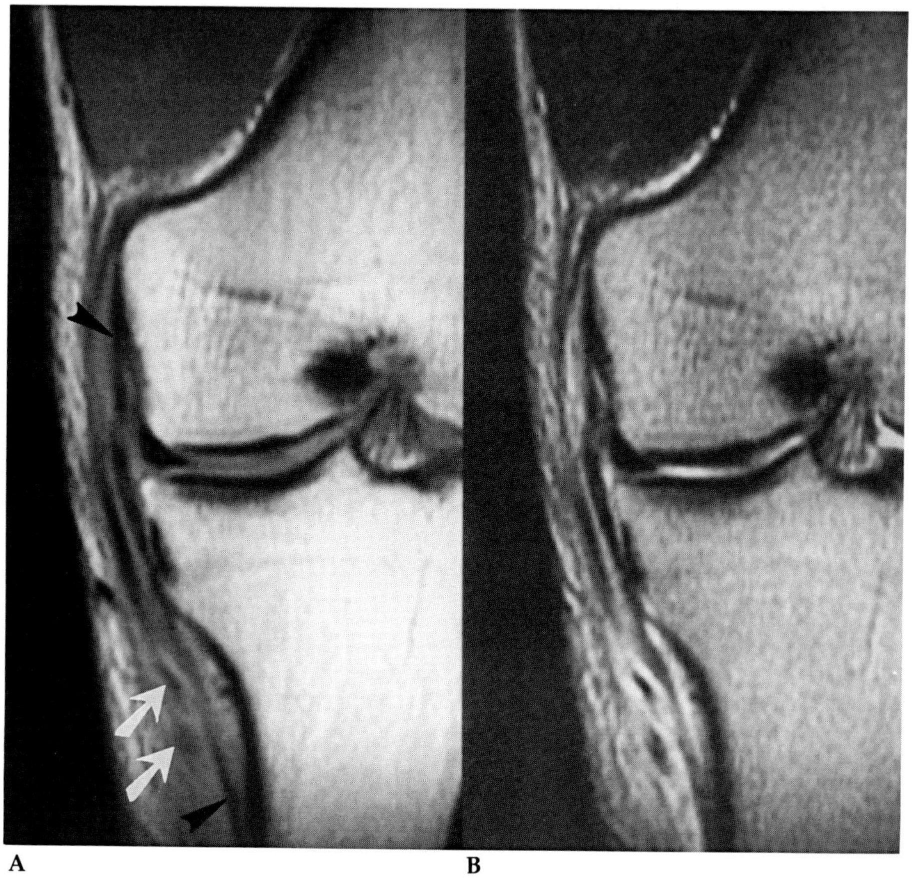

A B

FIGURE 37-1

DISCUSSION: The medial side of the knee can be identified from the images shown. The posterior cruciate ligament is round and always points to the medial side, while the linear fibers of the anterior cruciate ligament are directed toward to the lateral compartment.

The medial collateral complex (MCC) consists of (1) the superficial tibial collateral ligament (TCL), a semilunar, hypointense band concave medially, and (2) the deeper capsule, which is of intermediate signal intensity. The medial meniscus has tight capsular attachments; therefore, tears in the capsule are commonly associated with medial meniscal injuries.

MCC tears are graded on MRI in the following fashion:

Grade I: Capsular edema and/or hemorrhage (intermediate signal intensity).

Grade II: Capsular edema with interruption of only some TCL fibers.

Grade III: Capsular edema with complete TCL interruption.

Normally, in patients without arthropathy, a hyperintense fat pad lies medial to the medial meniscus. This pad may be obliterated by the hemorrhage of trauma, by granulation tissue, or by fibrosis from osteoarthritis. When this pad is obliterated by gray signal on T1-weighted sequences following trauma, we classify it as a grade I MCC injury. If there is associated disruption or fragmentation of some TCL fibers (white arrows in *A*) but others remain intact (arrowheads in *A*), a grade II MCC tear is diagnosed. Distally, at the injury site, hyperintense edema will circumscribe the injured fibers apparent in Figure 37-1*B*.

DIAGNOSIS: An MRI grade II MCC tear is present.

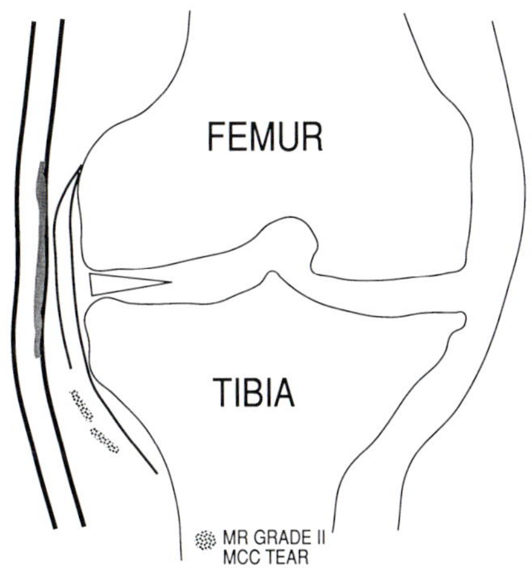

FIGURE 37-2

CASE 38

Differential Diagnosis of Knee Instability

HISTORY: A 21-year-old man sustained a valgus injury in rotational hyperextension during a college football game. What is the MRI diagnosis? (Fig. 38-1: coronal multiformat, multiecho proton-density (*A*) and T2-weighted (*B*) MR images.)

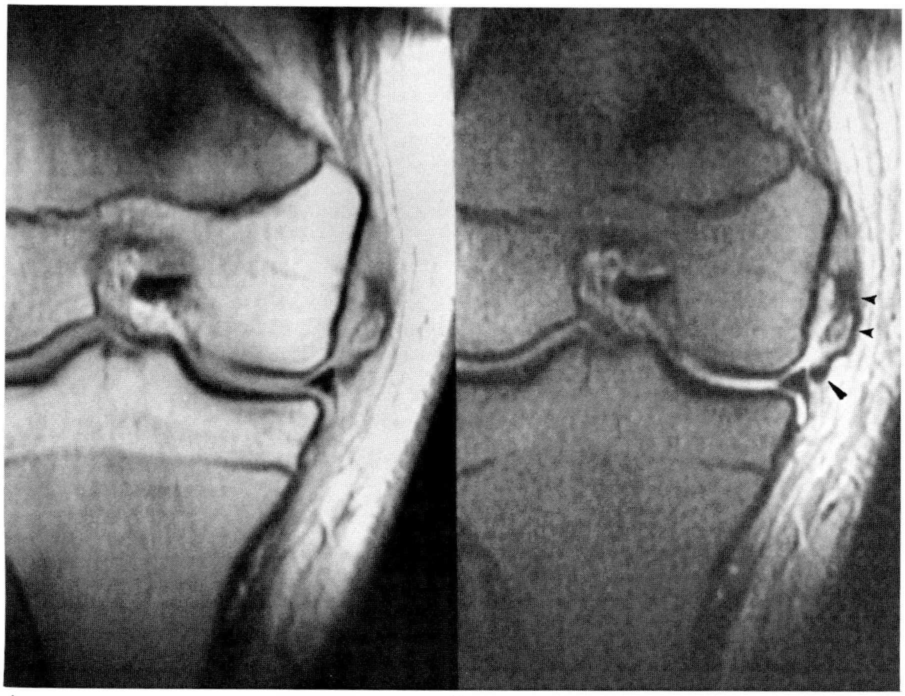

A **B**

FIGURE 38-1

DISCUSSION: The medial collateral ligament consists of a superficial component, the tibial collateral ligament (TCL), and a deeper, medial capsular ligament. The TCL component on MRI is a smooth, hypointense band that arises from the medial femoral condyle and inserts smoothly onto the medial aspect of the tibia 5.0 cm below the joint line. The superficial and deep ligamentous portions are separated by a bursa. The deep or capsular portion of the ligament attaches tightly to the body of the medial meniscus. The deep or fibrous capsule almost always tears before the superficial TCL fibers tear; therefore, a TCL tear implies capsular disruption. A third ligamentous component to give way is the anterior cruciate ligament (ACL). Frequently, tears of the TCL and capsule produce avulsion of the peripheral portion of the medial meniscus (single arrowhead in *B*). Note that the superficial or TCL component is not smooth, and its tibial insertion cannot be traced. Rather, the ligament is corrugated and has an accordian-like appearance (paired arrowheads in *B*). The apex of the torn medial collateral ligament terminates as a rounded or triangular hypointense focus that represents avulsion of the peripheral third of the meniscus. The combined occurrence of ACL tear, medial collateral complex injuries, meniscal tears, and bone contusions is known as the "terrible quadrad."

DIAGNOSIS: The patient has a medial collateral ligament tear, a medial meniscus midbody tear, and an anterior cruciate ligament tear (not shown).

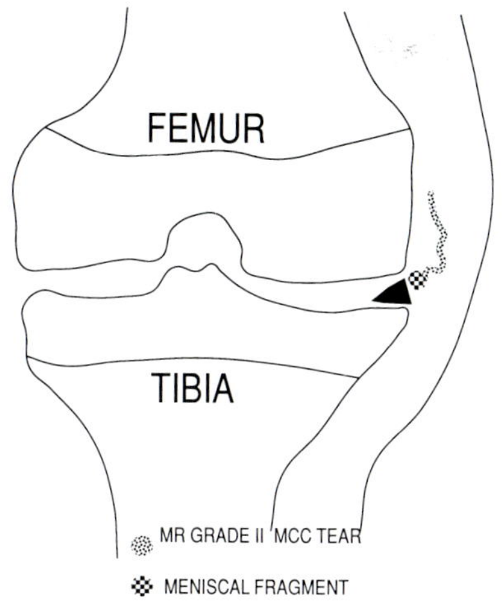

FIGURE 38-2

CASE 39

Differential Diagnosis of Acute Knee Pain

HISTORY: A 31-year-old man reported mild knee swelling and pain after a fall during a racquetball match. What is the MRI diagnosis? (Fig. 39-1: sagittal multiecho proton-density (*A*) and T2-weighted MR images, TR/TE 2,000/20, 80 msec, 16.0-cm FOV, 128 × 256 pixel matrix, 5.0-mm sections, 2 excitations.)

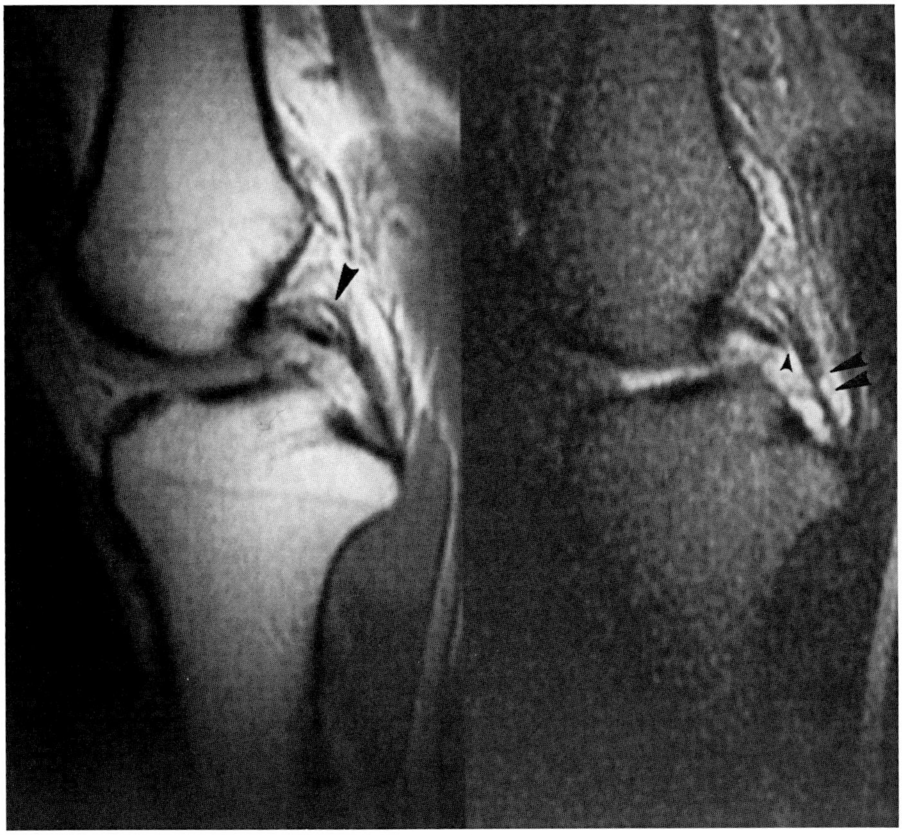

A **B**

FIGURE 39-1

DISCUSSION: The posterior cruciate ligament (PCL) is normally diminutive—approximately 13.0 to 20.0 mm thick in the sagittal plane. Smaller PCL diameters are seen in children. The ligament is normally invested by a circumferential sheath, and when a tear occurs, a pseudomass forms within the sheath. In this case, no such pseudomass was demonstrated. A small amount of fluid was noted in the dependent portion of the sheath (paired arrowheads in *B*). The T2-weighted image shows a small area of ligamentous discontinuity (small arrowhead in *B*).

This was called a PCL tear, and indeed, injury to 60% of the fibers of the PCL was present. This likely accounts for the signal alterations seen on the T2-weighted image. The ligament was also extremely small, and hypoplasia was diagnosed arthroscopically. Concomitant tear and congenital hypoplasia would be extremely difficult to differentiate from tear with secondary atrophy. However, this ligament was diminutive in size all the way to its proximal and distal insertions. PCL hypoplasia occurs in 1 in 600 cases.

The ligament of Wrisberg is seen in the sagittal plane behind the PCL (arrowhead in *A*).

DIAGNOSIS: The patient has a posterior cruciate ligament injury and hypoplasia.

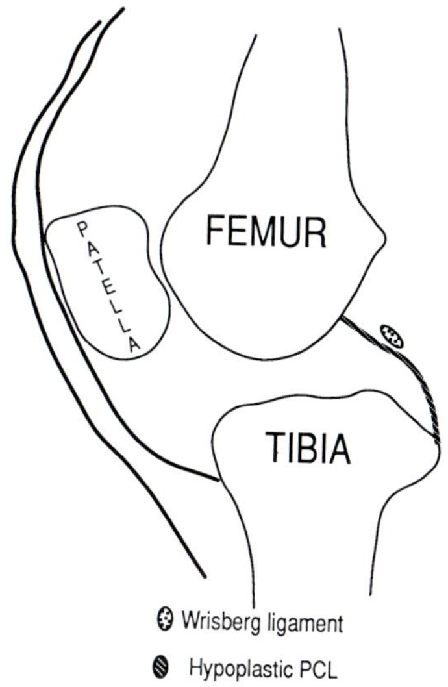

FIGURE 39-2

CASE 40

Differential Diagnosis of Knee Instability

HISTORY: A 27-year-old woman reported medial knee pain and knee instability after sustaining a medial twisting injury. What is the MRI diagnosis? (Fig. 40-1: sagittal proton-density MR image, TR/TE 1,000/20 msec.)

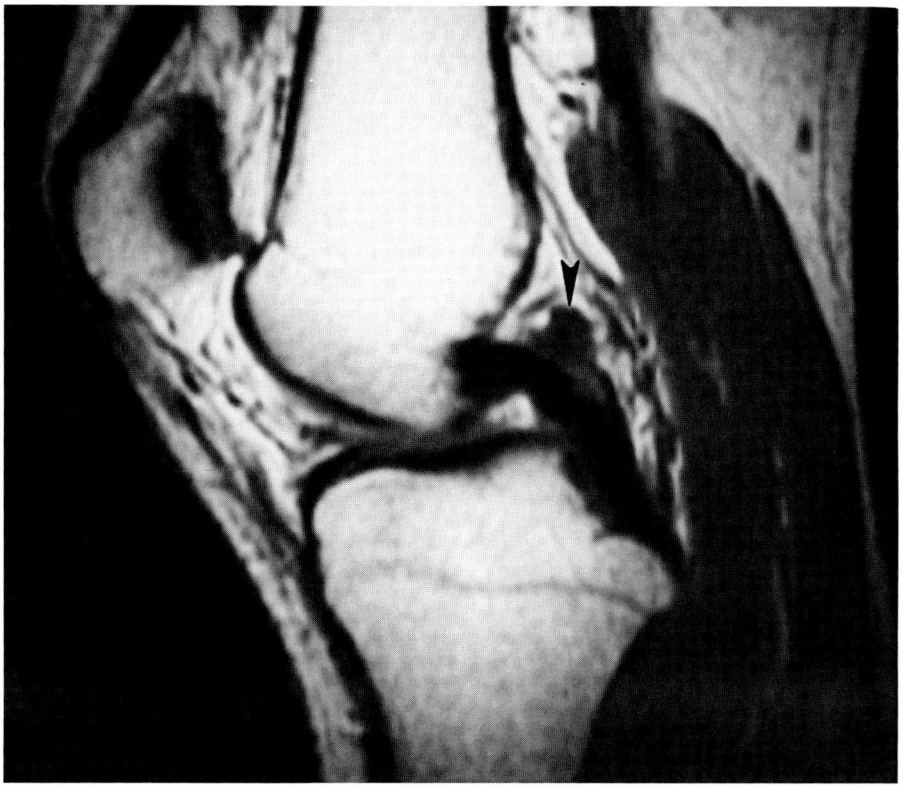

FIGURE 40-1

DISCUSSION: Behind the posterior cruciate ligament (PCL) is a globular area of intermediate signal intensity located at the intersection of the Wrisberg ligament. Occasionally, volume averaging of fibrous tissue or synovium (the PCL is extrasynovial and invested by a synovial covering) may produce intermediate signal intensity in or around the ligament (arrowhead), especially after arthroscopy. This signal will diminish with increased T2 weighting. Postarthroscopic signal alteration should not be misconstrued as a mass or tear.

Without discontiguity of the ligament or intraligamentous signal alteration, a diagnosis of PCL tear is unlikely. A prominent masslike bright intraligamentous T1 signal that is isointense or hypointense on T2-weighted sequences usually represents subacute hemorrhagic injury. Tear sites in or completely involving the PCL are not as masslike as the anterior cruciate ligament (ACL).

When bone avulsion occurs in association with PCL tear, it is usually at the tibial insertion. Therefore, discontiguity of ligament and bony surface is seen posteroinferomedially on MRI. From an anterior arthroscopic approach, only the femoral portion of the PCL is seen well when the ACL is intact—a distinct advantage of MRI over arthroscopy. The PCL is normally shorter, wider, and thicker than the ACL and of lower signal intensity. It is closely related to the attachment roots or insertion ligaments of the posteromedial meniscal horn.

DIAGNOSIS: The PCL is normal. A postarthroscopic synovial pseudomass is present.

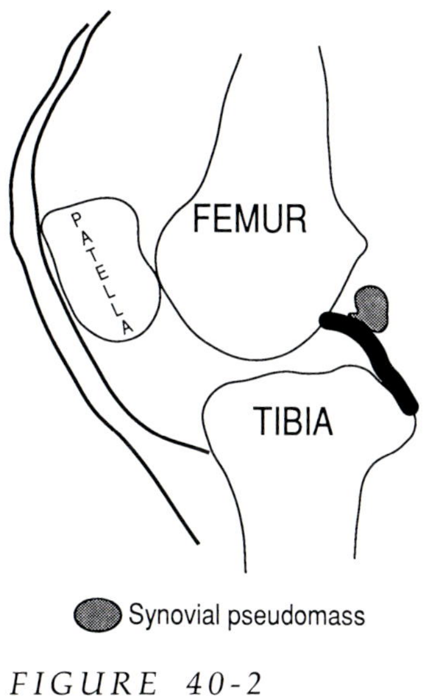

FIGURE 40-2

CASE 41

Differential Diagnosis of Ligamentous Disease of the Knee

HISTORY: A 56-year-old woman presented with posterior knee pain. What is the MRI diagnosis? (Fig. 41-1: sagittal multiecho proton-density (*A*) and T2-weighted MR images, TR/TE 1,400/20, 80 msec.)

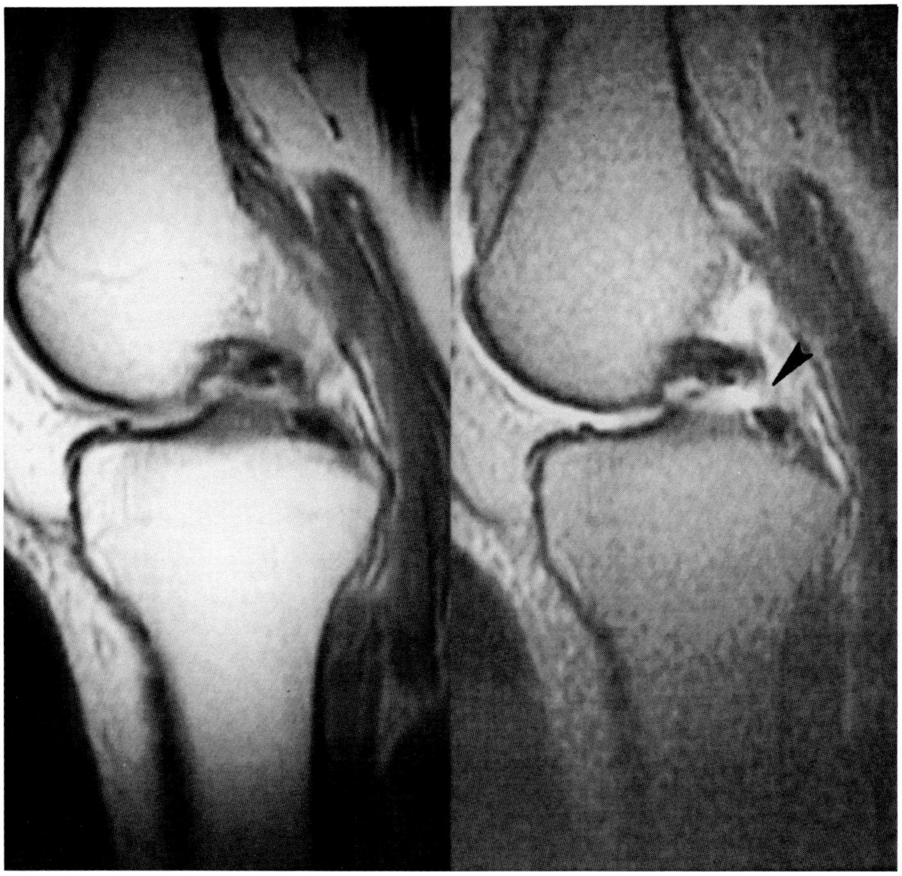

A B

FIGURE 41-1

DISCUSSION: The posterior cruciate ligament (PCL) is transected (arrowhead in *B*). Surrounding areas of T2 hyperintense edema or blood are noted in and about the ligament. The findings are compatible with complete tear of the PCL. The PCL is thicker, blacker, and less straight than the anterior cruciate ligament.

DIAGNOSIS: The patient has a complete tear of the PCL.

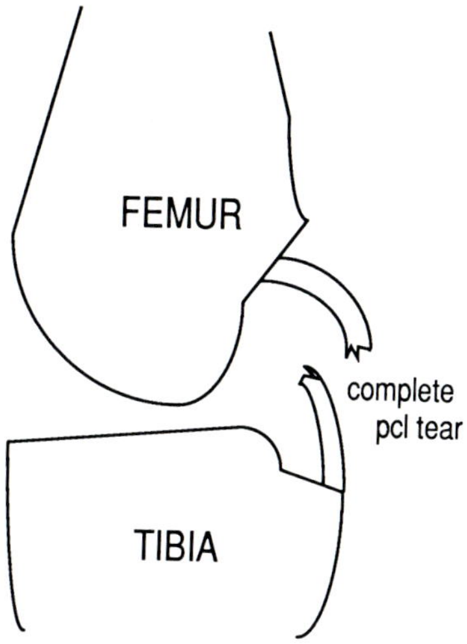

FIGURE 41-2

CASE 42

Differential Diagnosis of Posterior Knee Pain

HISTORY: A 26-year-old professional baseball player presented with posterior knee pain and difficulty running following a slide into third base with the knee in hyperflexion. The patient was referred for evaluation of posterior meniscus tear. What is the MRI diagnosis? (Fig. 42-1: sagittal, and Fig. 42-2: coronal T1-weighted MR images, TR/TE 900/20 msec.)

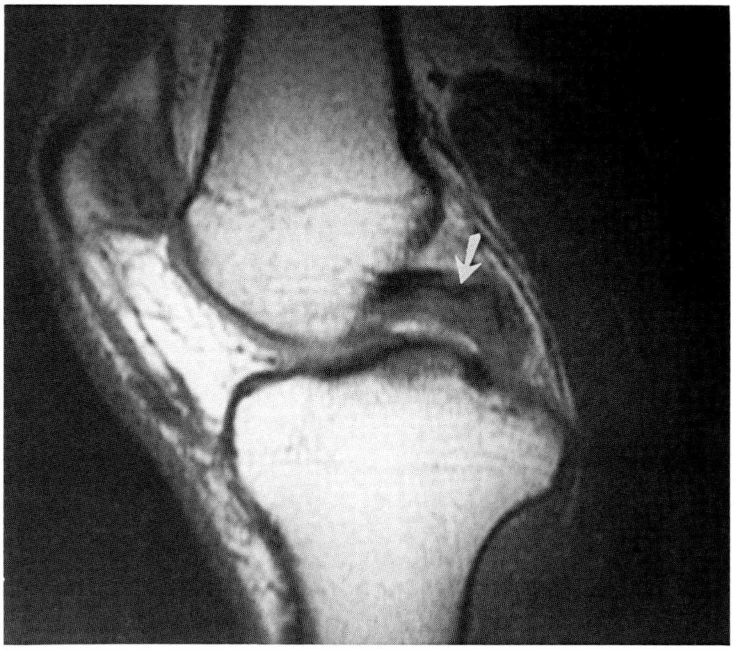

FIGURE 42-1

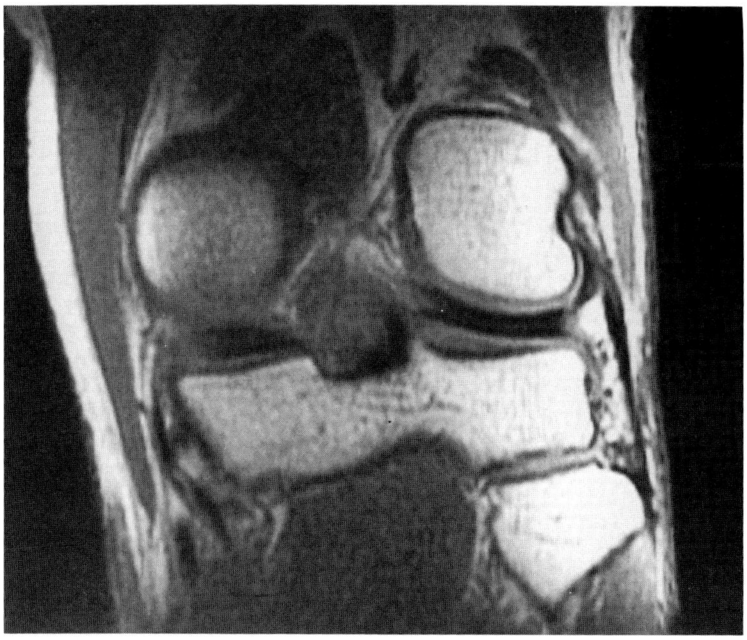

FIGURE 42-2

DISCUSSION: Normally the posterior cruciate ligament (PCL) is thicker and more hypointense than the anterior cruciate ligament (ACL), averaging 13.0 to 20.0 mm in cross-sectional diameter. The PCL is invested by a sheath and is extrasynovial. Rarely do the PCL proximal and distal fragments separate when torn, as the ACL fragments do. Usually the sheath contains an area of intermediate signal intensity hematoma that surrounds or bathes the cruciate fibers. Often the cruciate fibers can be seen coursing through this hematoma or area of contained edema; however, in this case the PCL fibers are barely visible (arrow in Fig. 42-1).

Most PCL injuries are a result of hyperflexion or a blow to the tibia with the knee in partial flexion. Extension-related PCL injuries occur but are rare. Although not as important as in evaluation of the ACL, examination of the PCL in the coronal projection is useful in confirming the extent of injury. A large round pseudomass of intermediate signal intensity may exist in the coronal projection, particularly near the posteroinferior tibial insertion.

DIAGNOSIS: The patient has a PCL tear and a coronal PCL hematoma pseudomass.

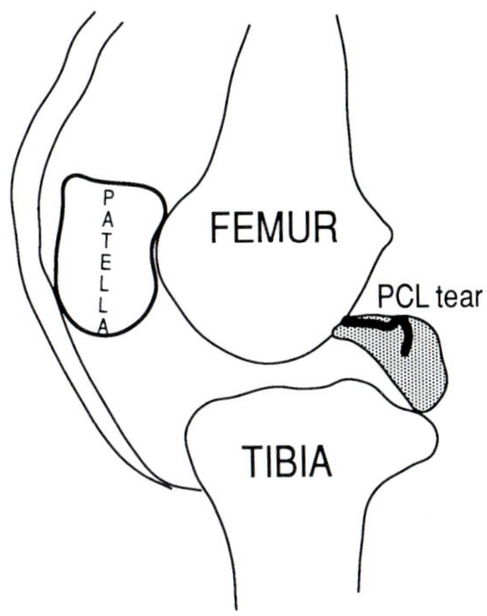

FIGURE 42-3

CASE 43

Differential Diagnosis of Osteocartilaginous Disease of the Knee

HISTORY: A 37-year-old former college soccer player presented with chronic bilateral knee pain, most severe laterally in the left knee. What is the MRI diagnosis? (Fig. 43-1: sagittal, and Fig. 43-2: coronal proton-density MR images.)

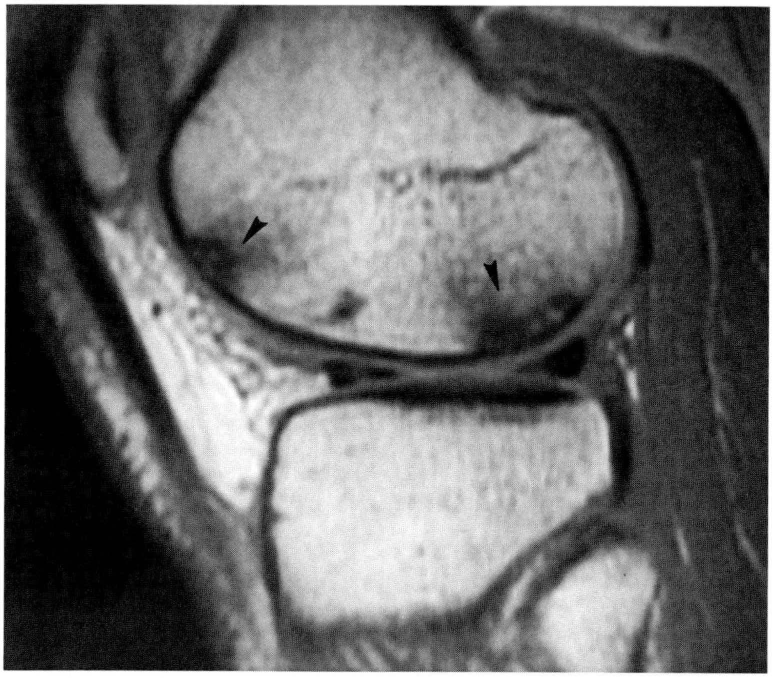

FIGURE 43-1

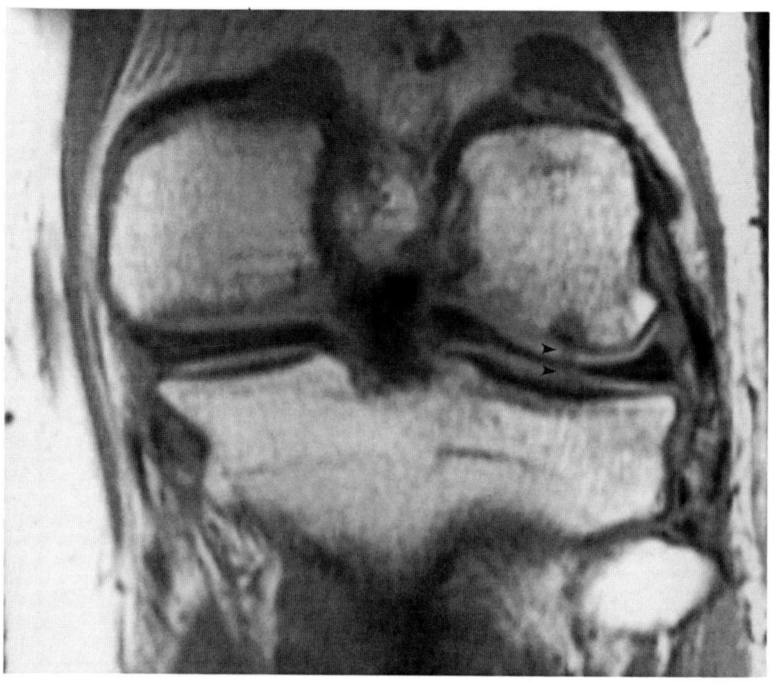

FIGURE 43-2

DISCUSSION: Multiple subchondral medullary bone foci of signal hypointensity are noted in the sagittal view (arrowheads in Fig. 43-1). These dark areas are surrounded by less hypointense and less well-demarcated bone edema. Although the cartilage appears intact in this projection, the coronal projection shows kissing ulcers (small arrowheads in Fig. 43-2) on the tibial and femoral surfaces. The femoral lesion extends through the cartilage and involves the subchondral bone. The cartilaginous involvement, multifocal nature of the process, and involvement of the weight-bearing surface make a diagnosis of grade IV chondromalacia absolute.

The most commonly used grading system for chondromalacia on MRI (see Fig. 43-3) is as follows:

- Grade I: Intracartilaginous signal hypointensity, the equivalent of cartilaginous softening.
- Grade II: Intracartilaginous signal hypointensity, contour alteration or blistering of the cartilaginous surface (caudal arrowhead in Fig. 43-1).
- Grade III: Broad areas of cartilaginous hypointensity extending to the surface and producing a serrated or crabmeat appearance to the chondral surface.
- Grade IV: Cartilaginous ulcers that produce signal alteration in the underlying bone and traverse the entire cartilaginous thickness.

On fast scan gradient-echo images, the normal hyaline cartilage appears smooth, homogeneous, and hyperintense. Ulcers appear as areas of thinning and signal hypointensity. Areas of sclerosis secondary to recurrent chronic trauma associated with degenerative chondromalacia must be differentiated from osteochondral fractures and osteochondritis dissecans. With acute injuries, soft tissue and/or bone edema, micro- or macrofracture lines, and frank bone displacement may be seen. Osteochondritis dissecans, a subset of osteochondral injury, is well demarcated, extremely hypointense, has typical non-weight-bearing distributions in its classic form, and may be displaced from its normal anatomic location.

DIAGNOSIS: The patient has grade IV chondromalacia.

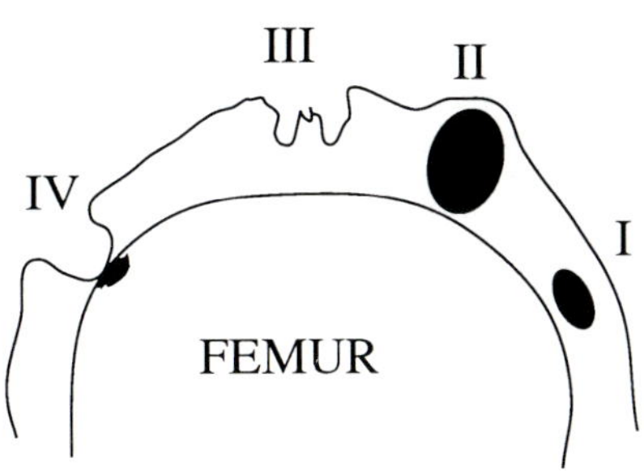

FIGURE 43-3

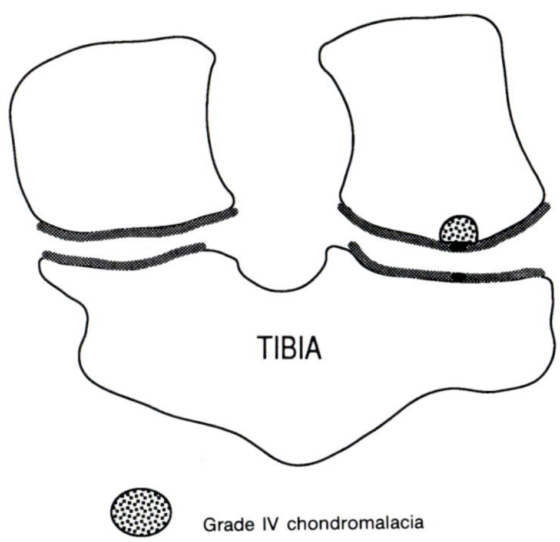

FIGURE 43-4

CASE 44

Differential Diagnosis of Osteocartilaginous Disease of the Knee

HISTORY: A 48-year-old woman with known chronic degenerative arthropathy but no history of recent trauma presented with acute knee pain and swelling. What is the MRI diagnosis? (Figs. 44-1 and 44-2: sagittal contiguous multisection single-echo proton-density MRI, TR/TE 1,400/20 msec, 14.0-cm FOV, 3.0-mm sections, 128 × 256 pixel matrix.)

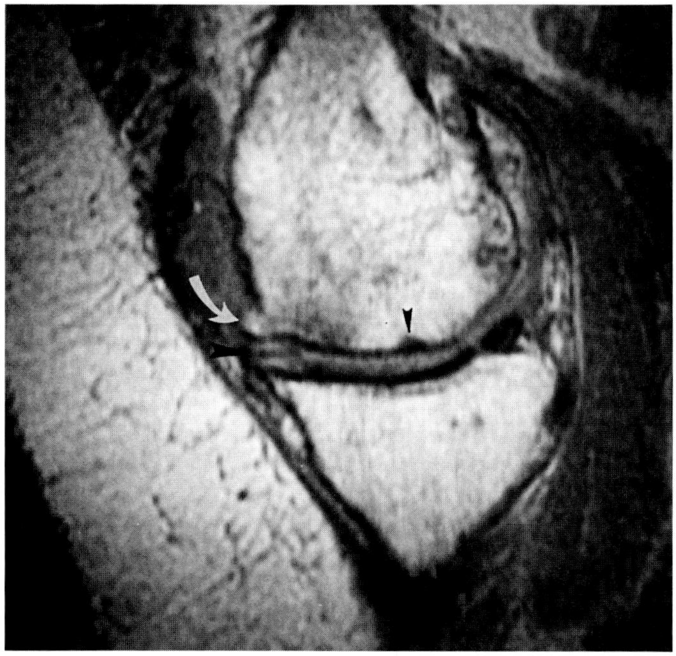

FIGURE 44-1

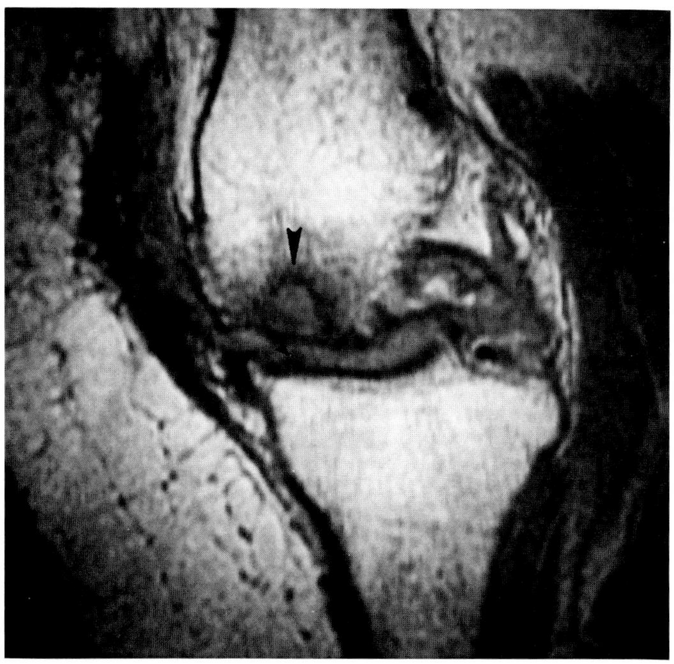

FIGURE 44-2

DISCUSSION: Cortical spurs (curved arrow in Fig. 44-1) as well as focal areas of decreased signal intensity within the intermediate signal intensity hyaline cartilage are present. Many of these hyaline cartilage ulcers extend to the bony surface and are evident posteriorly (vertical arrowhead in Fig. 44-1). A joint effusion is present. More anterior is a hypointense eliptical area (vertical arrowhead in Fig. 44-2) with a sharply marginated, hypointense rim and surrounding, poorly defined, hypointense edema. The lesion is larger than expected for simple grade IV chondromalacia ulcer.

Usually manifesting with acute pain, spontaneous osteonecrosis of the knee typically involves the weight-bearing segment of the mediofemoral condyle. Very occasionally the lateral femoral condyles are involved; rarely, the tibial plateaus (not necessarily their weight-bearing surfaces) are affected. This is a disease of older adults (most often women) aged 45 to 70 years and should not be misconstrued as osteochondritis dissecans or some other type of osteochondral injury or fracture. Osteochondritis dissecans most commonly occurs on non-weight-bearing surfaces and is more hypointense on T1-weighted or proton-density images than is early or midphase osteonecrosis. Chronic or acute trauma, intraarticular steroid injection, and loss of the normal meniscal pads owing to acute or chronic arthropathy have been implicated as etiologic factors.

In the setting of chronic arthropathy, these lesions do not overlie chondral ulcers. Typically the overlying meniscus is torn or absent (horizontal arrowhead in Fig. 44-1) due to degeneration as in this case. It is possible that loss of the normal meniscal pad results in local trauma and subsequent local ischemia predisposing to osteonecrosis. Subtle hypointense intracartilaginous foci are also present (vertical arrowhead in Fig. 44-1), representing earlier grades of chondromalacia.

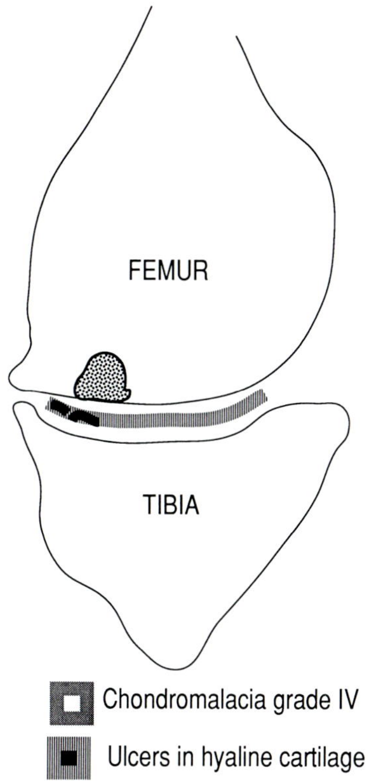

FIGURE 44-3

DIAGNOSIS: The patient has spontaneous osteonecrosis (adult type), degenerative arthropathy, chondromalacia, and degenerated menisci.

CASE 45

Differential Diagnosis of Osteocartilaginous Disease of the Knee

HISTORY: A 36-year-old man reported acute knee pain and swelling after sliding into third base. The patient was referred to rule out a diagnosis of medial meniscus tear. (Figs. 45-1 and 45-2: conventional anteroposterior radiographs of the knee. Fig. 45-3: sagittal proton-density (*A*) and T2-weighted (*B*) MR images, TR/TE 2,000/20, 5.0-mm sections, 16.0-cm FOV, 256 × 128 pixel matrix, 2 excitations.)

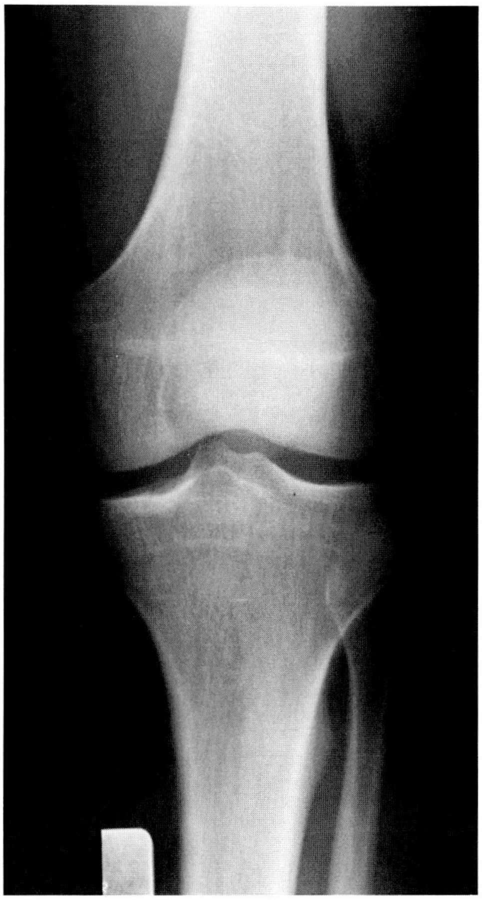

FIGURE 45-1

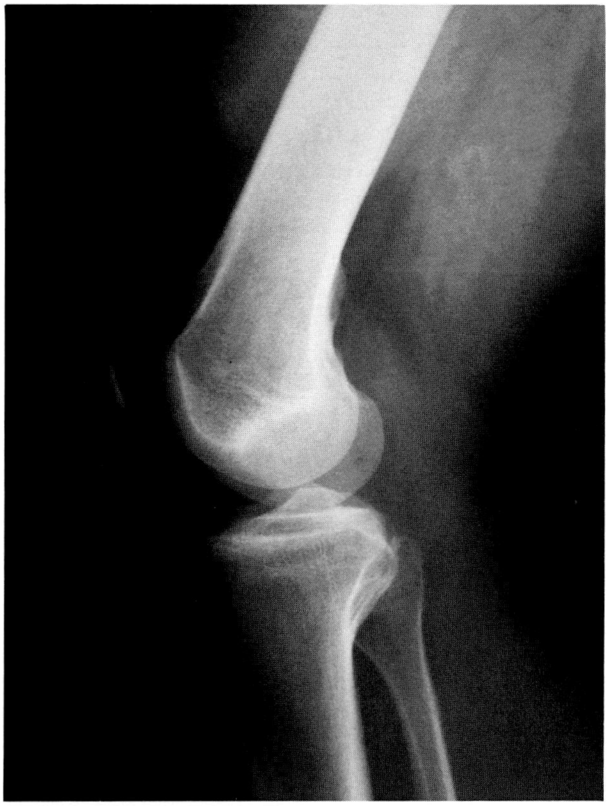

FIGURE 45-2

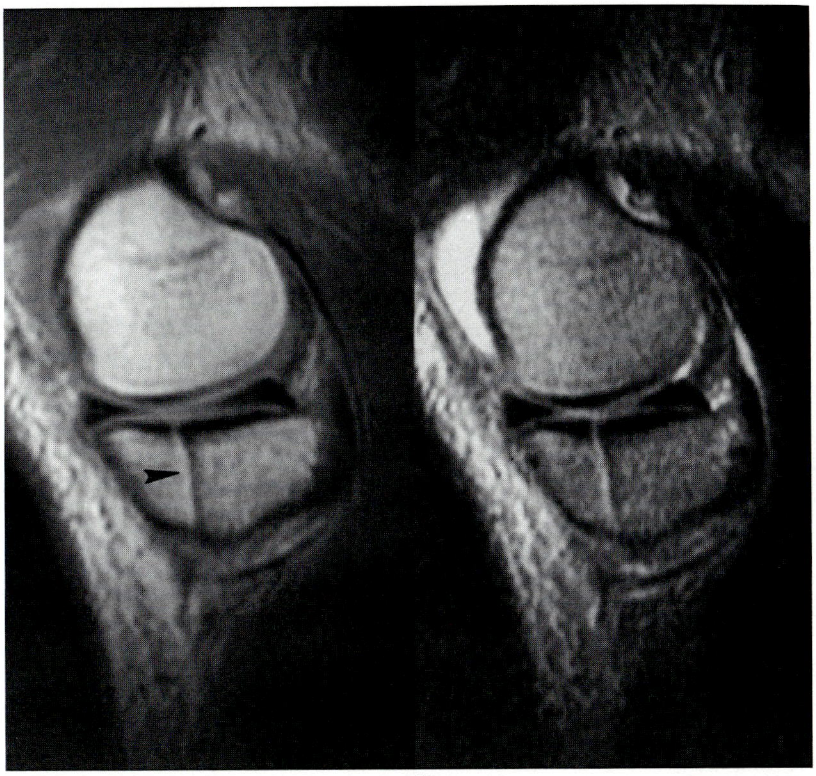

A B

FIGURE 45-3

DISCUSSION: A linear hypointense line extends to the cortical surface of the tibial plateau and has a linear hyperintense line adjacent and just anterior to it (arrowhead in Fig. 45-3*A*). The findings are typical of a relatively nondisplaced tibial plateau fracture. The intermediate signal intensity hyaline cartilage is intact, an important piece of clinical information. The parallel, thin, white-and-black fracture lines represent a frequency-shift artifact related to chemical shift: the fat/water interface created by edema and intramedullary fat from the tibia produces this parallel line artifact. Chemical shift occurs in the frequency encoding direction, which in this case is from posterior to anterior. In addition, the degree of shift depends on the size of the fat/water interface and the field strength of the unit in operation.

This fracture would be characterized as a pure wedge fracture that spares the fibula and is nondisplaced, a type I plateau fracture according to the classification of Müller (see diagrams). These fractures are rare but are more commonly seen on the lateral and posterior aspect of the tibia. A type II fracture consists of a local central depression. A type III fracture consists of a displaced wedge of tibial bone with a central depression and an associated fibular head fracture. A type IV fracture includes fractures of both plateaus which are displaced, comminuted, and associated with fibular fracture.

A hyperintense joint effusion is appreciated on the T2-weighted image.

DIAGNOSIS: The patient has a nondisplaced wedge medial tibial (type I) plateau fracture.

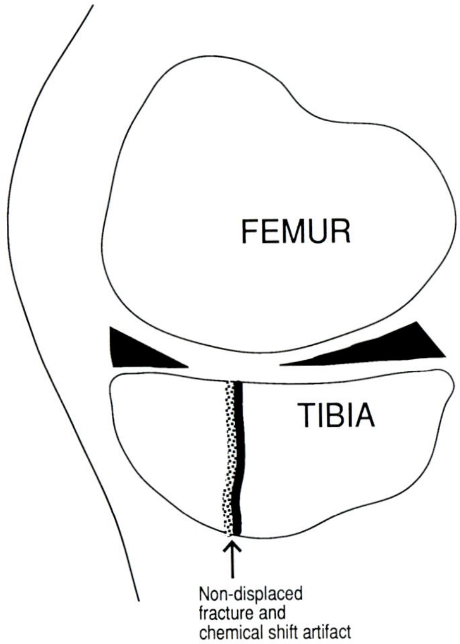

FIGURE 45-4

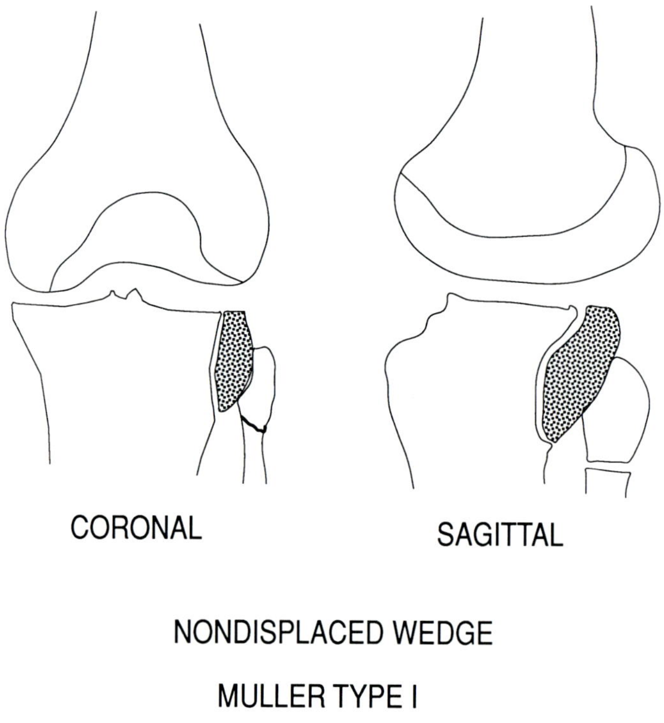

FIGURE 45-5

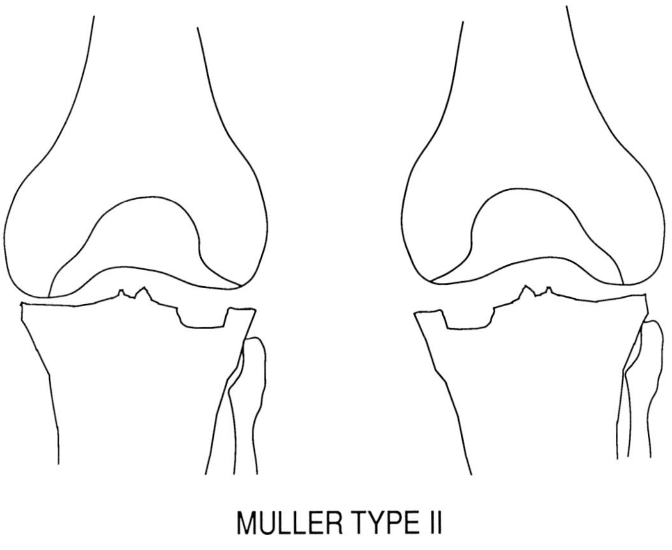

FIGURE 45-6

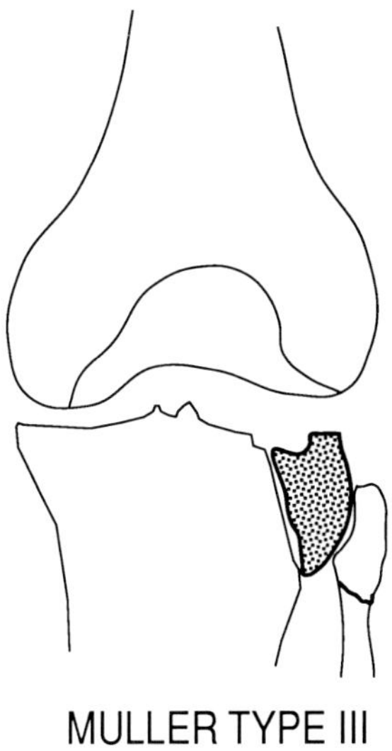

FIGURE 45-7

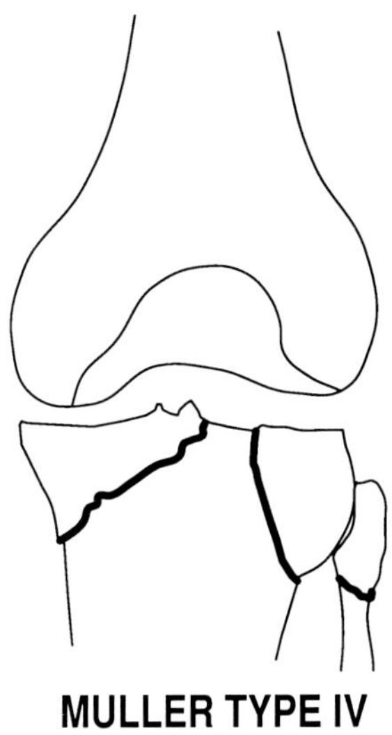

FIGURE 45-8

CASE 46

Differential Diagnosis of Osteocartilaginous Disease of the Knee

HISTORY: A 32-year-old man with lateral knee pain was referred for evaluation of a meniscal tear. (Fig. 46-1: coronal T1-weighted MR image.)

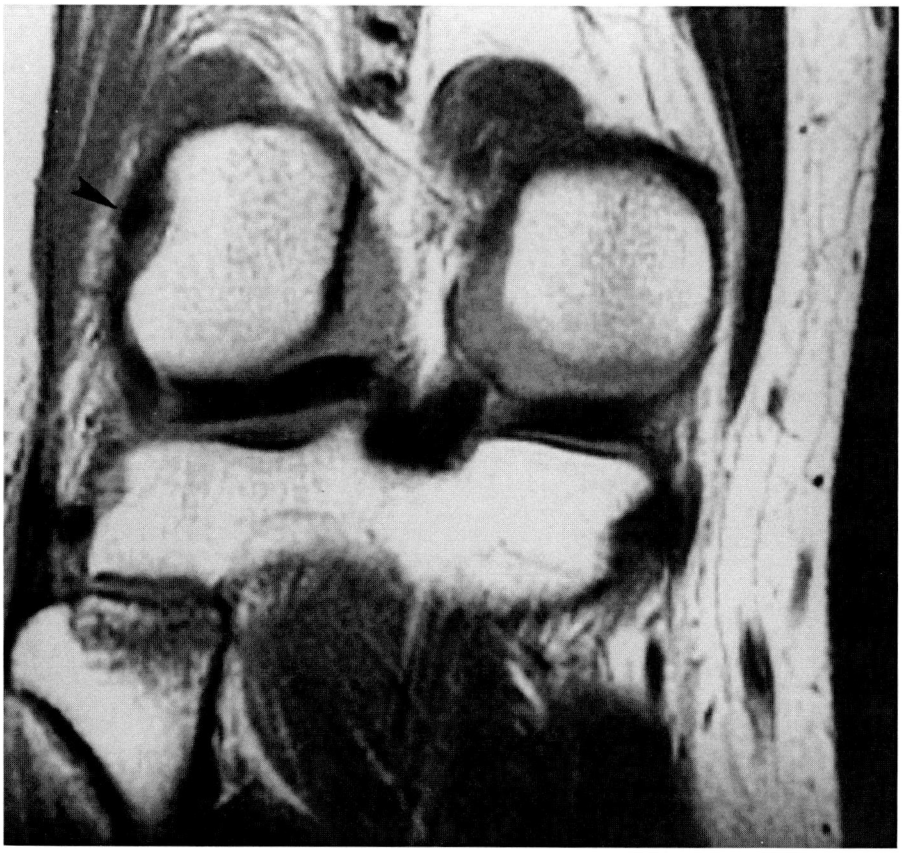

FIGURE 46-1

DISCUSSION: Both posterior meniscal horns are visible and have a rectangular shape. These will taper to a triangular shape on more anterior sections. The popliteus hiatus is seen as it originates from the lateral distal femur (arrowhead).

The menisci are of normal signal intensity and homogeneously hypointense. The patient's pain is not caused by meniscal disease; rather, the fibula exhibits hypointense signal in its most superior margin. The signal is moderately well demarcated and more hypointense than expected for a simple bone bruise. The signal is less hypointense than that seen with degenerative sclerosis, late-stage osteonecrosis, or osteochondritis dissecans. Both horizontal and vertical hypointense lines emanate from the proximal fibula.

DIAGNOSIS: The patient has a fibular stress fracture.

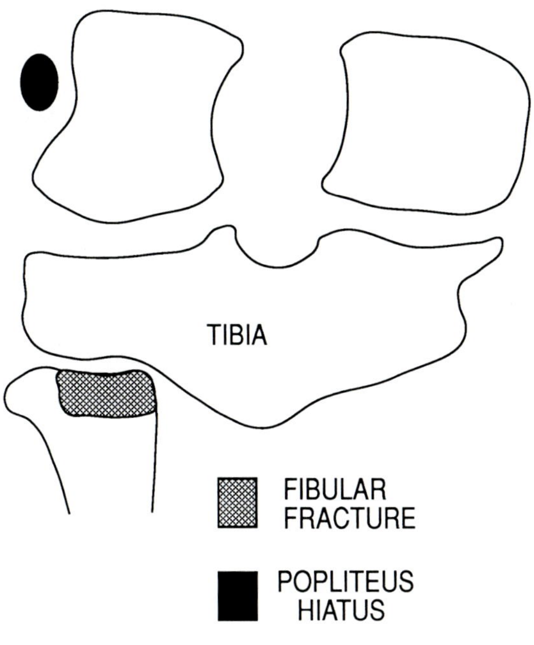

FIGURE 46-2

CASE 47

Differential Diagnosis of Osteocartilaginous Disease of the Knee

HISTORY: A 68-year-old patient presented with chronic bilateral knee pain of 2 years' duration. What is the MRI diagnosis? (Fig. 47-1: conventional anteroposterior radiograph of both knees. Fig. 47-2: sagittal multisection proton-density MR images, 4.0-mm sections.)

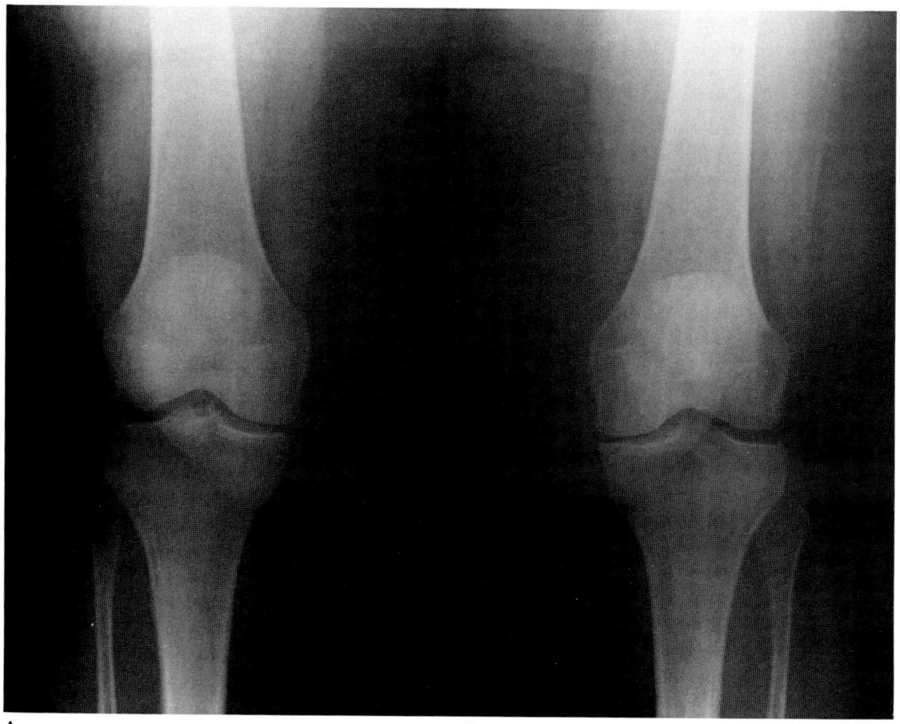

A **B**

FIGURE 47-1

A B

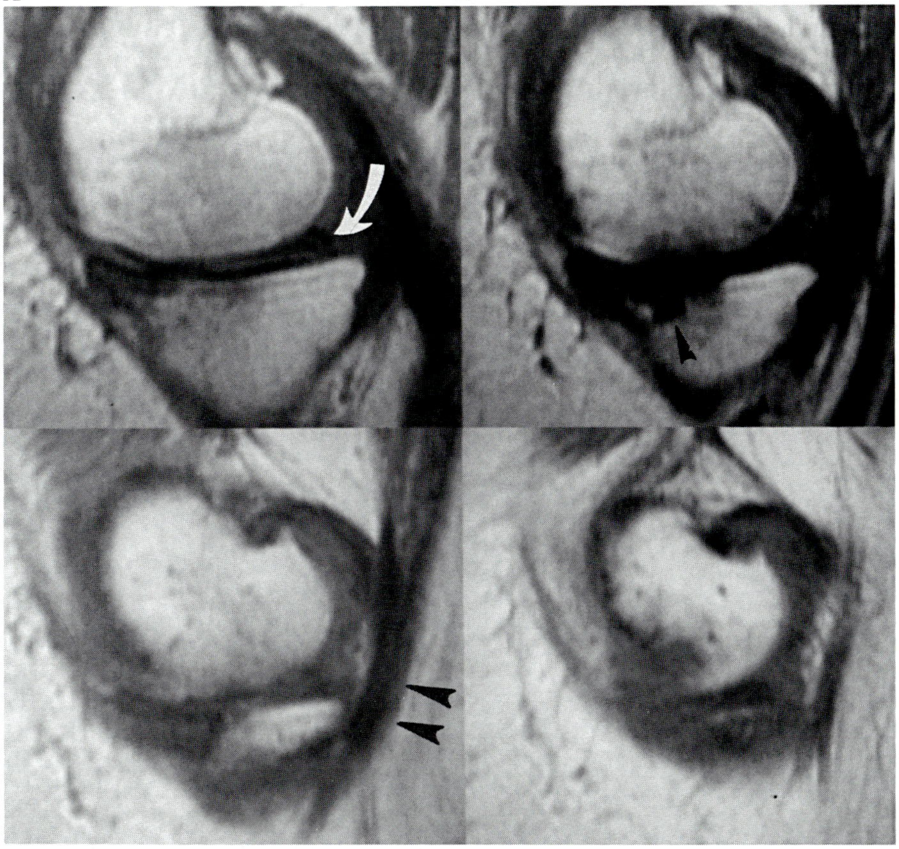

C D

FIGURE 47-2

DISCUSSION: The conventional radiograph, obtained with the patient standing, shows narrowing of the medial knee compartment bilaterally without evidence of bone disease. On the MR images the menisci appear small (curved arrow in Fig. 47-2*A*), a finding common with any form of arthropathy. The medial side of the knee is identified by the pes tendons anatomy (paired arrowheads in *C*). Focal areas of diminished signal intensity are present on both the tibial and femoral bone surfaces (*B*). The intermediate signal intensity hyaline cartilage pads appear small and thin. The subchondral location (arrowhead in *B*), marked hypointensity, multifocal nature, and relationship to a weight-bearing surface are typical of grade IV chondromalacia.

DIAGNOSIS: The patient has grade IV chondromalacia of the medial compartment.

CASE 48

Differential Diagnosis of Osteocartilaginous Disease of the Knee

HISTORY: A 17-year-old girl reported bilateral chronic knee pain of 8 months' duration. What is the MRI diagnosis? (Fig. 48-1: conventional and anteroposterior radiograph of both knees. Fig. 48-2: sagittal multisection proton-density MRI, and Fig. 48-3: coronal single-echo MRI of the left knee, 4.0-mm sections. Fig. 48-4: sagittal multisection proton-density MRI, and Fig. 48-5: coronal single-echo MRI of the right knee.)

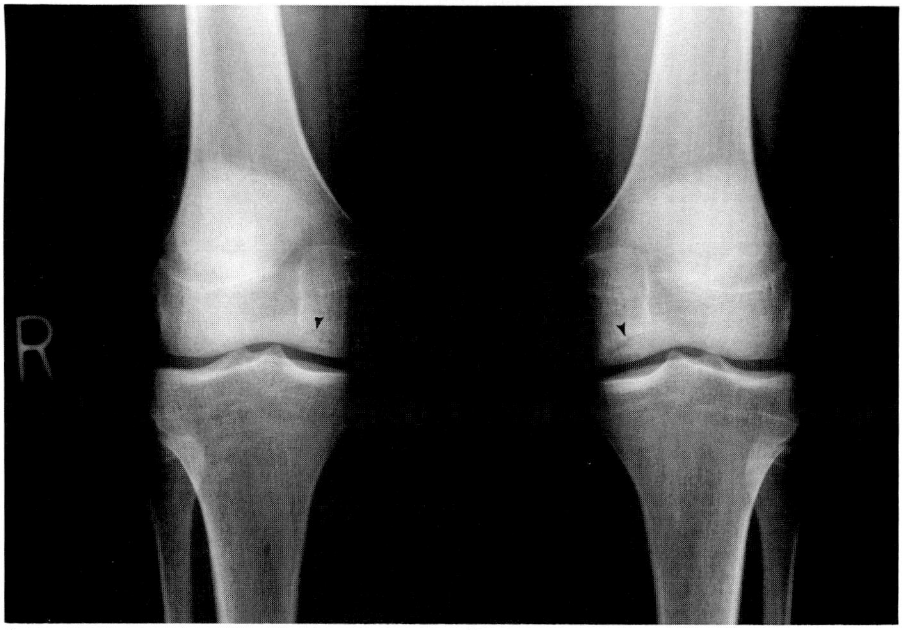

A B

FIGURE 48-1

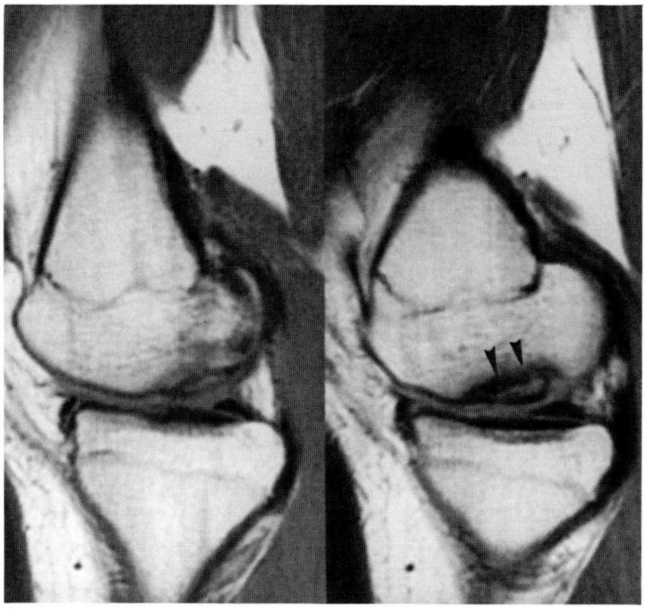

A B

FIGURE 48-2

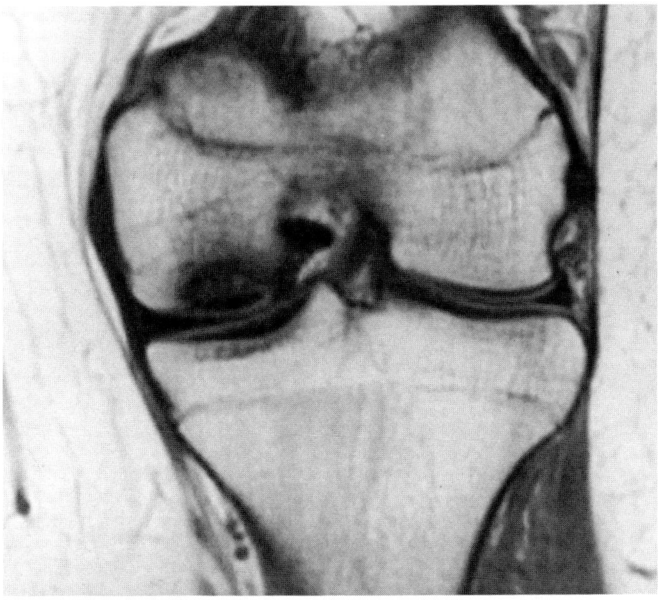

FIGURE 48-3

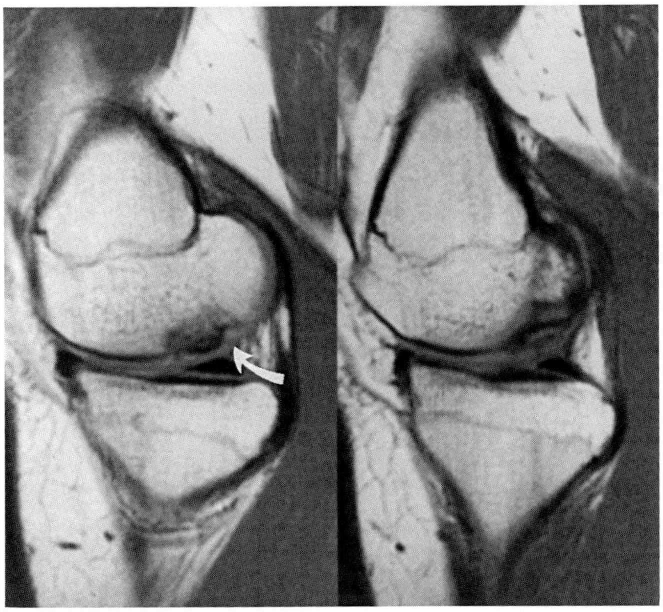

FIGURE 48-4

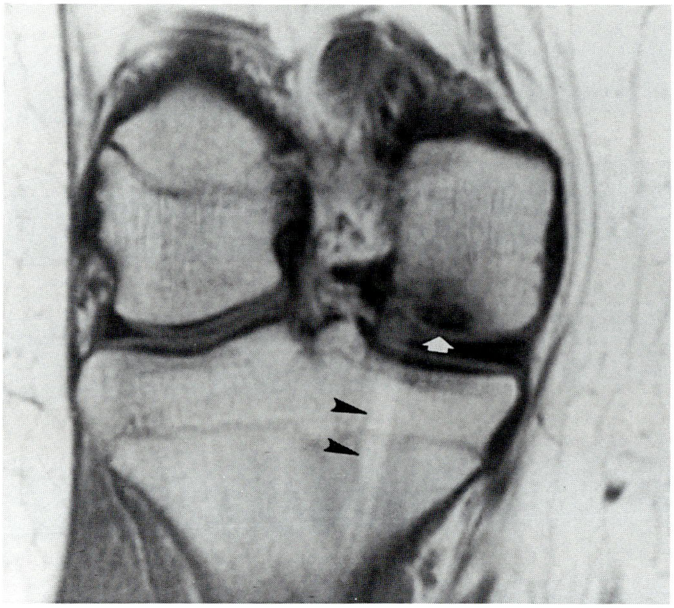

FIGURE 48-5

DISCUSSION: The conventional radiograph, obtained with the patient standing, shows subtle subchondral medial condylar irregularity (arrowheads). The bone irregularity involves the weight-bearing and non-weight-bearing portion of the medial femoral condyle, the "extended classic" form of osteochondritis dissecans.

The MR images show well-demarcated elliptical foci (paired arrowheads in Fig. 48-2*B*, white arrow in Fig. 48-5) of hypointense signal involving the medial femoral condylar apex (weight-bearing) and extending to the lateral portion of the medial condyle. The patient's young age, the bilateral nature of the process, and the absence of other systemic or focal arthropathies strongly support the diagnosis. Typical MRI findings of osteochondritis dissecans include the following:

1. Elliptical lesion shape,
2. Location (osteochondral, non-weight-bearing and weight-bearing),
3. T1 hypointensity,
4. Sharp demarcation,
5. Hypointense rim (paired arrowheads in Fig. 48-2*B*),
6. Paucity of surrounding edema,
7. Irregularity over overlying intermediate signal intensity cartilage.

Learning to evaluate cartilage abnormalities on T1 images can be difficult. Normally the hyaline cartilage is smooth, has a convex peripheral interface, and should not contain foci of punctate hypointense signal or linear hypointense signal (fissuring). In this case the intermediate signal alteration overlying the abnormal bone is variable in thickness, is irregular, and exhibits inhomogeneous signal, visible in the sagittal projection (white arrow in Fig. 48-4*A*).

Osteochondritis dissecans, a subset or complication of osteochondral injury, may be nondisplaced or displaced with regard to either its bone or cartilage component.

A foldover (aliasing) artifact is present (paired arrowheads in Fig. 48-5).

DIAGNOSIS: The patient has bilateral osteochondritis dissecans ("extended classic" type).

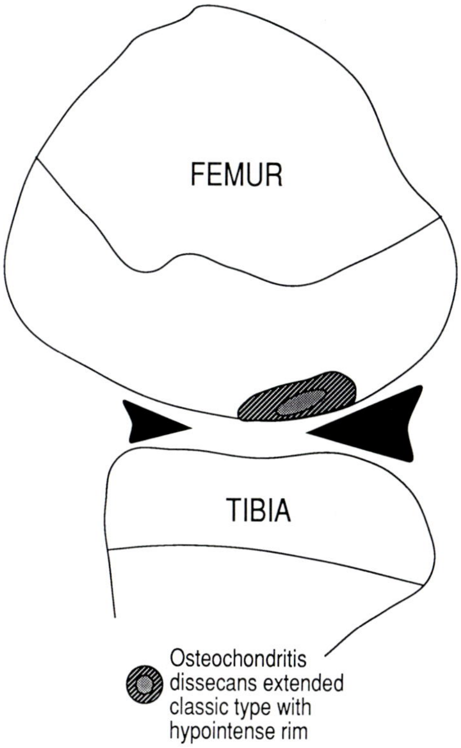

FIGURE 48-6

CASE 49

Differential Diagnosis of Osteocartilaginous Disease of the Knee

HISTORY: A 33-year-old patient described chronic anterior knee pain of 4 months' duration. What is the MRI diagnosis? (Fig. 49-1: sagittal, and Fig. 49-2: axial multisection single-echo proton-density MR images, 4.0-mm sections.)

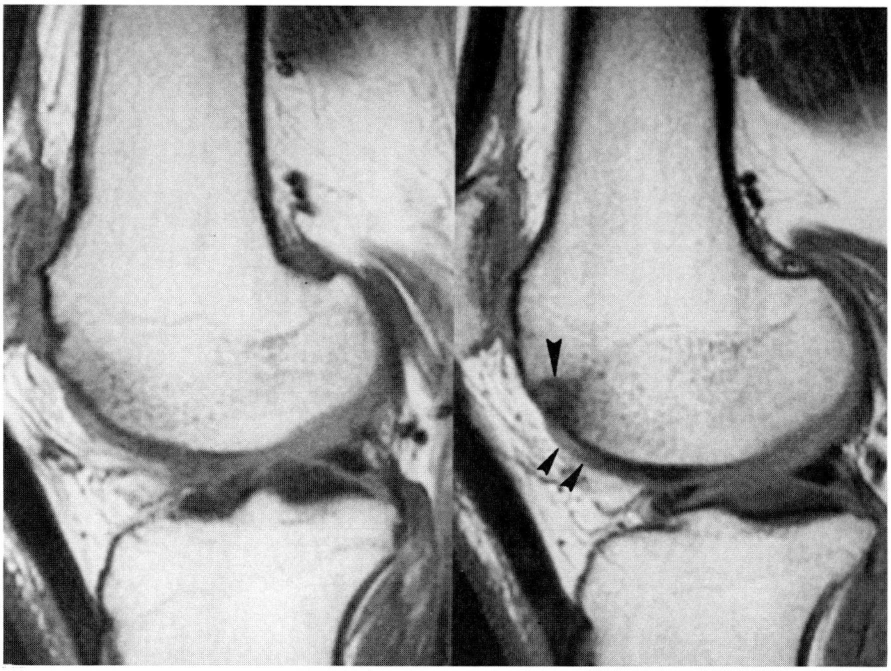

A B
FIGURE 49-1

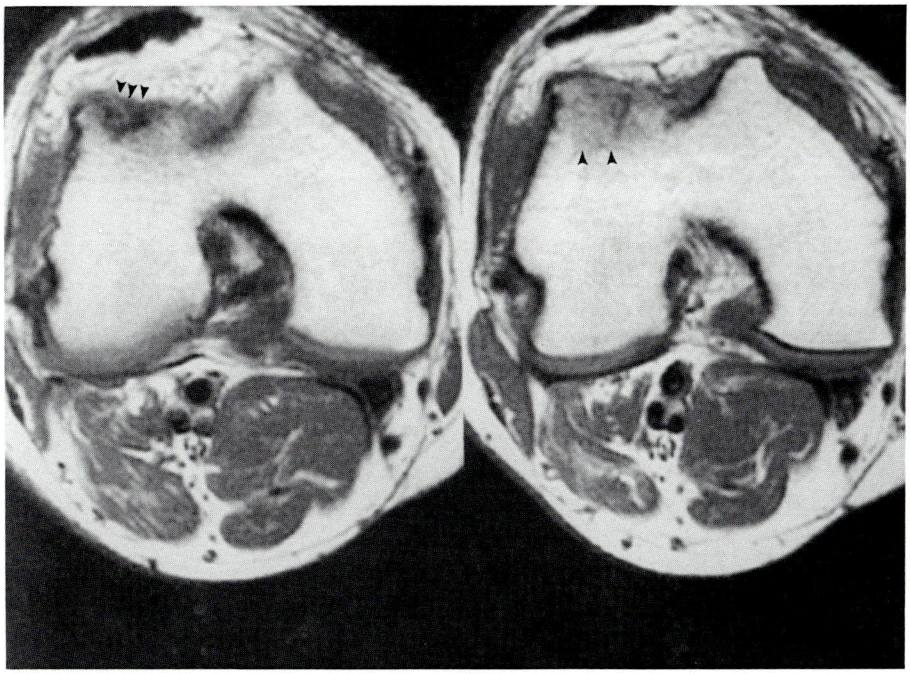

A B
FIGURE 49-2

DISCUSSION: A focal area of subcortical hypointense signal (large arrowhead in Fig. 49-1*B*) is noted along the anterior lateral femoral condyle. Surrounding areas of mild or nominal edema (small paired arrowheads in Fig. 49-2*B*) are located deep to the lesion. The normal hyaline cartilage thickness and signal are seen caudad to the lesion (paired arrowheads in Fig. 49-1*B*). The intermediate signal hyaline cartilage pad is interrupted over the lesion. Interruption of the overlying cortex (triple arrowheads in Fig. 49-2*A*) is also present. The findings are typical of an osteochondral injury (osteochondritis dissecans). The anterolateral location shown in this case is the least common location for this disease.

The differential diagnosis of subcortical lesions at the ends of bone can be divided into posttraumatic and nonposttraumatic etiologies. Both acute and chronic traumatic osteocartilaginous injuries about the knee can be subdivided into the following entities, based on their etiology and MRI findings:

ACUTE

1. Bone contusion or bruise: Vague, poorly defined hypointense foci on T1-weighted images that increase in signal with T2 weighting. No micro- or macrofracture lines are present, and the edema margin cannot be defined.
2. Micro- or stress fracture (bone involvement only): Bone edema with linear parallel or irregular but nondisplaced hypointense fracture lines.

3. Macrofracture (bone only): Can be subcategorized into displaced and nondisplaced types. Hypointense with T1 weighting, hyperintense with T2 weighting bone edema or bruise with a fracture line at least 1.0-mm thick, often apparent on conventional radiography.
4. Chondral bruise: Hypointense on T1-weighted and fast scans, with blistering or contour alteration of the normally smooth hyaline surface.
5. Chondral fissure or fracture: Linear hypointense T1 and discontiguous linear fast scan signal, often oblique.
6. Osteochondral fracture
   a. In situ. T1 hypointensity fracture lines without displacement and with normal medullary bone signal except for bone edema or bruising.
   b. Bone fragments are not displaced, but hypointense cartilage fragments migrate into the joint space.
   c. Both bone and cartilage are displaced from their normal location.

CHRONIC

1. Chondromalacia: Irregular, thinned cartilage with hypointense intracartilaginous foci. Unlike osteochondritis dissecans, multiple foci and involvement of weight-bearing articular surfaces predominate.

   Stage 1: Rounded or elliptical intracartilaginous areas of signal hypointensity with T1 weighting, often multifocal.

   Stage 2: Intracartilaginous areas of signal hypointensity on T1 weighting, with elevation of the cartilage surface.

   Stage 3: Broad, deep foci of intracartilaginous signal hypointensity sparing the underlying bone.

   Stage 4: Broad, deep foci of intracartilaginous signal hypointensity with underlying multifocal hypointense (with T1 weighting) bone erosions, areas of pannus, and geode formation.

2. Arthropathic subchondral cyst: Well-demarcated areas of signal alterations, hypointense with T1 weighting, hyperintense with T2 weighting, with both MRI signs (hyaline or fibrocartilage attenuation) and clinical signs of arthropathy. These lesions communicate with the joint space.
3. Intraosseous ganglion: Subcortical, eccentric, well-demarcated water-like signal on MRI. Does not communicate with the joint space. Most common along the medial tibial surface of the ankle rather than the knee.
4. Osteochondritis dissecans: Elliptical focus of signal hypointensity most common on a non-weight-bearing surface, well marginated, no or mild edema, normal or interrupted cartilage signal. This is a subset or chronic sequela of osteochondral injury.

DIAGNOSIS: The patient has osteochondritis dissecans, anterolateral type.

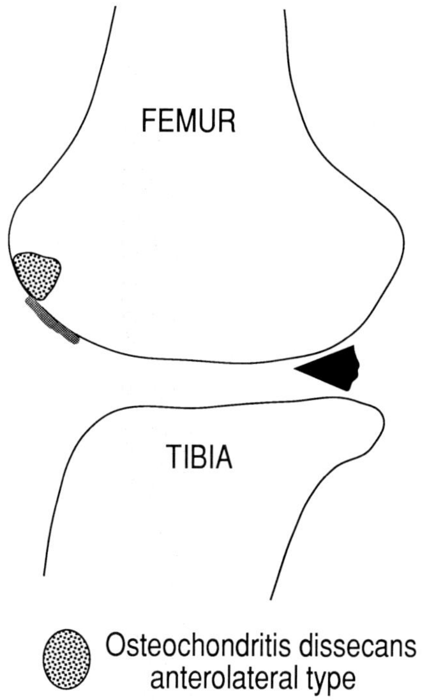

FIGURE 49-3

CASE 50

Differential Diagnosis of Osteocartilaginous Disease of the Knee

HISTORY: A 40-year-old man reported that his knee buckled under him in hyperflexion while he was mowing the lawn. The patient is now experiencing medial knee pain. What is the MRI diagnosis? (Fig. 50-1: sagittal multiecho proton-density (*A*) and T2-weighted (*B*) MR images.)

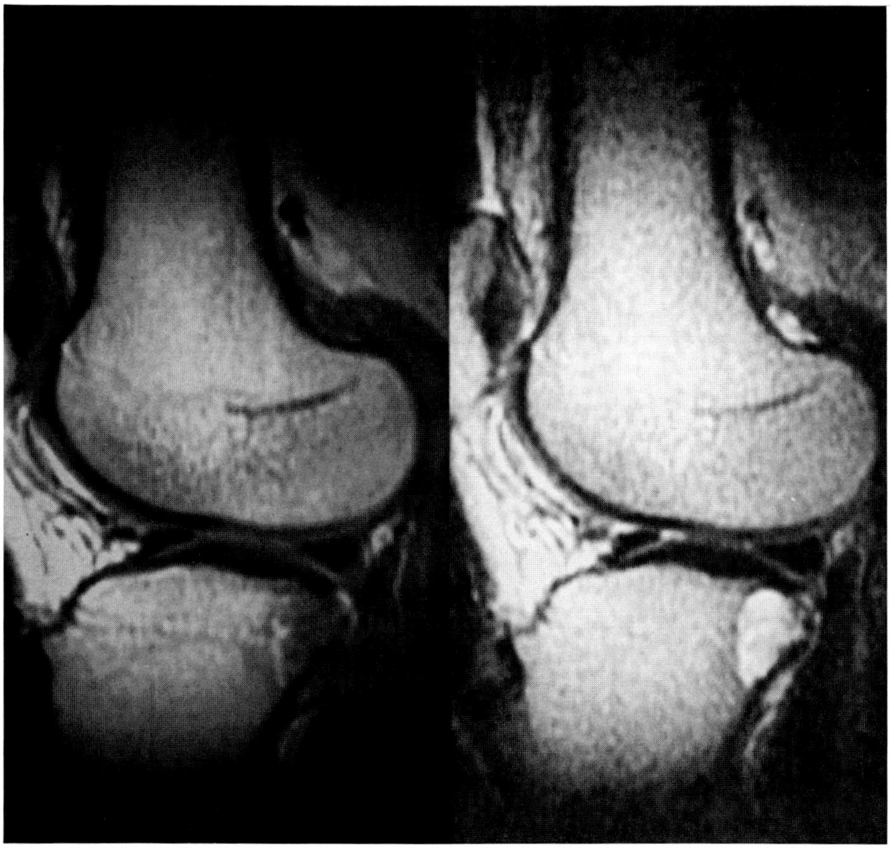

A **B**

FIGURE 50-1

DISCUSSION: Unlike cases of bone contusion or edema, in which signal alterations are poorly marginated, there is a focal, well-defined area of signal hypointensity on this study (smaller arrowhead in Fig. 53-1). The hypointense signal is not as dark as expected in a case of osteochondritis dissecans or frank necrosis (bone death). Areas of edema surround the trauma site and are hypointense on T1 weighting but are less well defined (larger arrowhead in Fig. 53-1). Notice the hypointense fissure within the cartilage in the sagittal projection (open arrow in Fig. 53-1). A focal osteocartilaginous fragment (small arrowhead in Fig. 53-2) appears as a punctate area of low signal intensity surrounded by intermediate signal intensity hyaline cartilage in the coronal projection. Interruption of the cortical bone with involvement of the underlying medullary bone (smaller arrowhead in Fig. 53-1) is compatible with the osseous portion of the injury.

Decreasing the likelihood of osteochondritis dissecans (a complication of osteochondral fracture) is the absence of sharp demarcation, the recent history of trauma, the presence of edema, and the poorly defined lesion margin. Although bone edema is present, the process is too focal to represent a simple bone contusion or edema. In addition, the chondral abnormalities preclude this diagnosis.

DIAGNOSIS: The patient has an acute femoral osteochondral fracture.

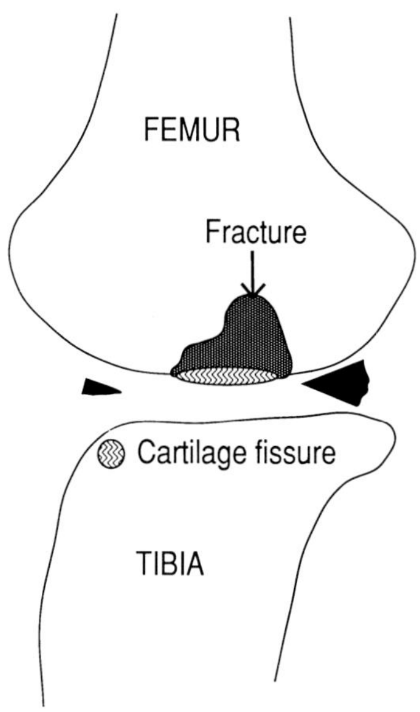

FIGURE 53-3

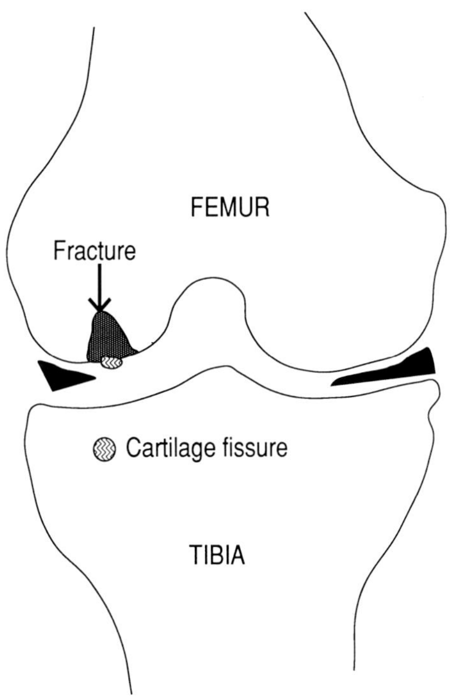

FIGURE 53-4

CASE 54

Differential Diagnosis of Osteocartilaginous Disease of the Knee

HISTORY: An 11-year-old Little League baseball player presented with chronic lateral knee pain of 1 year's duration. (Fig. 54-1: coronal T1-weighted MR image. Fig. 54-2: coronal fast scan gradient-echo MR image, TR/TE 250/15 msec, 18° flip angle.)

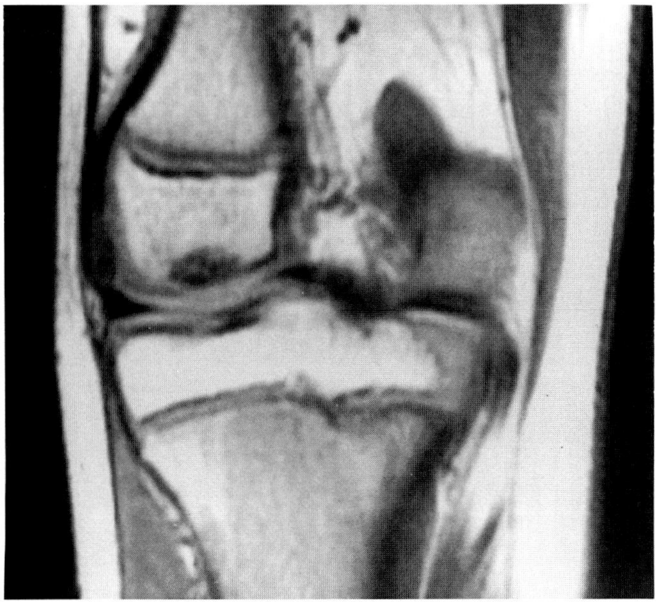

FIGURE 54-1

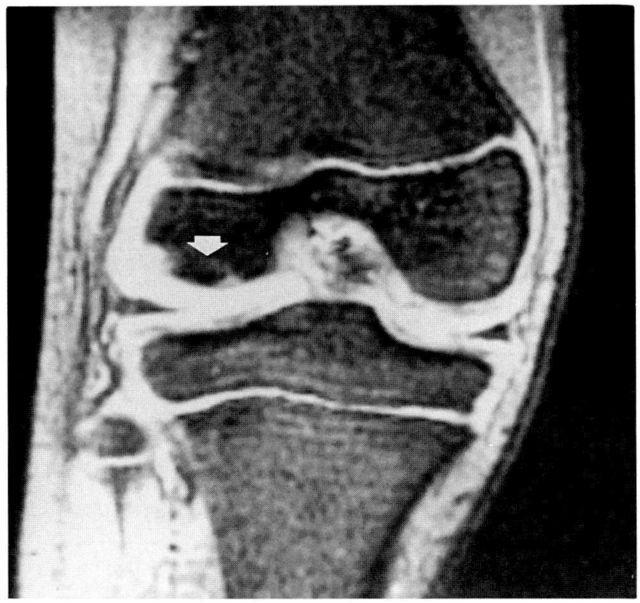

FIGURE 54-2

DISCUSSION: A confluent and well-demarcated hypointense subchondral crescenteric signal alteration is present in the posterolateral femur. The signal alteration on the coronal fast scan is barely visible in the bone (arrow in Fig. 54-2) and the overlying cartilage on all sequences is intact. The thick hyaline cartilage pad is homogeneous, smooth, hyperintense, and convex caudally on fast scan gradient-echo imaging. The lesion is well-demarcated, unlike a bone bruise. The normal hyaline cartilaginous appearance precludes grade IV chondromalacia as a diagnosis. The linear hypointense signal of stress fracture or recent macrofracture is not present. There is no bone or soft tissue edema, implying that the lesion is longstanding.

Typically, osteochondritis dissecans is hypointense on all pulse sequences, with a barely visible peripheral rim of increased signal intensity on fast scan images. The locations of osteochondritis dissecans are as follows:

1. lateral aspect of the medial femoral condyle (69%),
2. extended involvement of the medial femoral condyle from notch to apex (6%),
3. most medial aspect of the medial femoral condyle, or an inferocentral location (10%),

4. inferocentral lateral femoral condyle (13%), and
5. anterior lateral femoral condyle.

This is an inferocentral lateral condylar lesion. Since the cartilage is spared, this would be considered an in situ form of the disease. More advanced disease includes an osteocartilaginous flap that is partially attached (grade 2), an osteocartilaginous flap that is detached (grade 3), and an osteocartilaginous flap that is detached and has migrated (grade 4).

DIAGNOSIS: The patient has lateral femoral condylar osteochondritis dissecans.

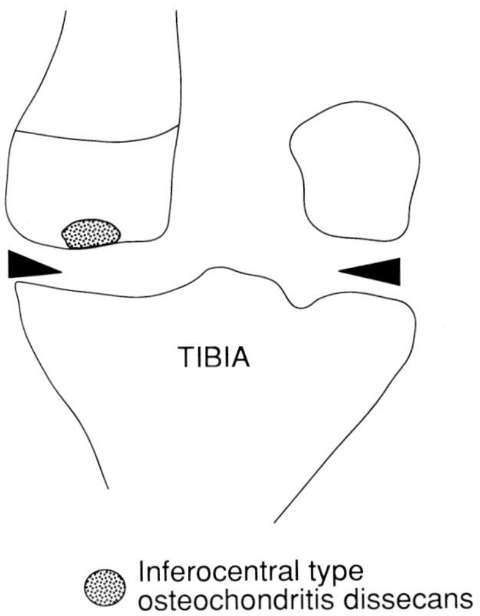

FIGURE 54-3

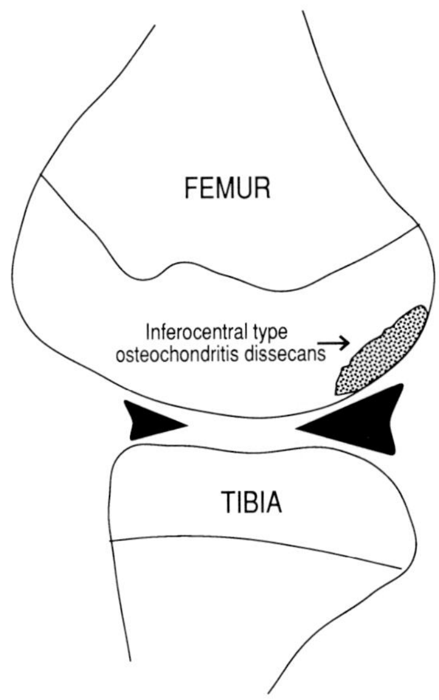

FIGURE 54-4

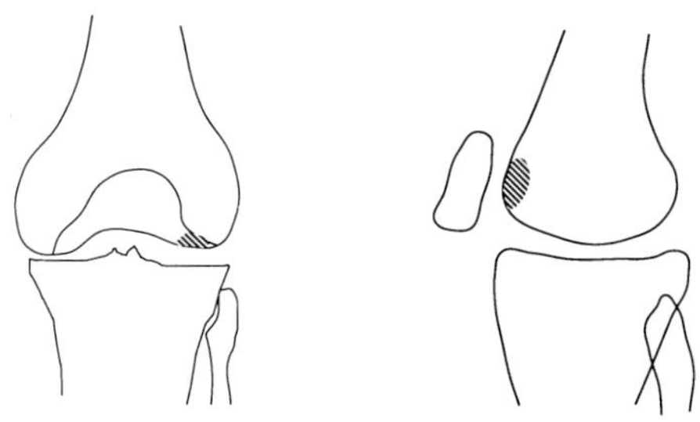

FIGURE 54-5

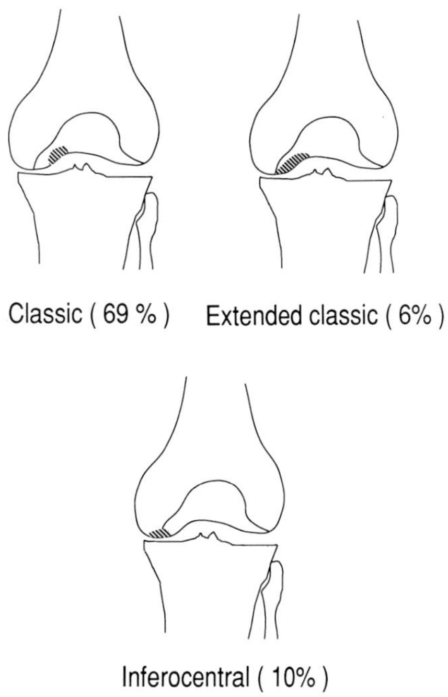

FIGURE 54-6

CASE 55

Differential Diagnosis of Osteocartilaginous Injury of the Knee

HISTORY: An 11-year-old child presented with chronic lateral knee pain. What is the MRI diagnosis? (Figs. 55-1 and 55-2: coronal contiguous multisection single-echo T1-weighted MR images of the right knee. Fig. 55-3: sagittal T1-weighted MR image.)

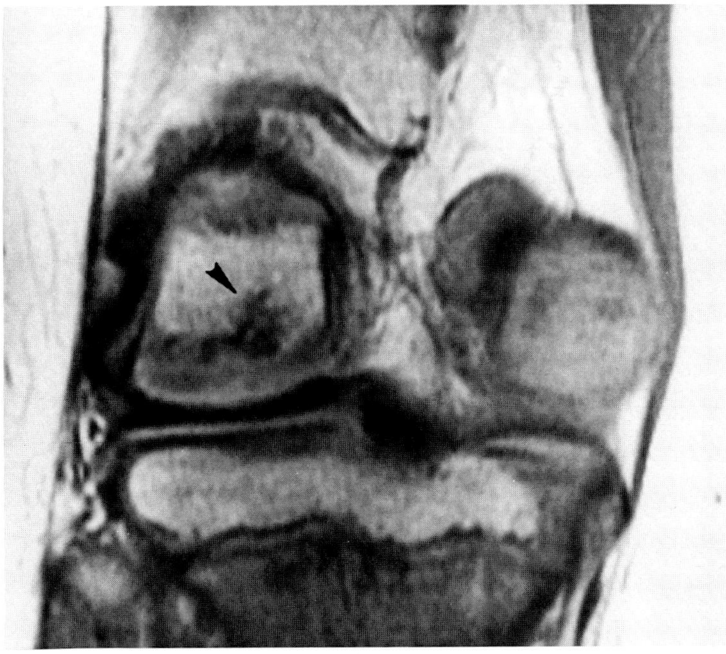

FIGURE 55-1

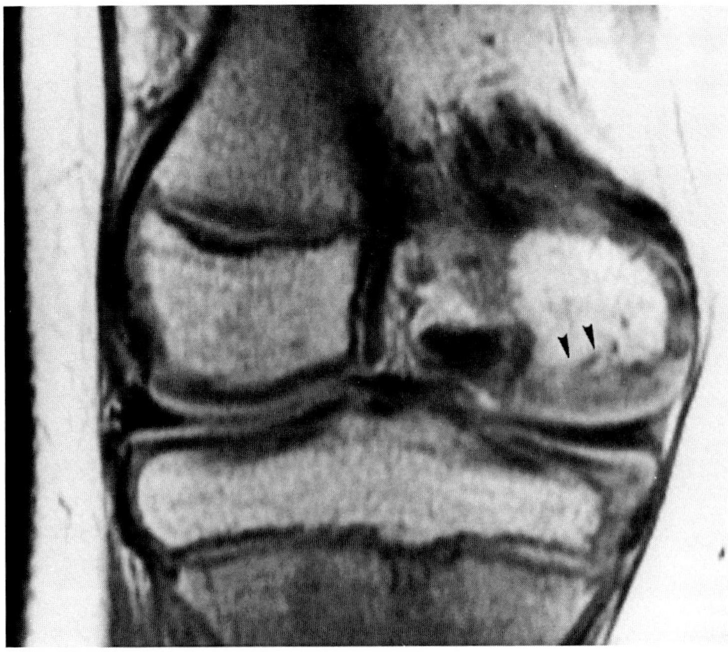

FIGURE 55-2

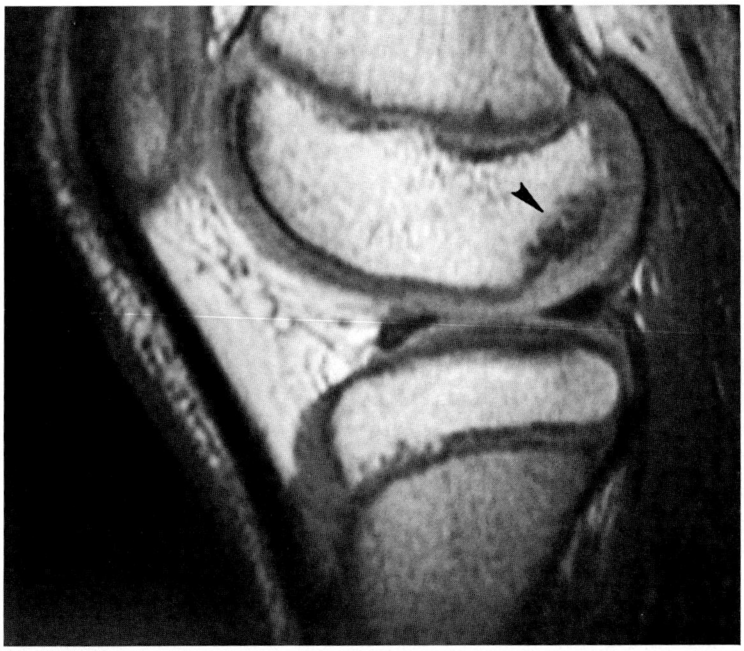

FIGURE 55-3

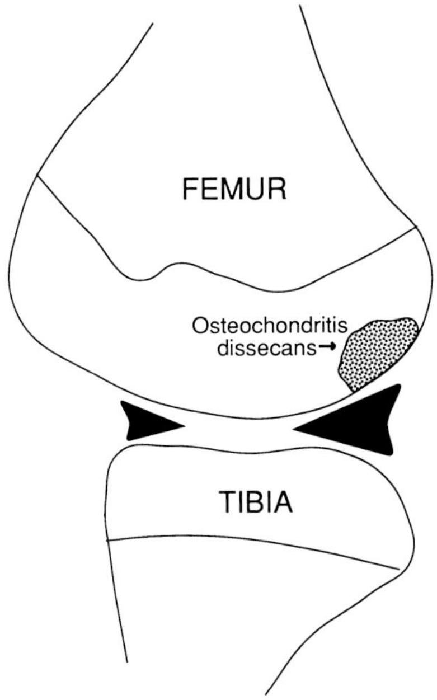

FIGURE 55-4

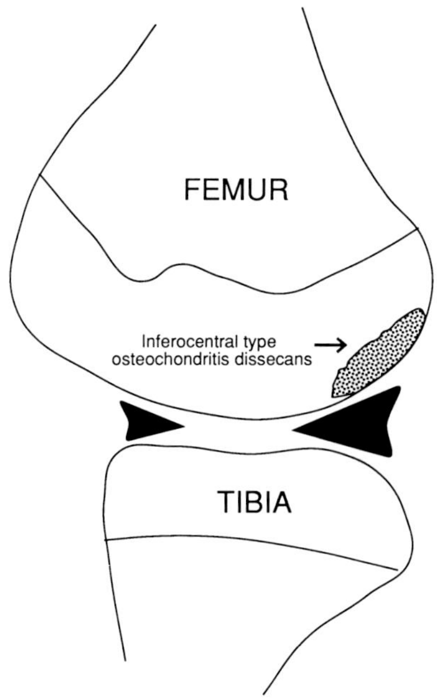

FIGURE 55-5

DISCUSSION: The critical information to be gleaned from this case is not the presence of osteochondritis dissecans (arrowhead in Figs. 55-1 and 55-3) of the inferocentral lateral femoral condyle, a disease site observed in 13% of patients with this disease. More important is the irregularity of the posterior subchondral bone of the femoral condyle on the normal side (arrowheads in Fig. 55-2). This is a normal variation and is often confused with true osteochondritis dissecans. Comparison of the two sides is extremely important when making this diagnosis, particularly in patients less than 12 years old. The femoral epiphyses are normally irregular along their distal margins in prepubescent patients, and these changes are most apparent on MRI, even more so than on conventional radiography.

The degree of hypointensity on the sagittal view is too pronounced and the area too large to represent a normal developmental irregularity. The weight-bearing surface is relatively spared and is the more posterior aspect of the femoral condyle. The overlying cartilage is not abnormal on these views.

It is critical to compare the sagittal and coronal projections with each other and with images of the contralateral normal knee, just as one would do with conventional radiographs.

DIAGNOSIS: The patient has inferocentral lateral femoral condylar osteochondritis dissecans with femoral cortical irregularity a normal variant in a preadolescent.

CASE 56

Differential Diagnosis of Osteocartilaginous Disease of the Knee

HISTORY: An 18-year-old man sustained a direct blow to the anteromedial femur while playing football. What is the MRI diagnosis? (Fig. 56-1: coronal T1-weighted MR image, TR/TE 900/20 msec, 18.0-cm FOV.)

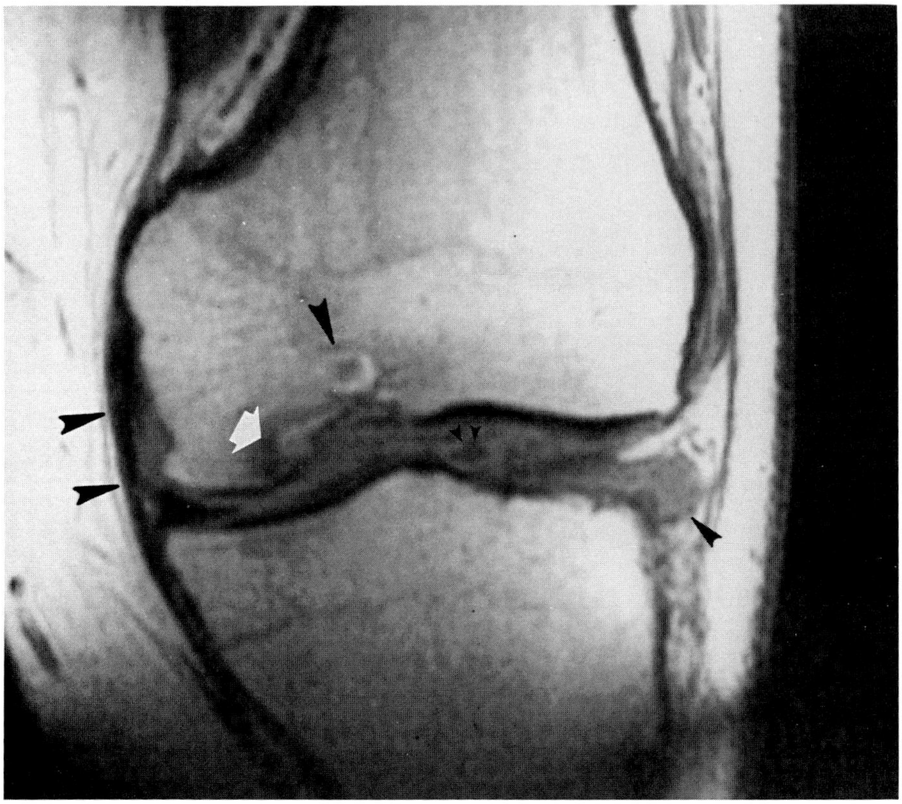

FIGURE 56-1

DISCUSSION: The medial collateral ligament is of normal thickness and normal contiguity (paired large arrowheads). The elliptical subchondral line in the medial femoral condyle represents a nondisplaced femoral fracture (white arrow). The coronal projection shows diffuse mottling and decreased signal intensity within the lateral compartment hyaline cartilage (paired arrowheads), compatible with hyaline cartilage fragmentation. A target-shaped area of hyperintense and hypointense signal (large arrowhead) represents a site of focal fat deposition as yellow marrow intervenes in this location during bone repair. Also identified is the usually large, redundant lateral meniscosynovial recess (medium arrowhead), now fluid-filled.

DIAGNOSIS: The patient has a nondisplaced femoral fracture with osteocartilaginous fragmentation.

CASE 57

Differential Diagnosis of Chronic Anterior Knee Pain

HISTORY: A 23-year-old man presented with chronic anteromedial knee pain and tenderness. (Fig. 57-1: coronal proton-density MR image, and Fig. 57-2: adjacent contiguous sagittal proton-density images, 3-mm sections.)

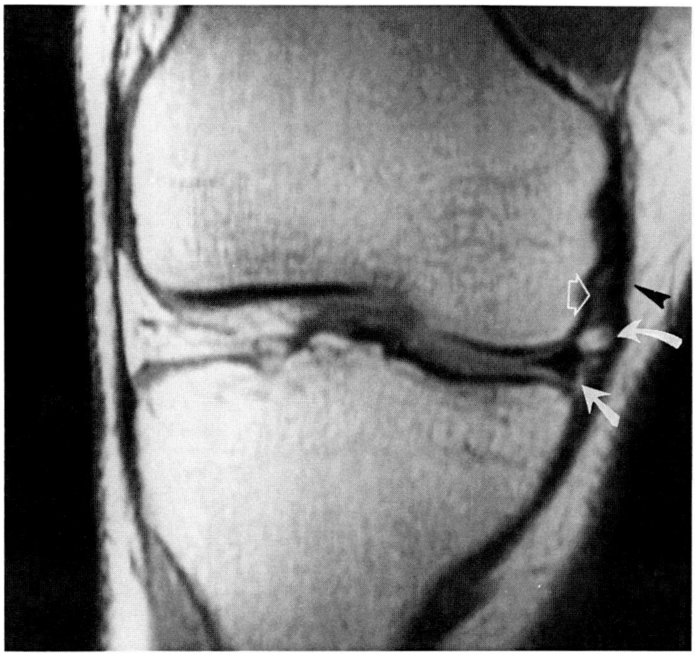

FIGURE 57-1

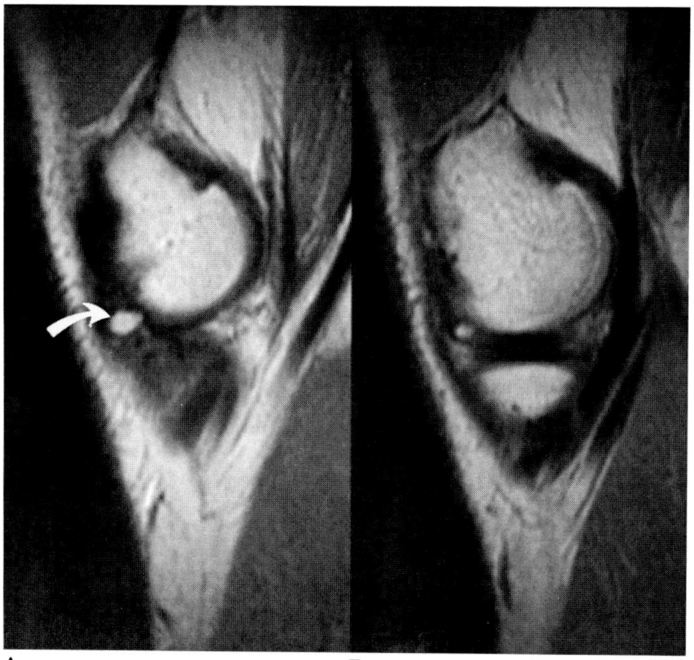

A B

FIGURE 57-2

DISCUSSION: The medial meniscus is visualized as a homogeneous black triangle. A slitlike thin, hyperintense fat pad (straight white arrow in Fig. 57-1) lies just lateral to the meniscus. Superficial to it is an intermediate signal intensity capsule that lies just beneath the hypointense tibial collateral ligament (arrowhead in Fig. 57-1). Within this gray capsule is a rounded hyperintense mass (curved white arrow) whose signal approximates that of medullary bone. It is surrounded by a faint hypointense rim and is therefore a corticated bone fragment. This could be easily confirmed with a conventional radiograph. Throughout this text we stress that all orthopaedic MRI examinations should be interpreted with the aid of plain radiographs.

The appearance of intraarticular calcific densities may vary from homogeneously hypointense to hyperintense with a corticated black rim. Occasional bone fragments and calcifications become hyperintense on T2-weighted images. These also exhibit a hypointense rim circumscribing a bright center. Areas of increased bulk-phase water, perhaps related to old hemorrhage, may produce this effect.

DIAGNOSIS: The patient has intracapsular calcification or a loose body.

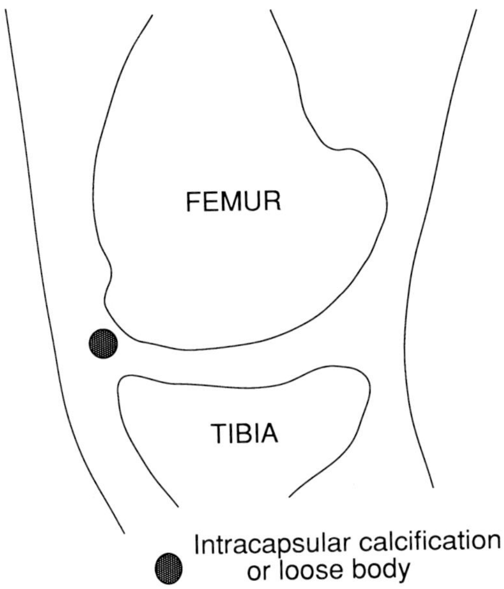

FIGURE 57-3

CASE 58

Differential Diagnosis of Acute Knee Pain

HISTORY: A 24-year-old man sustained an acute valgus stress injury of the left knee after receiving a direct blow to the anterolateral aspect of the knee. (Fig. 58-1: conventional anteroposterior radiograph. Fig. 58-2: coronal T1-weighted MR image. Fig. 58-3: sagittal T1-weighted MR image.)

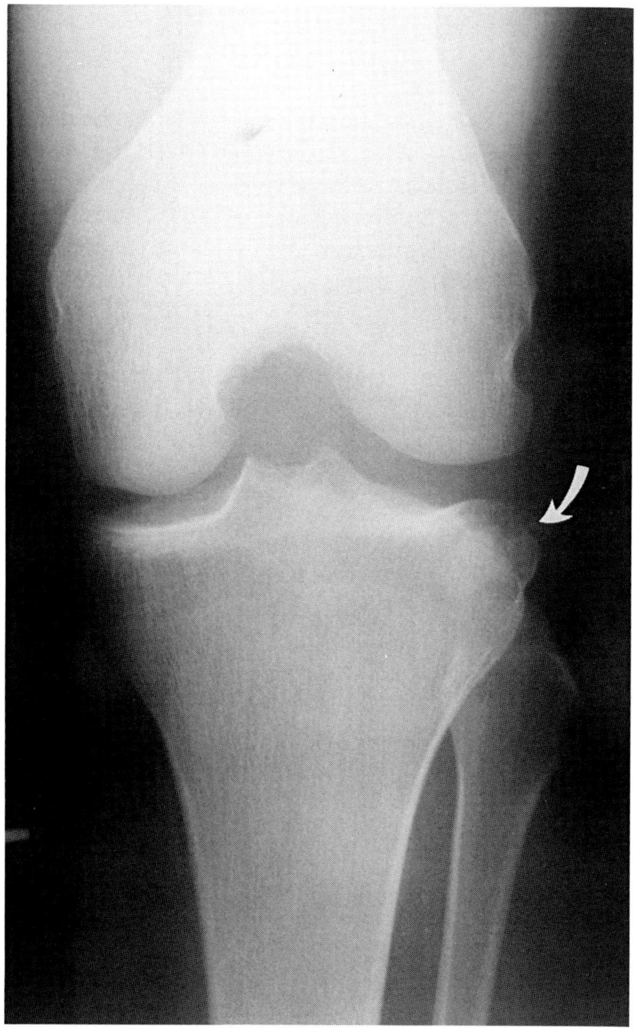

FIGURE 58-1

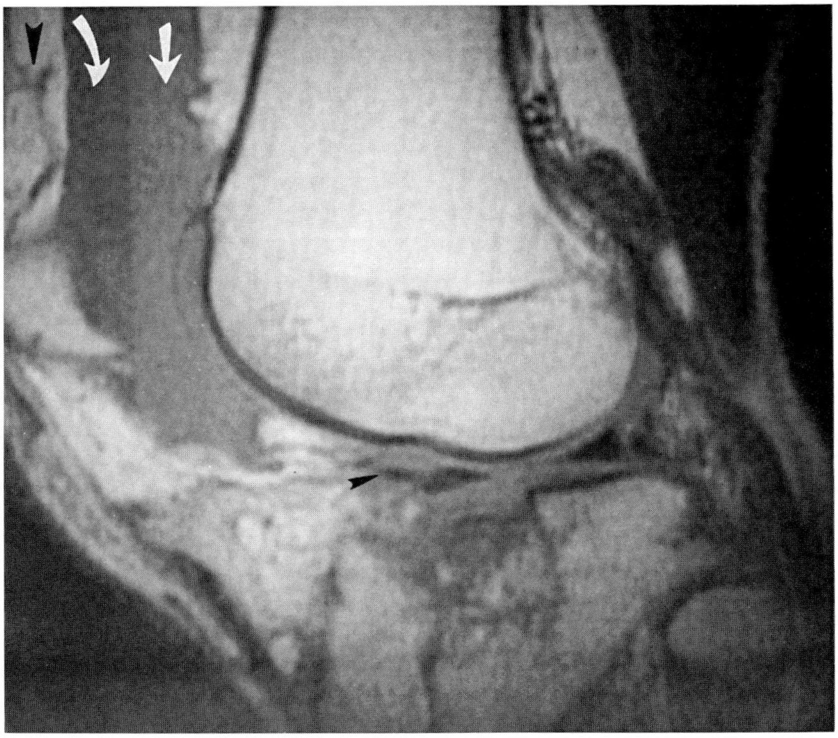

FIGURE 59-2

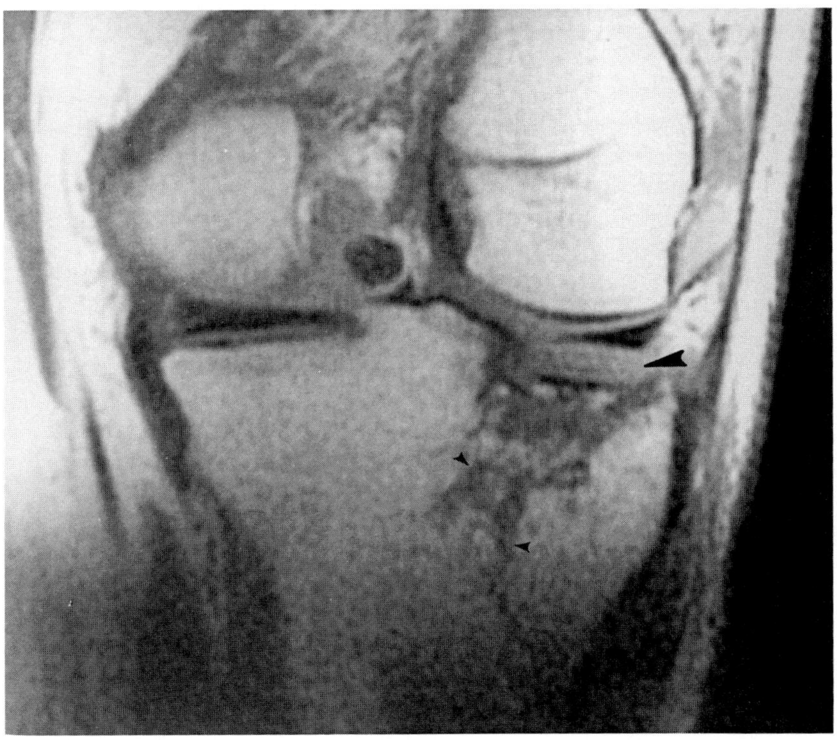

FIGURE 59-3

DISCUSSION: The plain radiograph shows a cleavage plane or fracture line through the lateral tibial plateau with 4 mm of diastasis. On the MR images the menisci are normal. Note the normal exit of the inferolateral geniculate artery and transverse ligament complex in the sagittal view (arrowhead in Fig. 59-3). A fat–fluid level is seen proximally, with the following layers identified: (1) the hemorrhagic and proteinaceous elements of a bloody effusion, layering dependently (straight white arrow in Fig. 59-2), (2) water elements, layering nondependently (curved arrow in Fig. 59-2), (3) the least dependent suprapatellar fat (arrowhead in Fig. 59-2).

The tibial plateau is interrupted by a cortical depression and underlying bone microfractures (small arrowheads in Fig. 59-3) and macrofractures that are linear in appearance. Since features of a type I plateau fracture (vertical fracture line) and type II fracture (central tibial depression) are present, this case is considered a type III fracture, according to the classification of Mueller (see case 45).

Another classification used in qualifying plateau fractures is that of Hohl. This system (see Fig. 59-5 *ff*) includes a nondisplaced fracture (type I), local compression (type II), split compression or depression (type III), displaced total medial plateau depression (type IV), nondisplaced anterior or posterior local split or wedge without depression (type V), and displaced comminution with both plateaus involved (type VI).

Open reduction of tibial plateau fractures usually is not attempted unless there is more than 8 mm of depression. In this case, 12 mm of depression exists. Thickened or edematous gray cartilage (horizontal arrowhead in Fig. 59-3) fills the depression site.

DIAGNOSIS: The patient has a tibial plateau depression fracture (type III of Hohl or Mueller) with acute hemarthrosis with a fat–fluid level.

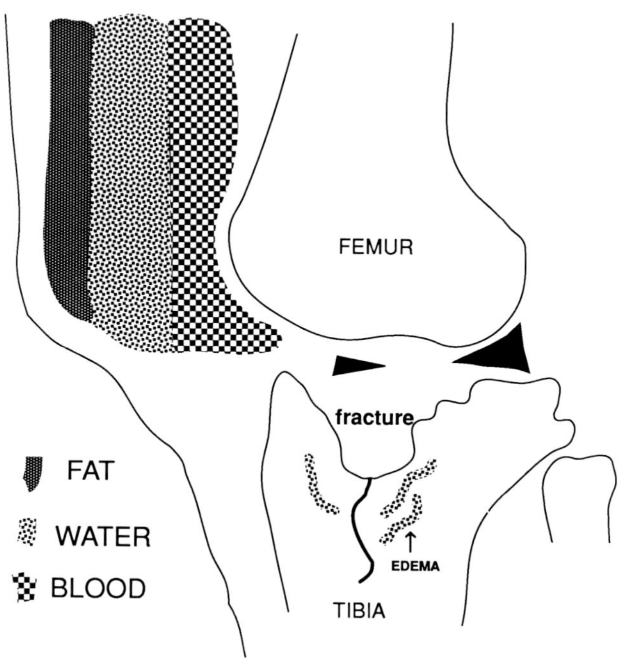

FIGURE 59-4

HOHL'S CLASSIFICATION OF TIBIAL PLATEAU FRACTURES

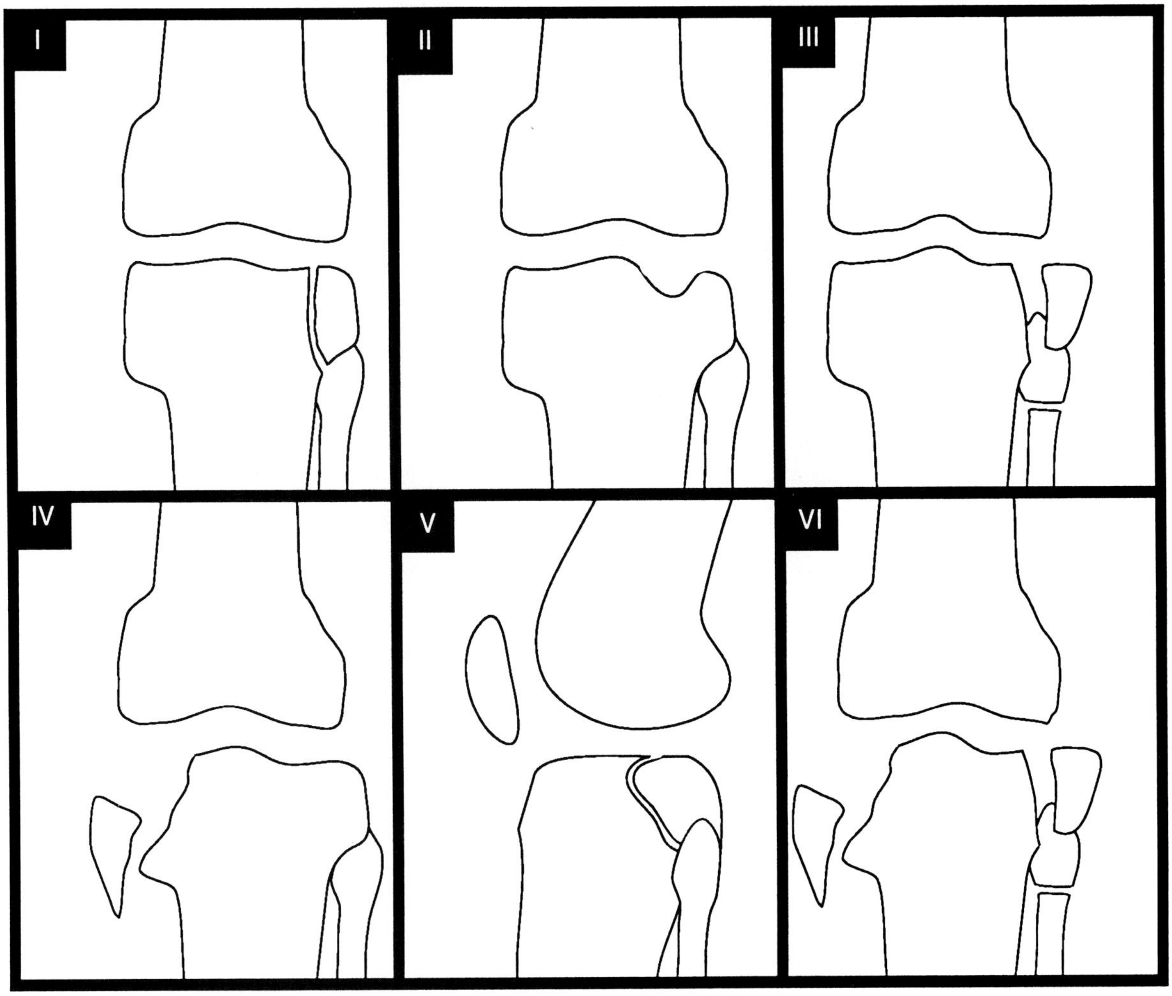

Type I: Nondisplaced split
Type II: Local central depression
Type III: Displaced local split depression
Type IV: Displaced, total depression of medial plateau (no comminution)
Type V: Nondisplaced posterior (or anterior) local split without depression
Type VI: Displaced, comminuted involving both plateaus

FIGURE 59-5

CASE 60

Differential Diagnosis of Osteocartilaginous Disease of the Knee

HISTORY: A 14-year-old girl experienced anterior knee pain after sliding into home plate during a softball game. What is the MRI diagnosis? Are any abnormalities other than bone lesions present? What does overflexion do to visualization of the anterior and posterior cruciate ligaments? (Fig. 60-1: sagittal, and Fig. 60-2: coronal multisection single-echo multiformat (four-on-one) T1-weighted MR images.)

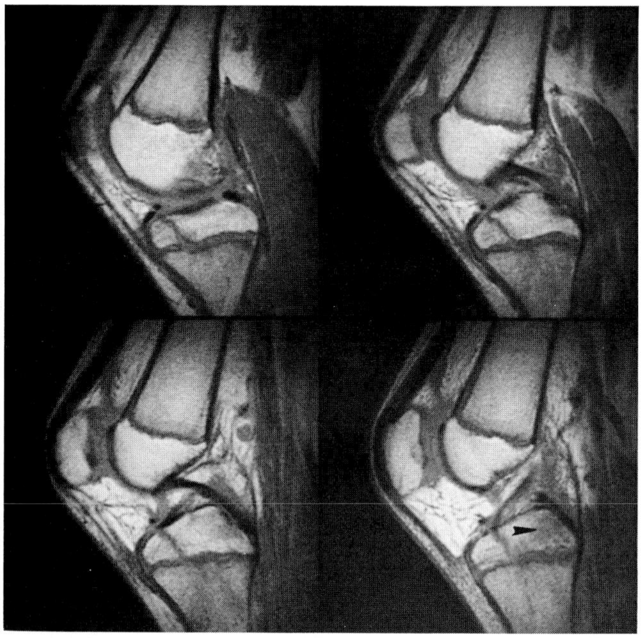

A B C D

FIGURE 60-1

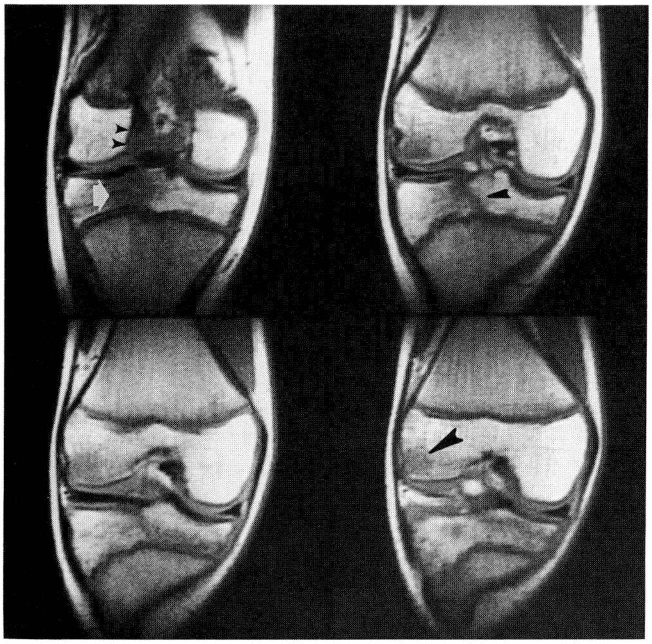

A B C D

FIGURE 60-2

DISCUSSION: An oblique fracture line in the tibial epiphysis courses superomedially to inferolaterally (medium arrowhead). The lesion is too wide and too well-defined to represent a stress fracture. Posteriorly in the tibial epiphysis a less well-defined rounded area of hypointense signal is compatible with a bone contusion (white arrow in Fig. 60-2*A*, arrowhead Fig. 60-1*D*). A similar area of poorly defined hypointensity is visible (arrowhead in Fig. 60-2*D*) in the medial femoral condyle (the medial side is identified by the superficial or tibial component of the medial ligamentous complex).

Also apparent in the sagittal view is a joint effusion, and in the coronal view a gray pseudomass (paired small arrowheads in Fig. 60-2*A*) surrounding the anterior cruciate ligament (ACL), a partial ACL injury.

Overflexion of the knee during MRI has two important effects. First, it may give the posterior cruciate ligament (PCL) a stretched appearance and suggest PCL thinning. Second, the ACL may appear corrugated, folded, or lax, or may be completely hidden from view. This will create the false impression of ACL tear or partial injury. Remember that most ACL injuries are a result of hyperextension during valgus stress, while most PCL injuries arise from hyperflexion injuries, particularly in internal rotation.

Our grading system for acute cruciate injuries is as follows:

Grade I: Intraligamentous signal only, without thickening of the ACL or PCL sheath (nominal injury).

Grade II: Ligamentous thinning or diffuse sheath thickening with residual continuous hypointense fibers still seen (partial tear).

Grade III: Complete interruption of the normal hypointense ACL or PCL band, with or without a pseudomass of fluid and blood at the rupture site (complete tear).

Grade IV: Findings identical to those of grade III injury with associated tibial or femoral bone fragment avulsion.

DIAGNOSIS: The patient has femoral and tibial bone contusions, a tibial epiphysis macrofracture, joint effusion, and a partial tear of the ACL.

CASE 61

Differential Diagnosis of Osteocartilaginous Disease of the Knee

HISTORY: A 31-year-old woman reported anterior knee pain after a professional beach volleyball game. No obvious injury had occurred during the competition. What is the MRI diagnosis? (Fig. 61-1: lateral plain radiograph of the left knee. Fig. 61-2: coronal T1-weighted MR image. Fig. 61-3: lateral conventional radiograph of the tibia and fibula. Fig. 61-4: axial multiecho, multiformat proton-density (*A*) and T2-weighted MR images. Fig. 61-5: magnification view, axial T2-weighted MR image.)

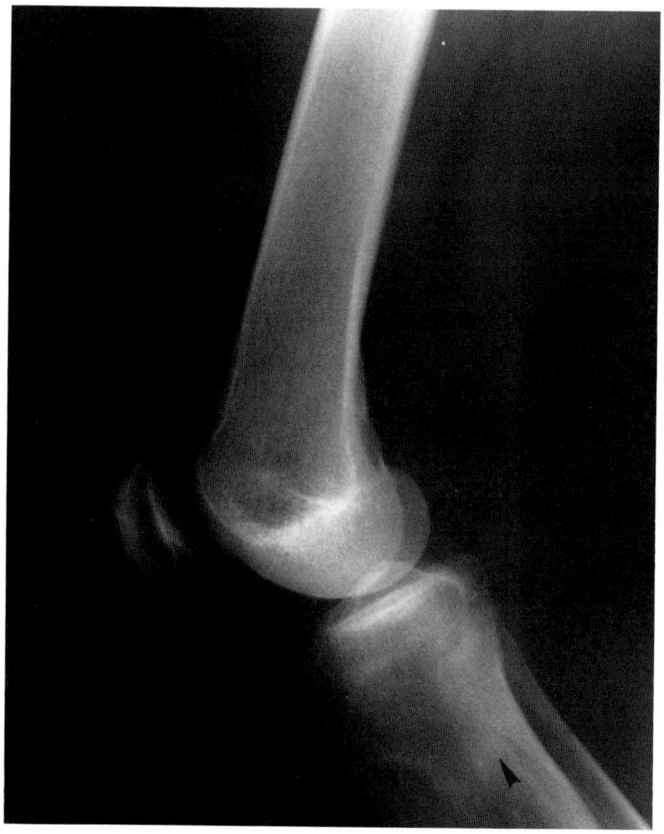

FIGURE 61-1

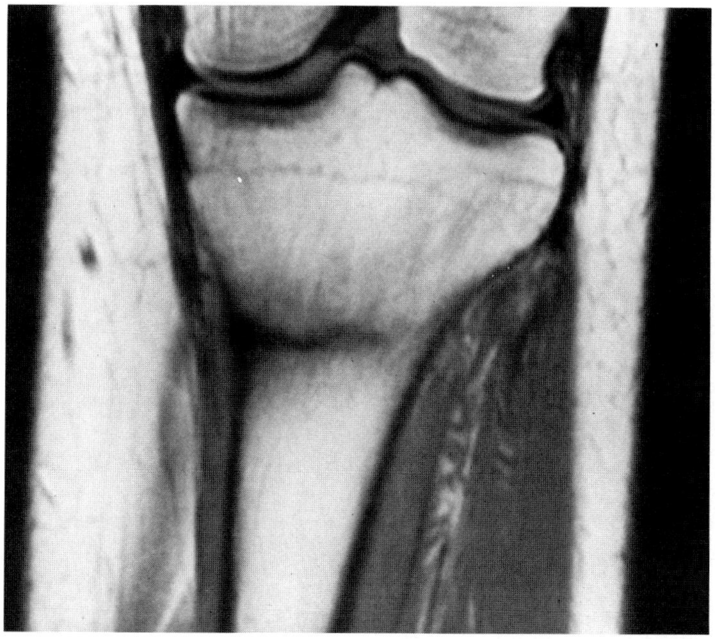

FIGURE 61-2

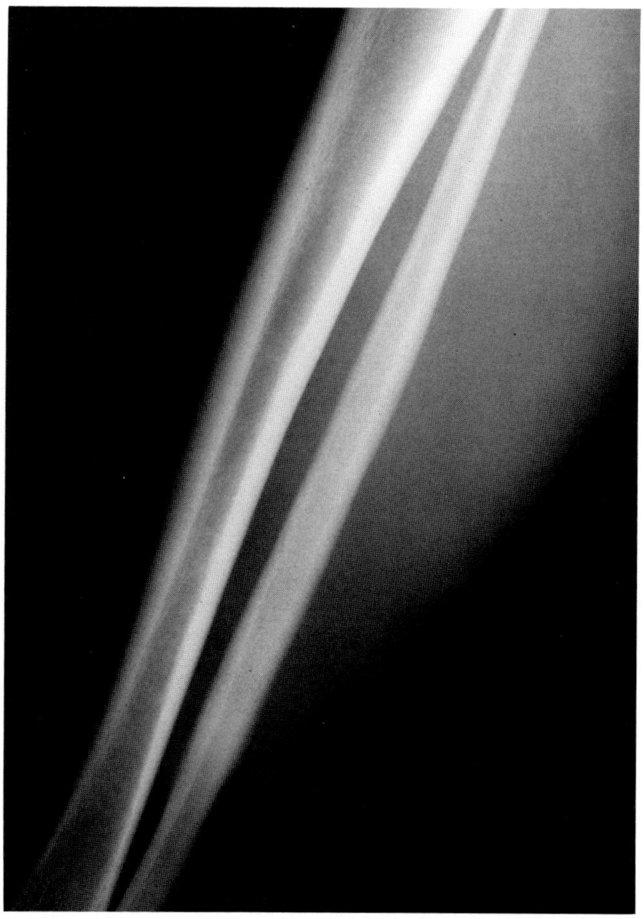

FIGURE 61-3

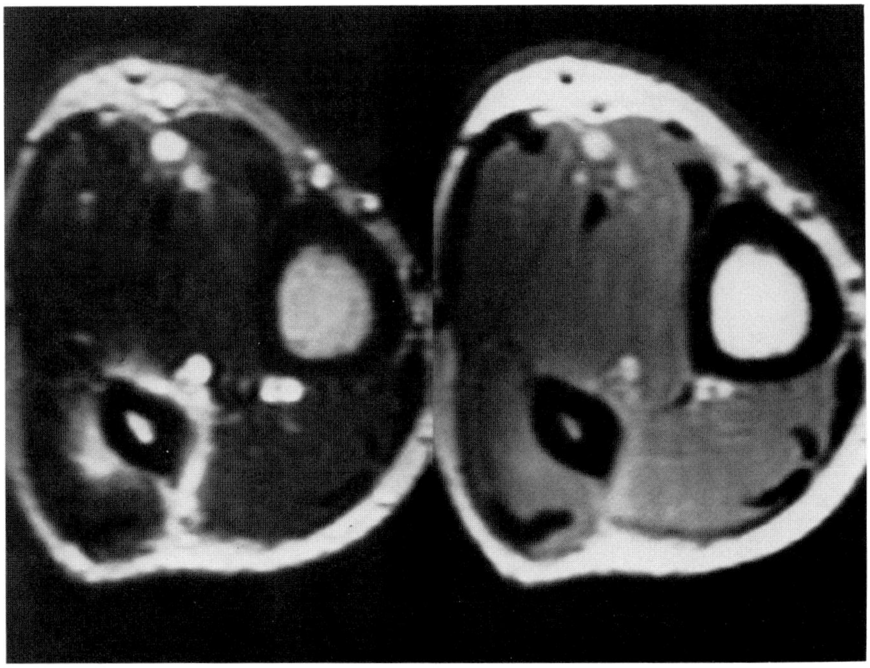

A B

FIGURE 61-4

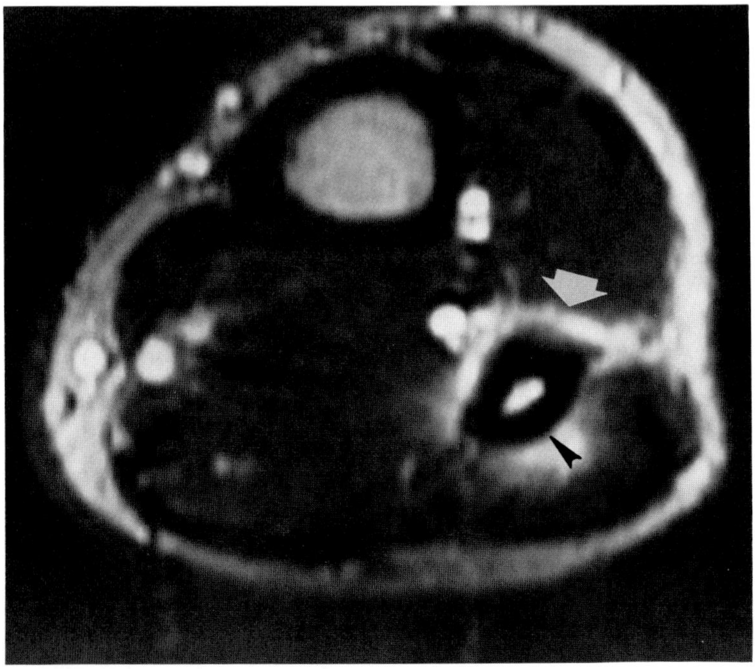

FIGURE 61-5

DISCUSSION: A subtle area of sclerosis on the lateral plain film has a linear shape but poorly defined margins (arrowhead in Fig. 61-1). A similar area of linear hypointense signal, surrounded by less hypointense, poorly defined edema, is visible on the MR images. This is the typical appearance of a stress fracture. The signal intensity alteration on T1 (hypointense) or on T2 gradient-echo or short-time inversion-recovery sequences (hyperintense) is apparent early, as it is on radionuclide scintigraphy. MRI has the additional capability of distinguishing soft tissue, tendinous, ligamentous, cartilaginous, cortical, and medullary injuries, which radionuclide imaging does not. MRI also differentiates microfractures from macrofractures and can demonstrate lesions that communicate with the joint spaces. The advantage of radionuclide scintigraphy is its ability to image large fields of view and to screen large volumes of skeletal tissue. However, the spatial resolution of this modality is limited. An indirect sign of stress fracture, occasionally the only sign, is a circumferential hypointense signal surrounding the hypointense cortical bone (arrowhead in Fig. 61-5) symmetrically and without soft tissue mass (white arrow). Sclerosis and cortical buttressing are seen on the conventional radiograph of the fibula (Fig. 61-3).

DIAGNOSIS: The patient has tibial and fibular stress fractures.

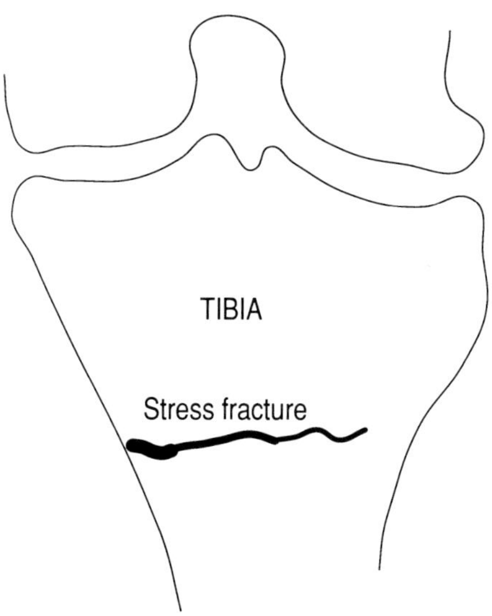

FIGURE 61-6

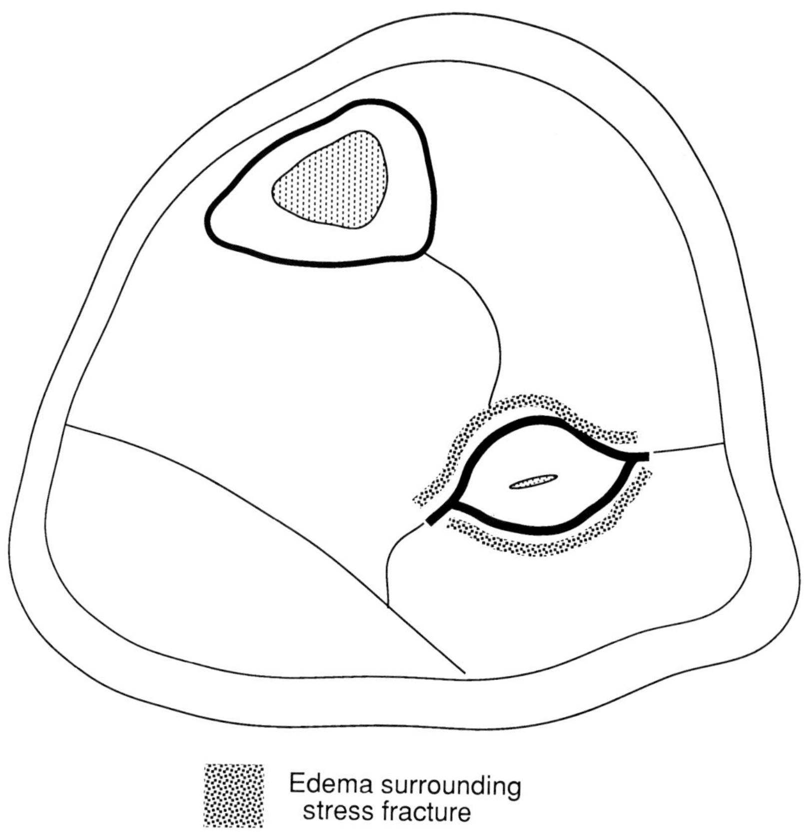

FIGURE 61-7

CASE 62

Differential Diagnosis of Osteocartilaginous Injury to the Knee

HISTORY: A 30-year-old woman with known systemic disease underwent MRI. What is the diagnosis? (Fig. 62-1: coronal T1 MR image of the knees.)

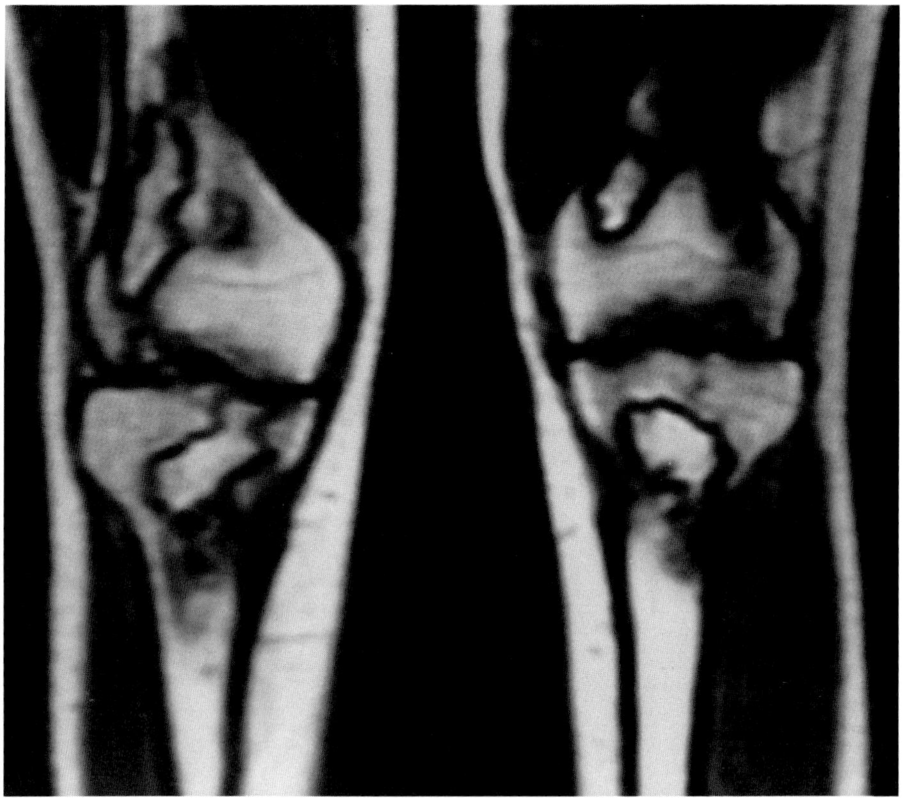

FIGURE 62-1

DISCUSSION: Both femora and tibiae have ring-like areas of diminished signal intensity that are typical of the ring pattern of infarction avascular necrosis. The earliest phase of avascular necrosis is characterized by a ring (MR stage I) or crescenteric T1 hypointensity that maintains the normal homogeneous medullary fat signal. Eventually this area fills in and appears hypointense centrally (MR stage II). Further progression results in microfractures, areas of bone repair, and finally bone fibrosis, necrosis, and irreversible bone injury (MR stages III and IV). These stages are discussed in greater detail in Part III.

At age 30, sickle cell disease is unlikely to have caused these changes since the marrow does not exhibit reconversion (red marrow) and appears to represent predominantly yellow marrow. Red marrow would be of intermediate signal intensity on T1- and T2-weighted imaging. This is also true in Gaucher's disease, which commonly produces this pattern of avascular necrosis and multiple ringlike bony infarcts in the extremities. However, Gaucher's disease is characterized by marrow replacement or myelophthisis, which appears as intermediate diffuse intramedullary T1 signal that spares the epiphyses and apophyses. Caisson's disease and pancreatitis might cause such infarcts; however, they would be unusual presentations of these diseases. Immune-related disorders such as systemic lupus erythematosus or polyarteritis nodosa often produce severe multifocal ischemic disease even if the patient has received steroids. Steroid administration alone, however, would rarely produce such extensive bone disease in the long bones.

DIAGNOSIS: The patient has systemic lupus erythematosus with multifocal bone infarcts and avascular necrosis of the hips (not shown).

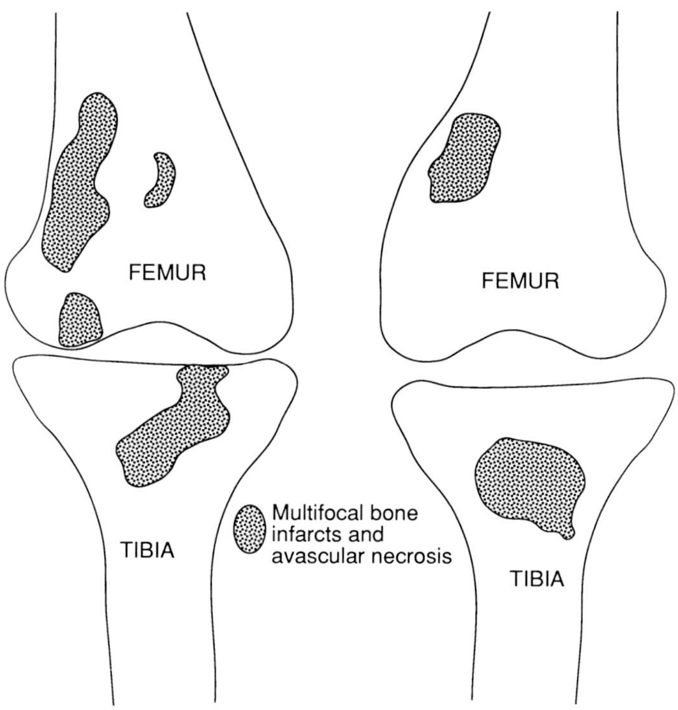

FIGURE 62-2

CASE 63

Differential Diagnosis of Osteocartilaginous Injury to the Knee

HISTORY: A 39-year-old man underwent radiologic evaluation for chronic knee pain and intermittent swelling. The conventional radiograph was initially interpreted as normal. Is that interpretation correct? (Fig. 63-1: lateral conventional radiograph of the left knee. Fig. 63-2: sagittal, and Fig. 63-3: coronal T1-weighted images.)

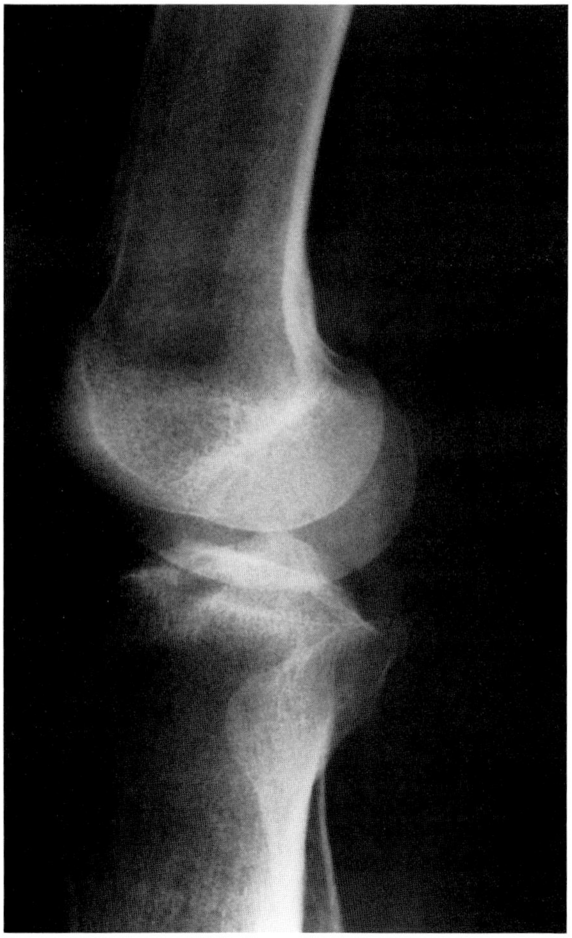

FIGURE 63-1

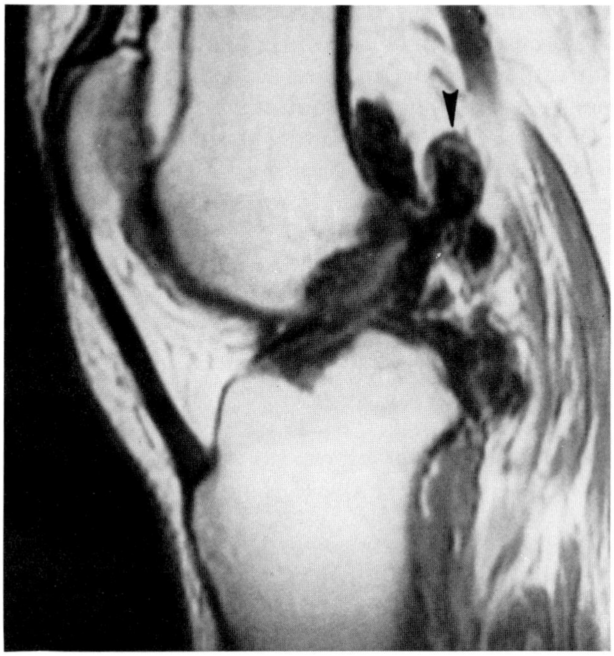

FIGURE 63-2

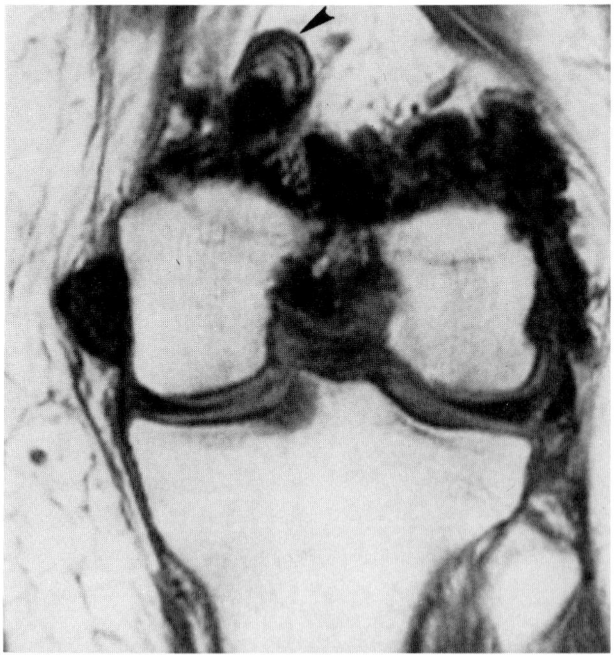

FIGURE 63-3

DISCUSSION: Posterosuperior to the joint line are subtle foci of increased density relative to the soft tissues and fat. Comparison of the MRI views will help identify these abnormalities. In the sagittal view, multiple foci of rounded hypointense signal (arrowhead in Fig. 63-2), approximately 1 to 2 cm in size, lie behind the knee; they also circumscribe the knee in the coronal projection. The findings are pathognomonic of idiopathic or primary synovial chondromatosis, a disorder produced by synovial metaplasia. This condition must be differentiated from the acquired disorder of osteocartilaginous loose bodies, or secondary chondromatosis. The latter condition results from osteochondral fracture or injury in which cartilage, bone, or osteocartilaginous fragments may be present. The following criteria may be used to differentiate these two conditions:

1. The fragments are more numerous in the idiopathic disorder.
2. Osteocartilaginous bone defects are less common and occur later on MRI in idiopathic synovial chondromatosis than secondary chondromatosis early in the disease. When these changes do occur in the idiopathic disease they are diffuse, multifocal, and secondary to degenerative joint disease, whereas in secondary chondromatosis they are focal and often large.
3. Idiopathic synovial chondromatosis more commonly affects males than females.
4. The fragment MRI signal in idiopathic disease is usually hypointense, whereas in secondary chondromatosis the fragments often have a hyperintense center and a hypointense rim. However, the latter appearance may be seen in idiopathic disease, owing to fatty marrow in the nodule centers.

The nodules in idiopathic synovial chondromatosis are usually round, uniform, and up to 2 to 3 cm in size. As in this case, they may not appear calcified on conventional radiographs, but their hypodensity or hypointensity may be obvious on computed tomography or MRI.

The treatment for idiopathic synovial chondromatosis is synovectomy and debridement. For secondary chondromatosis, loose body removal only is the accepted therapy.

Other conditions to be differentiated from idiopathic synovial chondromatosis include the following:

synovial sarcoma: heterogeneous hyperintense T2 signal with a mass effect often arising adjacent to rather than in the joint space.

pigmented villonodular synovitis: lamellated or alternating areas of hyperintense signal (edema or capsular inflammation) and hypointense signal (hemosiderin) on T2-weighted imaging.

synovial hemangioma: mixed hyperintense foci with pinpoint calcification on plain radiographs and tubular or rounded foci of intermediate or increased signal intensity on T1- and T2-weighted images (flow studies).

synovial redundancy or inflammation: irregular, homogeneous areas of waterlike signal on MRI that prolapse into the Hoffa fat space and posterior to the joint line.

DIAGNOSIS: The patient has primary synovial chondromatosis.

CASE 64

Differential Diagnosis of Anterior Knee Pain and Patellofemoral Disease

HISTORY: A 30-year-old man, an avid tennis player and gardener, presented with prepatellar tenderness and pain of 7 weeks' duration. What is the MRI diagnosis? (Fig. 64-1: sagittal proton-density MR image, TR/TE 1,000/20 msec, 14.0-cm FOV, 4.0-mm sections, 192 × 256 pixel matrix, 2 excitations.)

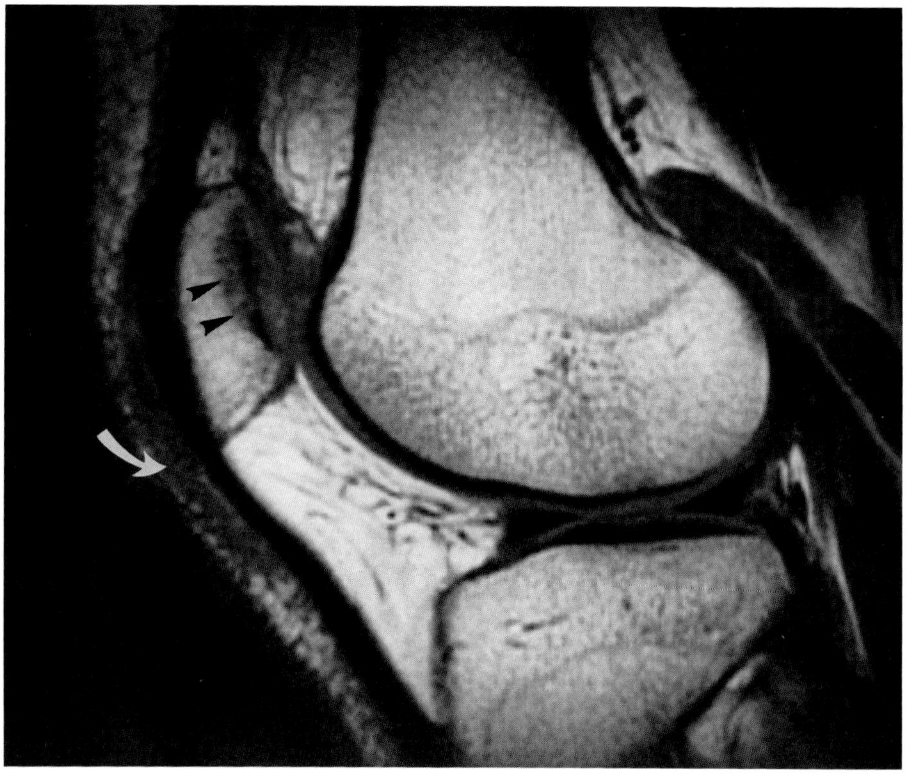

FIGURE 64-1

DISCUSSION: Anterior to the patellar tendon and patella are areas of subcutaneous intermediate signal intensity (curved arrow) that became hyperintense on T2-weighted images. The patient had no prior history of soft tissue trauma. Just anterior to the patella is a very thin bursa that may become inflamed and filled with fluid. This often occurs in patients who must kneel in their work or who have known systemic arthropathy or joint effusion. The absence of a history of trauma and the patient's love of gardening, in conjunction with the MRI findings, might suggest the diagnosis. An inflamed bursa is often indistinguishable from edema in the overlying soft tissues. Prepatellar hematoma formation may occur intrinsic or extrinsic to this prepatellar bursa. Acute hematomas are hypointense on T2-weighted images. Intratendinous signal involving the infrapatellar tendon is a different disorder, common in athletes, called "jumper's knee." Note the hypointense signal (paired arrowheads) along the posterior patellar margins. The curved patellar interface produces a volume averaging artifact that is often confused with chondromalacia.

DIAGNOSIS: The patient has prepatellar tendinitis.

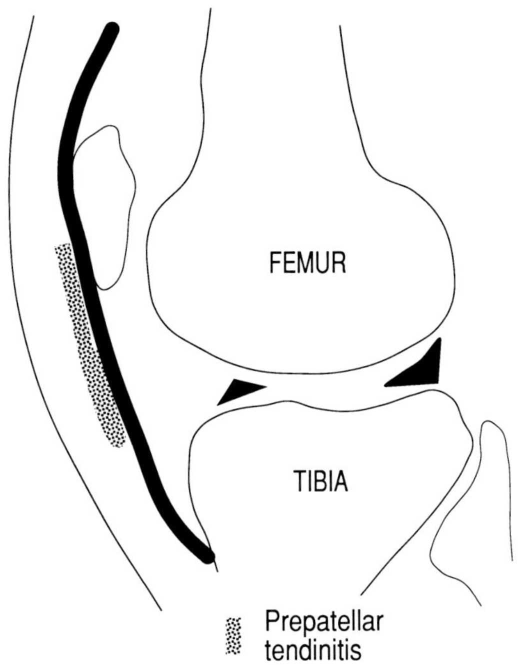

FIGURE 64-2

CASE 65

Differential Diagnosis of Chronic Anterior Knee Pain

HISTORY: A 22-year-old man underwent radiologic evaluation for chronic anterior knee pain and joint swelling. What are the MRI findings? (Fig. 65-1: sagittal contiguous multisection, multiecho proton-density (*A*) and T2-weighted (*B*) MR images.)

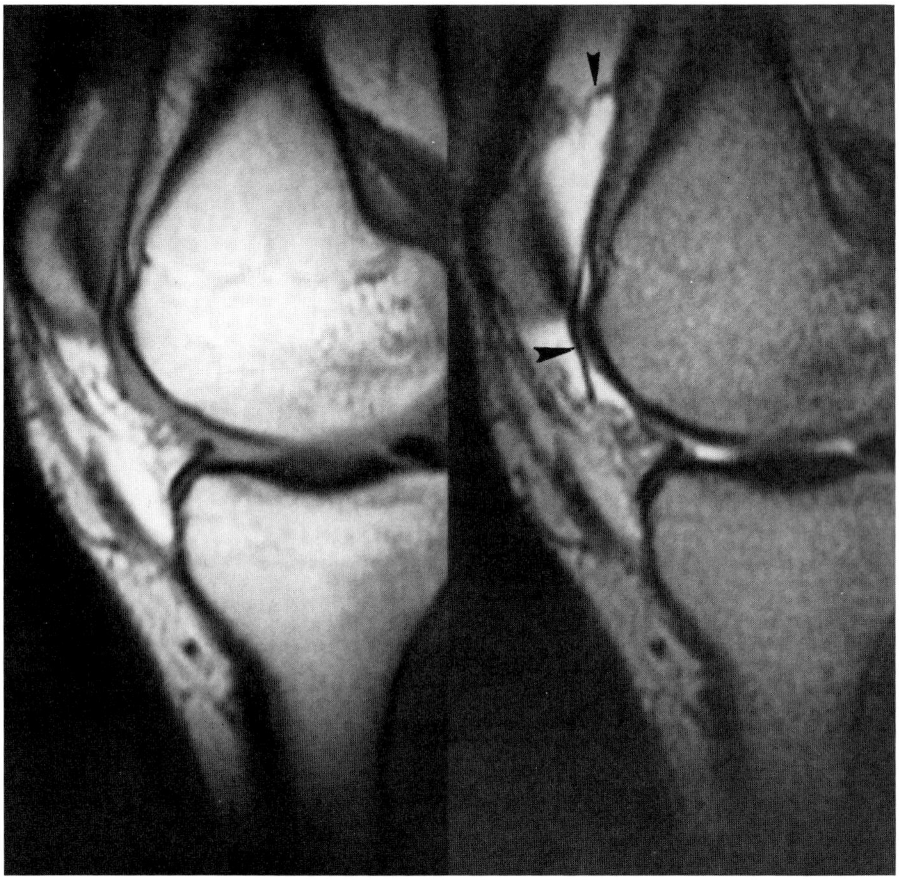

FIGURE 65-1

DISCUSSION: Synovial plicae are embryologic remnants of septa that divide the knee into three compartments. They appear as a normal variant on MRI in a majority of cases. The superomedial joint space adjacent to the patella (upper arrowhead in *B*) is the most common site of plica visualization on MRI, with medial or paramedian patellar and infrapatellar sites (lower arrowhead) less common. Plicae located above the patella, as in this case, are best seen in the sagittal projection, whereas medial patellar plicae are visualized in the axial projection. Although suprapatellar and medial patellar plicae are most frequently visualized on MRI, pathologically, infrapatellar plicae are most common. Symptomatic suprapatellar plicae and infrapatellar plicae are rare. Orthopaedic surgeons require prior knowledge of plica formation, since it may impede insertion of the arthroscopy instrument.

DIAGNOSIS: The suprapatellar and infrapatellar plica band is normal.

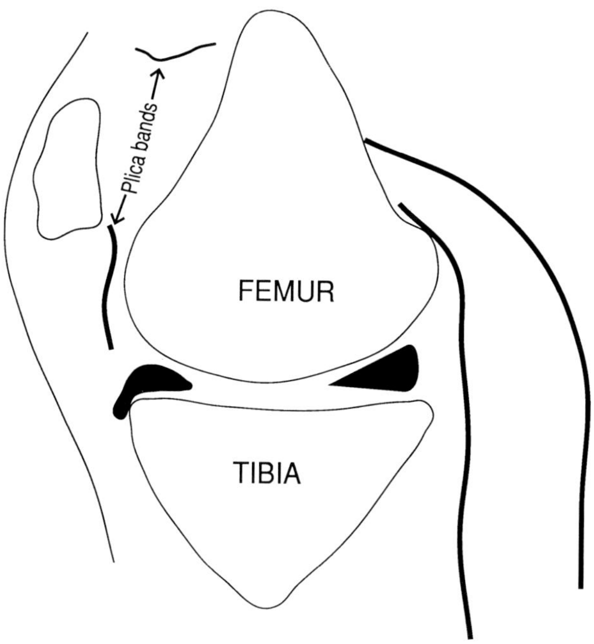

FIGURE 65-2

CASE 66

Differential Diagnosis of Chronic Anterior Knee Pain and Patellofemoral Disease

HISTORY: A 26-year-old woman underwent radiologic evaluation for chronic anterior knee pain of 3 years' duration that was exacerbated by exercise. (Fig. 66-1: axial multiformat contiguous (four-on-one) T1-weighted MR images. Fig. 66-2: axial, and Fig. 66-3: sagittal multisection, single-echo T1-weighted MR images.)

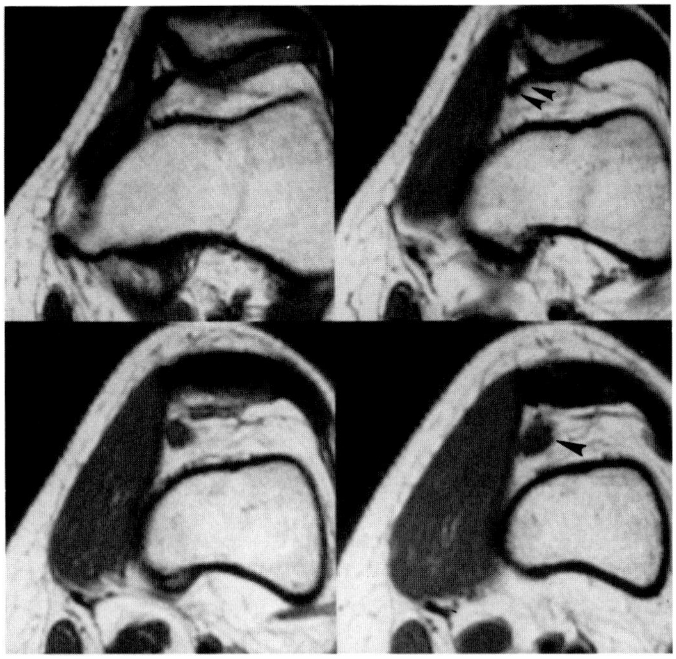
A B C D

FIGURE 66-1

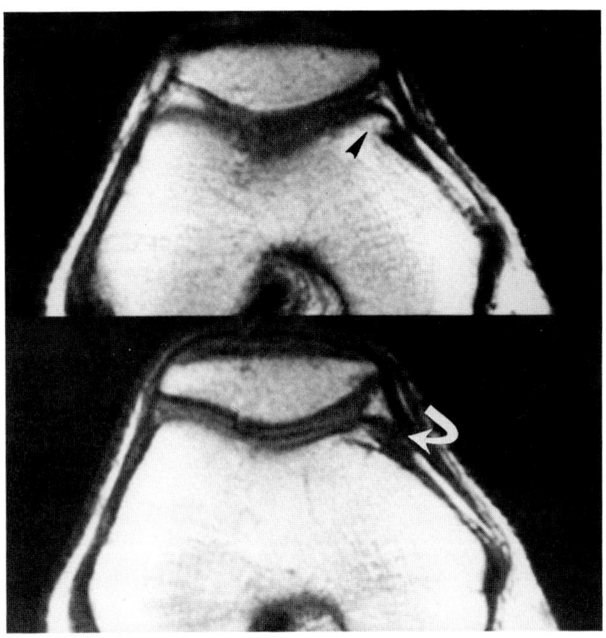
A B

FIGURE 66-2

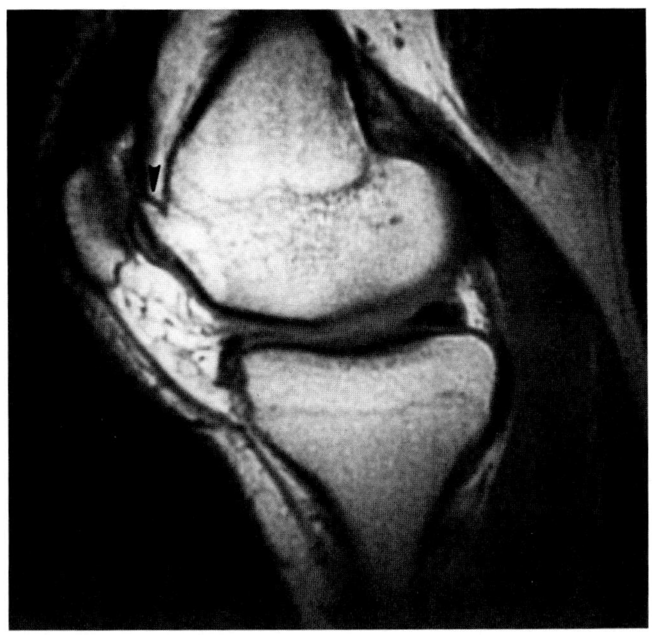

FIGURE 66-3

DISCUSSION: The synovial plica is a redundant fold of the synovial knee joint lining. It represents a vestigial septum and is an embryologic remnant. It extends from the infrapatellar fat pad medially, is crescent-shaped, and crosses the medial femoral condyle near the quadriceps tendon in the suprapatellar region. It then passes laterally over the laterofemoral condyle to the lateral retinaculum. The synovial plica is visualized in almost every axial image set and can be seen in 60% to 70% of sagittal and coronal high-resolution images as well.

When the synovial plica is inflamed or fibrotic, the patient experiences anterior knee pain that worsens with sitting or knee flexion and produces an aching sensation. When the patient rises and begins walking, pain is excessive for the first five or ten steps, then lessens. With the knee in flexion, the synovial plica is draped over the femoral condyles and is held in tension. With extension, the articularis genu muscle extracts the plica, preventing it from being entrapped in the patellofemoral joint. With a weak articularis genu muscle, eight to ten steps may be needed to extract the plica or elevate it out of the patellofemoral joint. Therefore, the initial phase of ambulation should be done from the sitting position.

With severe fibrosis, the plica may remain entrapped or folded in the joint, a finding visible on MRI as a redundant hypointense band within the joint space (arrowheads in Fig. 66-1*B*). A scarred or fibrotic plica may remain permanently entrapped in the patellofemoral joint and appears as a thickened iso- or hypointense band or rounded structure best seen in the axial projection (arrowhead in Fig. 66-1*D*). Occasionally the plica may appear edematous, exhibiting high signal intensity on T2 imaging. With marked thickening, a prominent hypointense linear band results (curved arrow in Fig. 66-2*B*), and the patient may report popping or snapping with knee flexion and extension that reduces the sensation of pain or discomfort. Occasionally, focal spur formation (arrowhead in Figs. 66-2*A* and 66-3) contributes to plica entrapment. Accompanying MRI findings include quadriceps muscle atrophy and modest or nominal joint effusion. Hamstring tightness may predispose to synovial plica syndrome.

DIAGNOSIS: The patient has synovial plica syndrome.

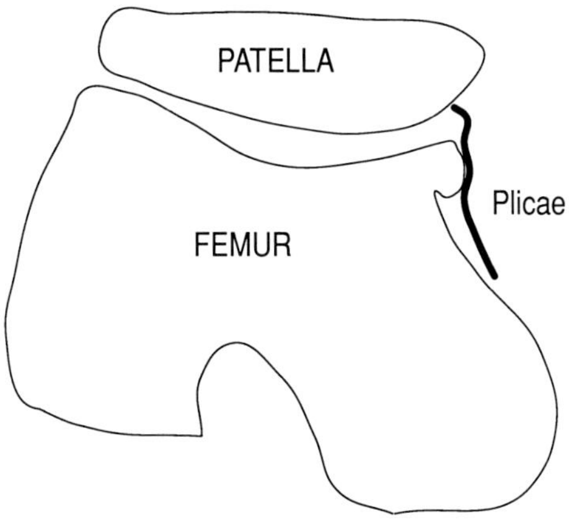

FIGURE 66-4

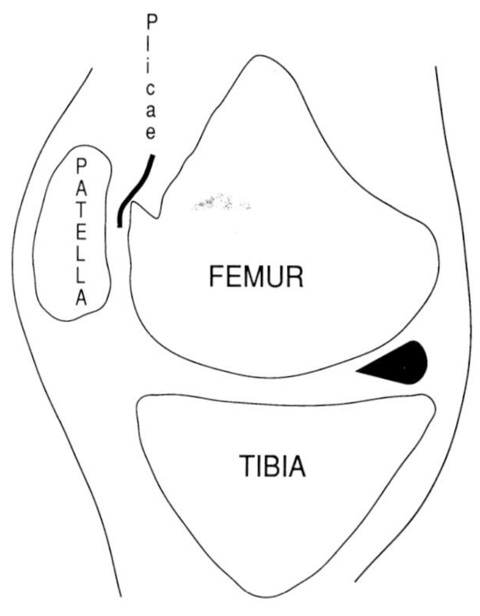

FIGURE 66-5

CASE 67

Differential Diagnosis of Anterior Knee Pain and Patellofemoral Disease

HISTORY: A 20-year-old patient with a chronic history of anterior knee pain, swelling, and pain exacerbated by squatting, jumping, or resistive knee extension underwent radiologic evaluation. What is the MRI diagnosis? (Fig. 67-1: lateral conventional radiograph. Fig. 67-2: sagittal T1-weighted MR image.)

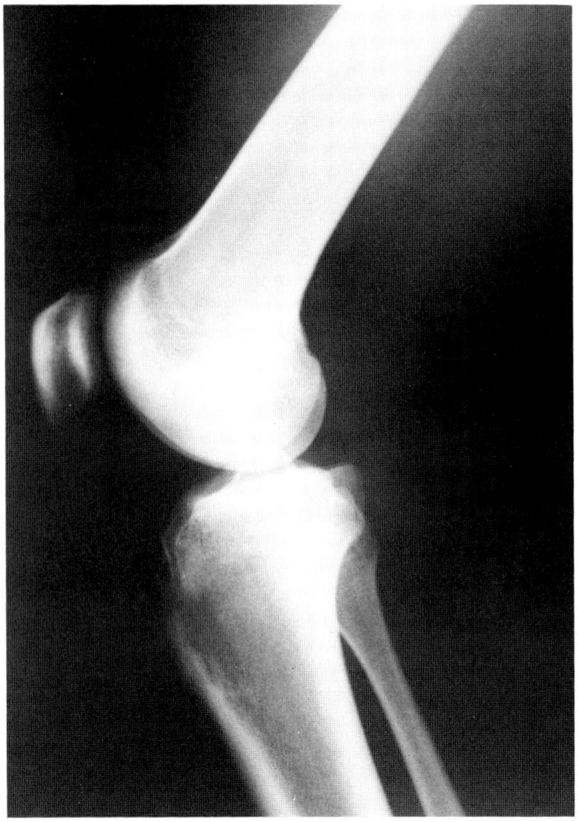

FIGURE 67-1

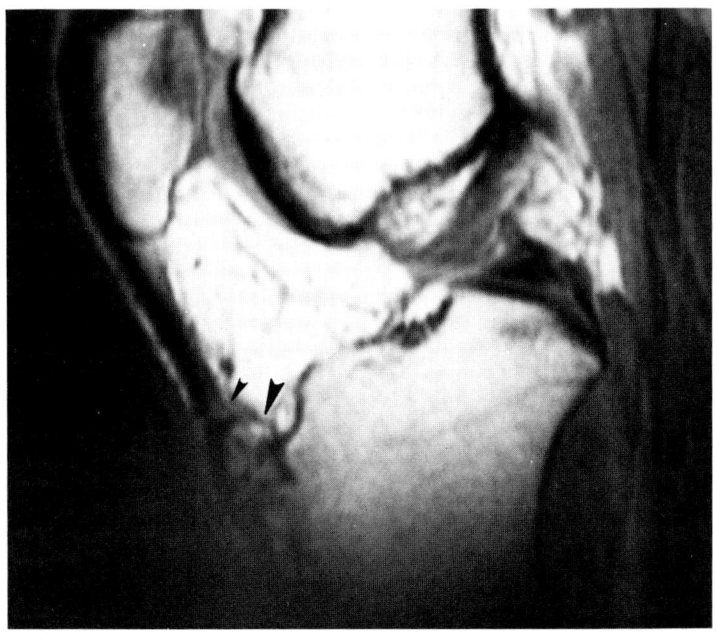

FIGURE 67-2

DISCUSSION: A sagittal, single-echo T1-weighted image and a conventional radiograph faintly demonstrate an irregular configuration and segmented appearance to the tibial tubercle (large arrowhead in Fig. 67-2) typical of Osgood-Schlatter disease. Boys are more frequently affected than girls, in a 3:1 ratio. This irregular tubercle may be accompanied by intermediate increased T1 signal or intermediate to hyperintense T2 signal in the adjacent infrapatellar tendon (small arrowhead) and remaining extensor tendon mechanism. Normally the apophysis of the tibial tubercle bonds with the upper tibial epiphysis at age 13. However, in young, active patients, chronic tensile stress of the patellar tendon may avulse this apophysis, producing chondro-osseous separation. The pain worsens with exercise and is relieved by rest and aspirin. Falling and tenderness are common. Often rest, anti-inflammatory agents, and application of ice following exercise are the cornerstones of treatment. After excessive activity, jumping, or squatting, frank edema may develop in the adjacent infrapatellar tendon.

The MRI findings can be summarized as follows:

1. edema of the upper end of the patellar tendon, intermediate in signal intensity on T1 and hyperintense at times on T2 spin-echo or gradient-echo sequences,
2. peritendinous signal hypointensity relative to fat,
3. hypointense signal in the underlying tibial medullary bone (30% of cases), and
4. chondro-osseous bone fragments adjacent to the tibial tubercle.

This condition must be differentiated from "jumper's knee," or primary infrapatellar tendinitis, and Larsen-Johansson disease. In Larsen-Johansson disease an avulsion type of injury due to traction of the tendon on the inferior patellar surface results in bone fragmentation of heterotopic ossification at this proximal tendon insertion. A fragmented infrapatellar appearance may also be seen in patients with spastic paralysis, and in rare variants of patellar segmentation (<2%).

DIAGNOSIS: The patient has Osgood-Schlatter disease.

CASE 68

Differential Diagnosis of Acute Anterior Knee Pain and Patellofemoral Disorders

HISTORY: A 46-year-old man sustained acute trauma to the anterior knee in an automobile accident. What is the MRI diagnosis? (Fig. 68-1: sagittal multiformat (two-on-one) multisection, single-echo T1-weighted MR images, TR/TE 900/20 msec, 14.0-cm, FOV, 192 × 256 pixel matrix, 4.0-mm sections, 2 excitations.)

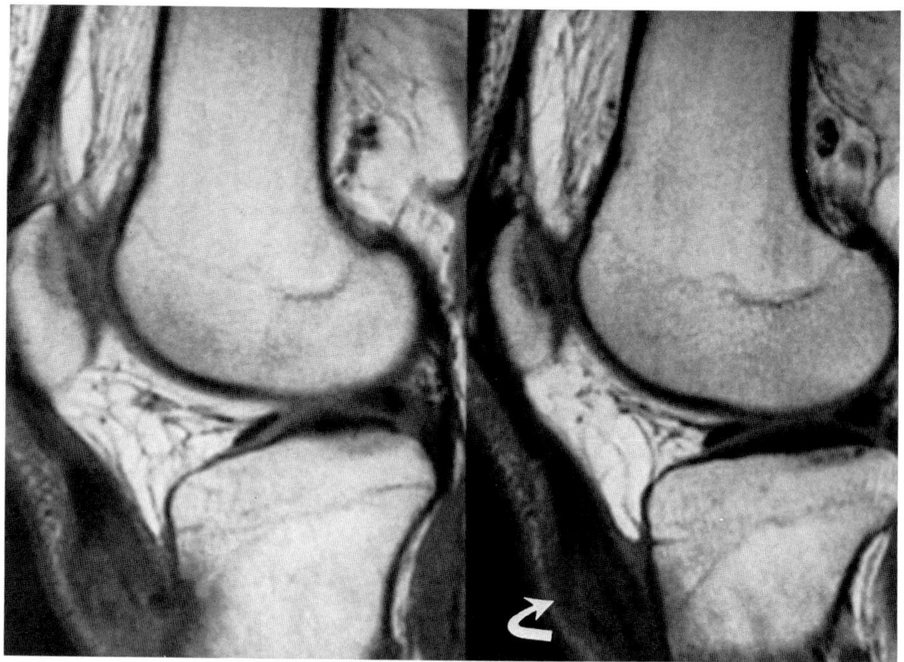

A **B**

FIGURE 68-1

DISCUSSION: This patient had a posterior cruciate ligament injury and lateral collateral ligament injury (not shown). In addition, a post-traumatic synovial cyst or rent in the synovium was also present laterally. The sagittal images show edema and hemorrhage within the infrapatellar tendon at its tibial insertion. In addition, there is diffuse edema and acute hemorrhage (intermediate signal) at the site of detachment of the patella to the tibial tuberosity (curved arrow in *B*). The inferior or distal patellar tendon is markedly thickened. A prepatellar intermediate signal intensity contusion is noted in the subcutaneous fat anterior to the hypointense tendon. Acute hemorrhage is intermediate in signal intensity on T1-weighted images at high or low field strengths.

DIAGNOSIS: The patient has intrapatellar tendon injury with partial avulsion of the distal patellar tendon and prepatellar soft tissue hematoma.

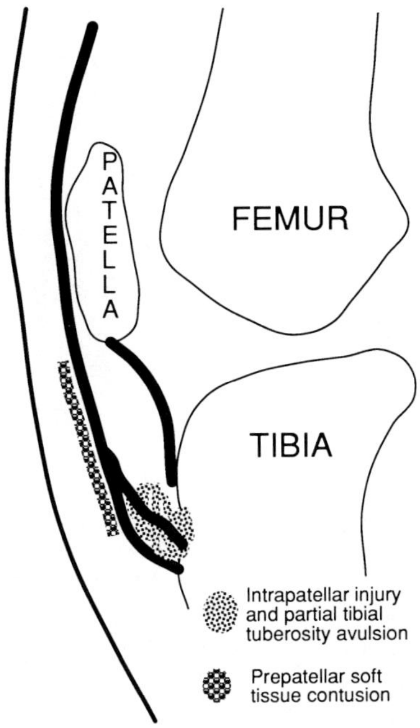

FIGURE 68-2

CASE 69

Differential Diagnosis of Chronic Anterior Knee Pain and Patellofemoral Disorders

HISTORY: A 27-year-old woman reported anterior knee pain and tenderness of 1 year's duration. What is the MRI diagnosis? For comparison, an MR image of the knee of a professional basketball player is shown. (Fig. 69-1: conventional radiograph. Fig. 69-2: axial proton-density MR image. Fig. 69-3: axial proton-density MR image of the knee of a 22-year-old professional basketball player.)

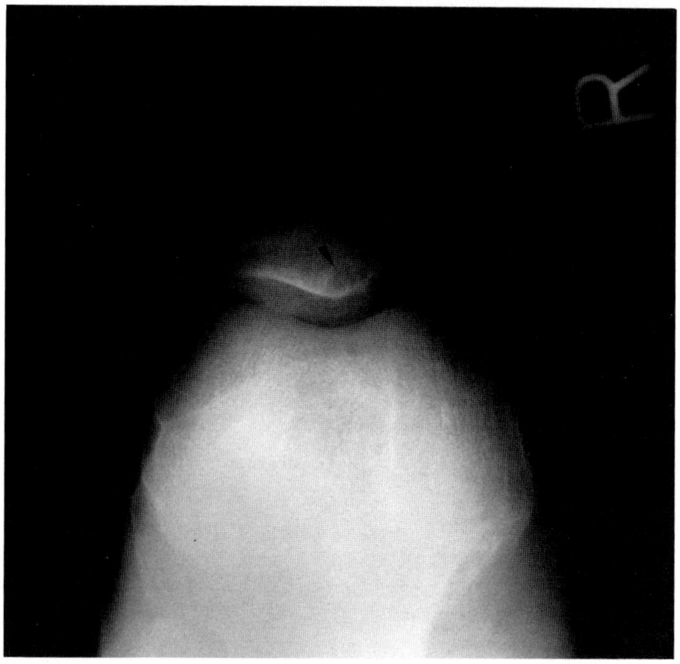

FIGURE 69-1

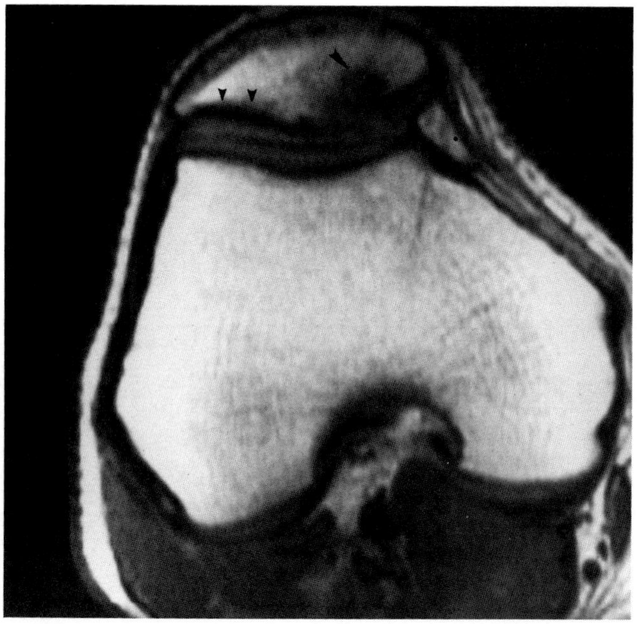

FIGURE 69-2

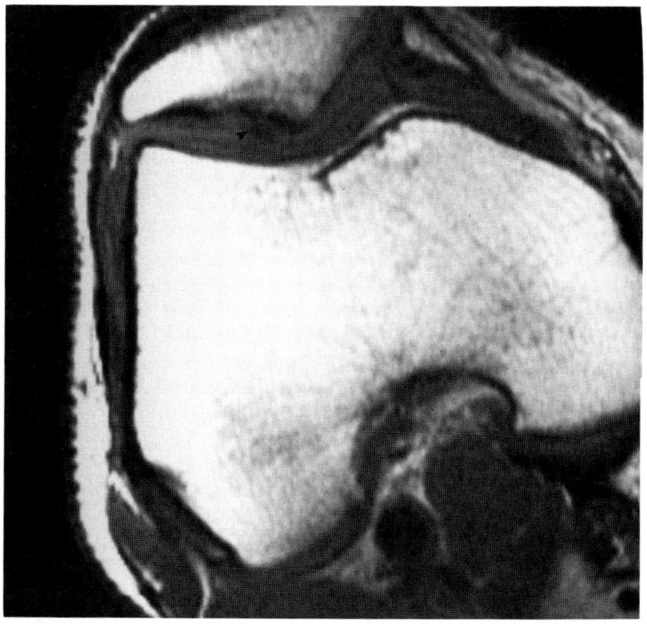

FIGURE 69-3

DISCUSSION: The axial spin-density image (Fig. 69-1) was obtained at the level of the midpatella. All MRI examinations of the knee should be accompanied by an axial scout or diagnostic axial set of images. In the sagittal plane, the patella should be evaluated for:

- cartilaginous homogeneity and smoothness, with attention to the signal of the underlying bone, which should be homogeneous and hyperintense on T1-weighted imaging
- patellar rotation (clockwise or counterclockwise)
- patellar height in the sagittal projection, either alta (elevated) or baja (depressed)
- proximal or distal patellar tilt
- anterior or posterior patellar displacement
- presence or absence of joint effusion and plica formation

Many of these individual parameters will be discussed in other cases.

The posterior patellar margin exhibits irregularity and discontiguity, with a focal area of hypointense signal (large arrowhead in Fig. 69-2) interrupting the intermediate signal intensity of the cartilage, the hypointense cortical bone, and the hyperintense underlying bone. This posterior patellar ulcer is apparent on the plain radiograph (arrowhead in Fig. 69-1). The normal isointense hyaline cartilage and the normal smooth cortical bone margin anterior to it (paired arrowheads in Fig. 69-2) are visible along the lateral patellar facet. Chondromalacia of the patella is a syndrome consisting of irregularity of the patellar undersurface, clinical evidence of crepitation, and retropatellar pain, or "movie sign."

Chondromalacia can be categorized as a subset of one of three subtypes of patellofemoral disease:

1. chondromalacia,
2. malalignment and/or subluxation, and
3. instability and/or subluxation.

Malalignment and instability can be diagnosed from MR images. Instability refers to a susceptibility to displacement from the femoral sulcus. Patellar malalignment refers to displacement of the patella through all or a portion of the range of the flexion. These functional changes can be assessed with cine MRI or MRI movies.

Crepitus is present in 50% of patients upon knee flexion. Isolated ulceration of the lateral patellar facet appears in 5% of cases. Medial and lateral facet ulcers are seen in 55%, and isolated medial knee ulcers (as in this case) occur in 40% of patients.

On MRI, grade 1 chondromalacia appears as a simple, poorly defined hypointensity within the intermediate signal intensity patellar cartilage (small arrowhead in Fig. 69-3). Grade 2 chondromalacia produces hypointensity within the patellar cartilage that deforms the posterior patellar chondral surface. Grade 3 chondromalacia causes deformation of the posterior patellar surface, which then appears broad, irregular and pathologically has a crabmeat appearance. Grade 4 chondromalacia is characterized by diffuse, broad signal hypointensity on spin-density, T1, and fast scan images that extends to the bony surface with associated hypointensity within the medullary bone and a serrated appearance to the retropatellar surface (see Fig. 69-4).

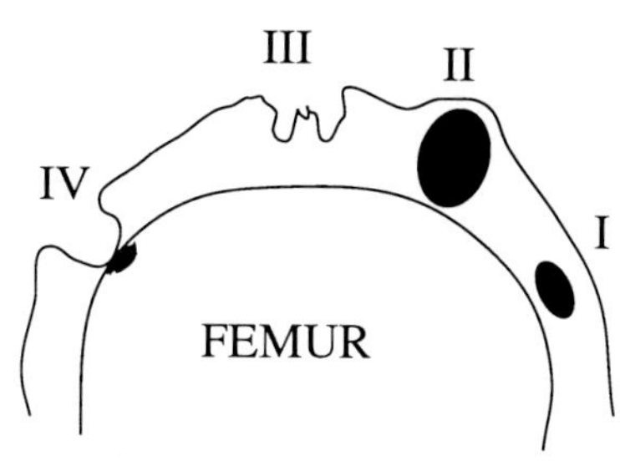

FIGURE 69-4

DIAGNOSIS: The patient has grade 4 chondromalacia.

CASE 70

Differential Diagnosis of Acute Anterior Knee Pain and Patellofemoral Disease

HISTORY: A 16-year-old boy reported acute knee pain and swelling after a blow from a football helmet to the right knee. The clinician suspected a giant joint effusion and possible fracture or internal derangement. What structures are called out in this image? (Fig. 70-1: sagittal multiecho proton-density (*A*) and T2-weighted MR images.)

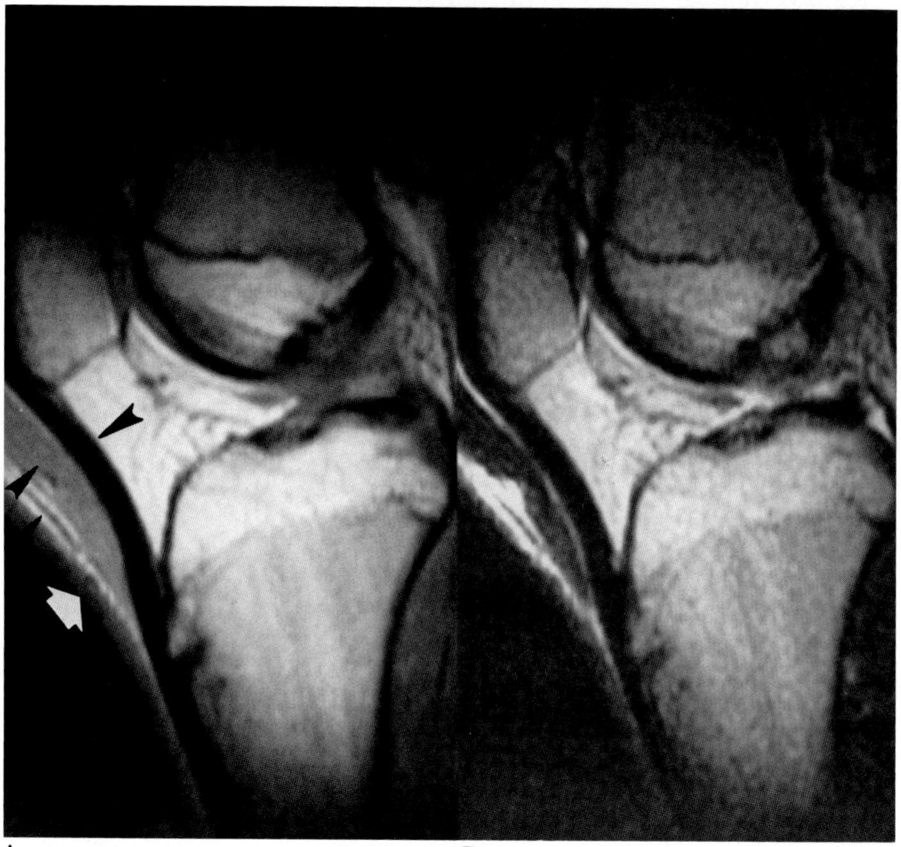

A B

FIGURE 70-1

DISCUSSION: In the prepatellar space, an area of intermediate signal intensity is visible on the proton-density sagittal image (intermediate arrowhead in Fig. 70-1*A*); however, on the T2-weighted image this area appears almost as hypointense as the adjacent patellar tendon. In the setting of acute injury, this represents a large prepatellar soft tissue acute hematoma. The hypointense signal of blood on the T2-weighted image is related to a susceptibility effect, shortened relaxation time due to intracellular methemoglobin and deoxyhemoglobin. This effect is field dependent. However, preferential T2 shortening (PT2PRE) is less consistent and less pronounced than in the closed environment of the brain.

Superficial to the dependent components of the prepatellar bursa hematoma is a layer of T2 signal and hyperintensity, intermediate in signal on the proton-density image (small arrowhead in Fig. 70-1*A*). This supernatant represents the waterlike component of this layering hematoma. The most superficial layer, of intermediate signal intensity (white arrow in Fig. 70-1*A*), represents the normal dermal and epidermal layers. The infrapatellar tendon is spared. There is no evidence of joint effusion, and the bony structures are normal.

The primary differential diagnosis is a prepatellar hematoma located outside (either superficial or deep to) the prepatellar bursa. Hematomas outside the bursal space are not contained or well-marginated, as in this case.

DIAGNOSIS: The patient has a giant prepatellar bursa hematoma.

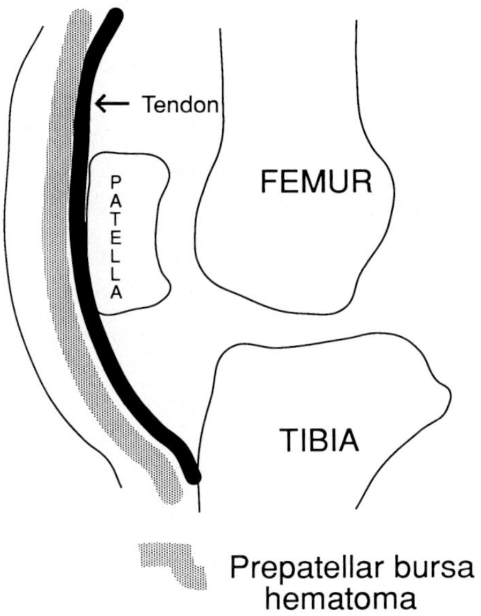

FIGURE 70-2

CASE 71

Differential Diagnosis of Anterior Knee Pain and Patellofemoral Disease

HISTORY: A 22-year-old man reported chronic anterior knee pain, nontender and without knee swelling. (Fig. 71-1: plain radiograph of left patella, axial view. Fig. 71-2: axial multisection, single-echo T1-weighted MR images. Fig. 71-3: anteroposterior radiograph. Fig. 71-4: coronal multisection, single-echo T1-weighted MR images.)

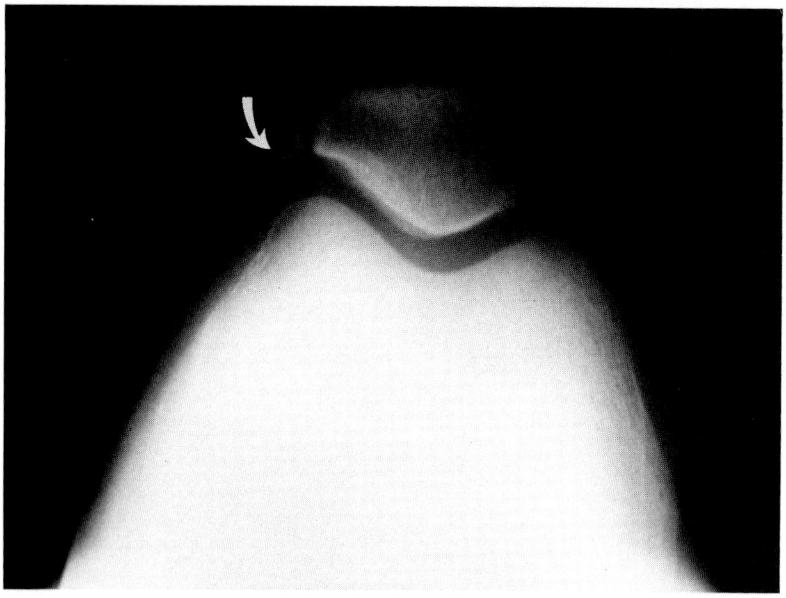

FIGURE 71-1

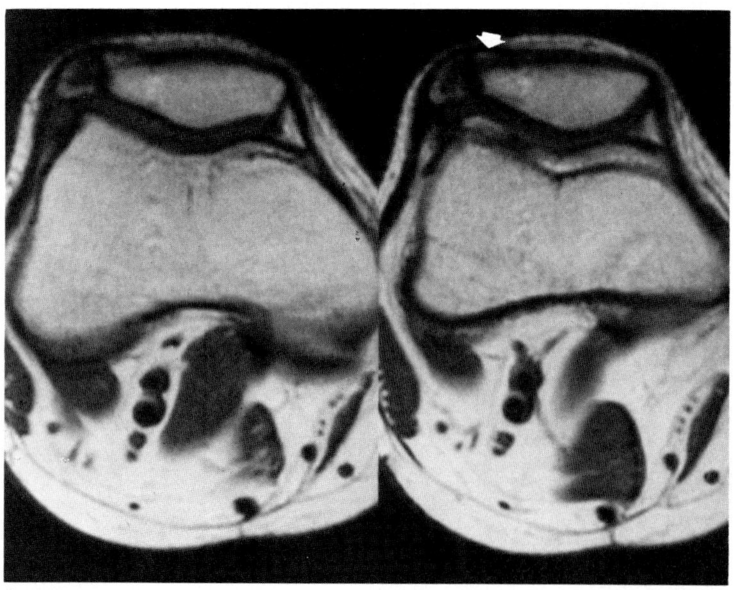

A **B**

FIGURE 71-2

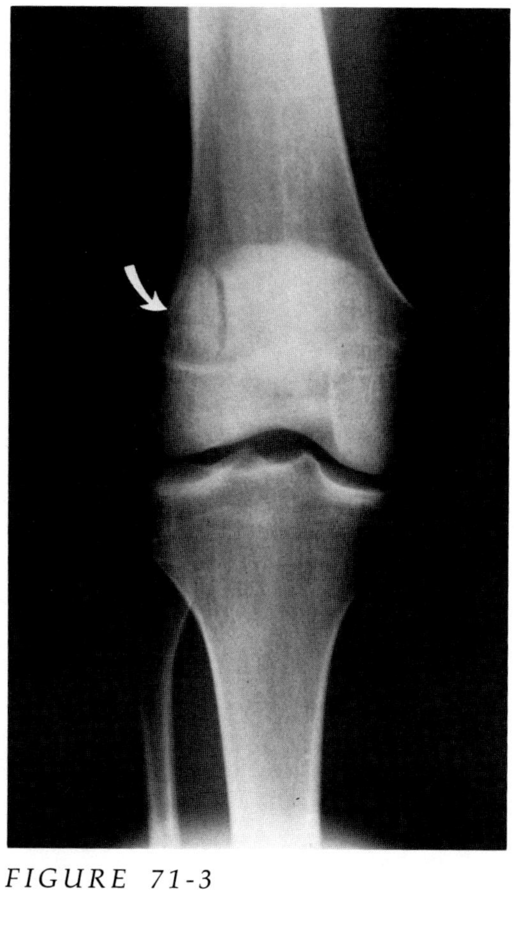

FIGURE 71-3

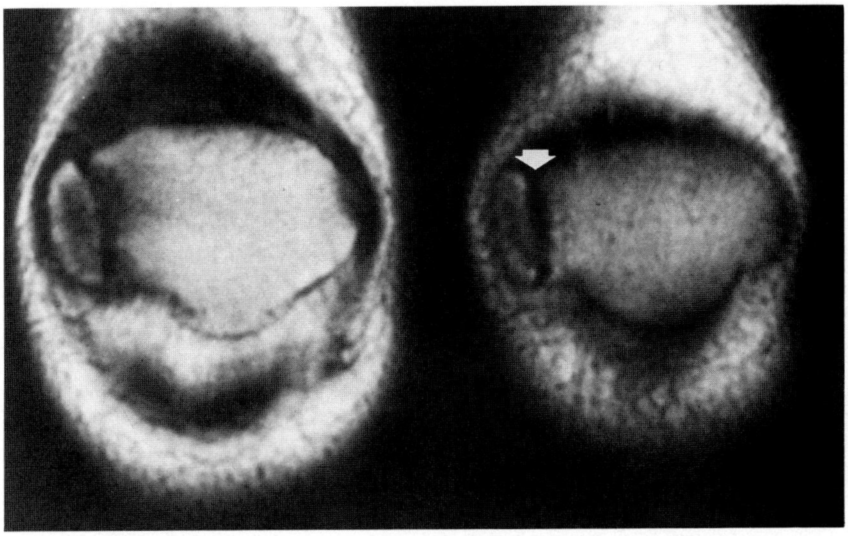

A B

FIGURE 71-4

DISCUSSION: The patella normally begins to ossify between ages 5 and 6 years. Ossification occurs centrifugally, with some accessory foci. Because the margin between an expanded ossification center and the overlying cartilage is weak in growing young adults, chronic chondro-osseous separation may occur, resulting in a painful, fragmented or segmented patella (bipartite or tripartite).

Painful bipartite or tripartite patellas are common in young persons and affect boys more often than girls (ratio of 9:1). Approximately 50% of these lesions are unilateral. Involvement of the superior pole (5%), lateral pole (20%), and superolateral pole (75%) is the approximate anatomic distribution. Some bi- and tripartite patellas actually occur secondary to fracture in adulthood. They may occur in adolescent athletes with no previous symptoms, as a result of violent quadriceps contraction or forced flexion of the knee against a contracted quadriceps muscle. The same phenomenon may also produce spontaneous rupture of the patellar tendon. Nevertheless, any patient with acute pain after trauma and with radiographs consistent with a segmented bi- or tripartite patella is treated with immobilization.

The segmented appearance of the superolateral patella is apparent on the conventional radiographs (arrows in Figs. 71-1 and 71-3). A cleft of separation exists on the MR images, without evidence of hypointense edema or hemorrhage in bone or soft tissues on T1-weighted imaging.

DIAGNOSIS: The patient has a tripartite patella.

CASE 72

Differential Diagnosis of Anterior Knee Pain and Patellofemoral Disease

HISTORY: A 31-year-old patient presented with chronic anterolateral knee pain. What is the MRI diagnosis? (Fig. 72-1: axial T1-weighted MR image.)

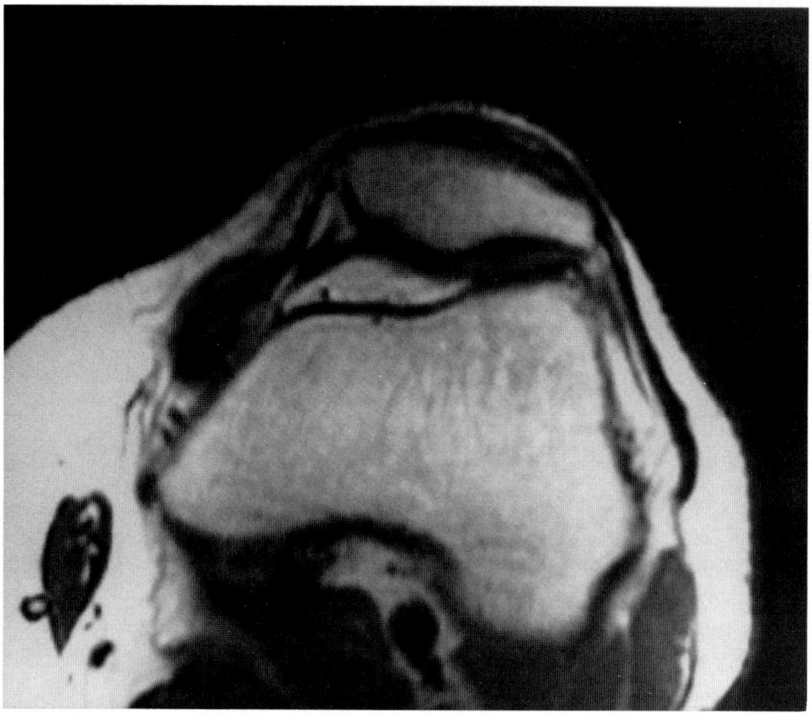

FIGURE 72-1

DISCUSSION: Axial sections at the level of the midpatella are obtained with the knee in 20° of flexion. The patella appears tilted or rotated counterclockwise. On axial views of the patella the lateral patellar facet normally appears larger than the medial facet by an average ratio of 1.4 to 1.0. The thickest articular cartilage (6.5 mm) is found on the median patellar ridge. The lateral facet is concave and the medial patellar facet varies from concave to convex. MR evaluation of the patellofemoral joint must take into account (1) knee flexion angle, (2) knee rotation, and (3) the presence or absence of joint effusion. Joint effusion may produce exuberant patellar tilt.

In the normal state, the lateral patellofemoral or tilt angle (angle *OOP* in the Patella II diagram) is an open angle greater than 8°. When this angle becomes less than 6° to 8°, lateral pressure on the femoral ridge may occur. Abnormal patellar tilt need not be accompanied by patellar subluxation or dislocation. However, abnormal patellar tilt exists in 10% of patients with idiopathic chondromalacia but in only 2% of asymptomatic patients. When accompanied by lateral patellar displacement where the lateral patellar facet overrides the lateral femoral ridge, patellar subluxation is more common. This is particularly true in patients with Weiberg 3 patellofemoral configurations when the lateral ridge is diminutive. Tilt rather than subluxation or instability is more commonly associated with lateral patellar osteophytes; therefore, axial patellofemoral evaluation can be subcategorized into lateral displacement or subluxation without tilt or with tilt, or tilt alone without subluxation, as shown in the Patella I diagram.

Diagnostic signs of patellar subluxation or displacement include the following:

1. lateral patellar posture and patellar alta,
2. dysplasia of the vastus medialis obliquus, as indicated by concavity of the medial aspect of the distal thigh when the leg is actively extended against gravity at 45°,
3. lateral concavity, indicating retinaculum contraction,
4. vastus lateralis muscle hypertrophy (visible on MRI),
5. lateral passive hypermobility or subluxation of the patella (best evaluated in 45° of flexion),
6. medial patellar pain and a snapping sensation felt by the patient when the patella is pushed laterally, representing the plica catching between the patella and the medial femoral condyle.

Patellar tilt and displacement can be accurately assessed on MRI with as little as 10° of knee flexion. Methods of measuring lateral displacement or shift of the patella and tilting angle are outlined in the diagrams Patella I, Patella II, and Patella V.

DIAGNOSIS: The patient has a lateral pressure syndrome with a closed patellar tilt angle.

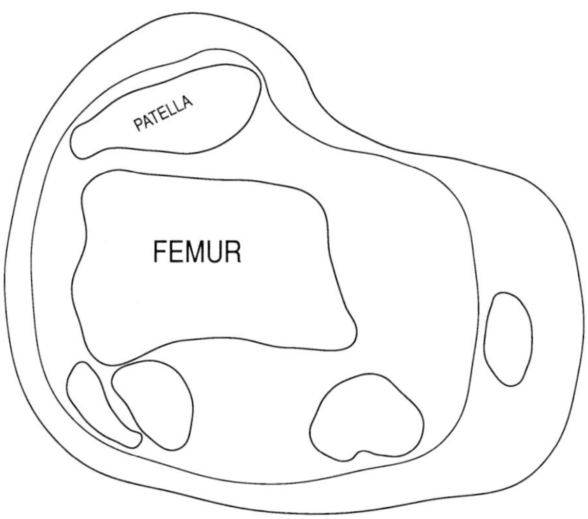

FIGURE 72-2

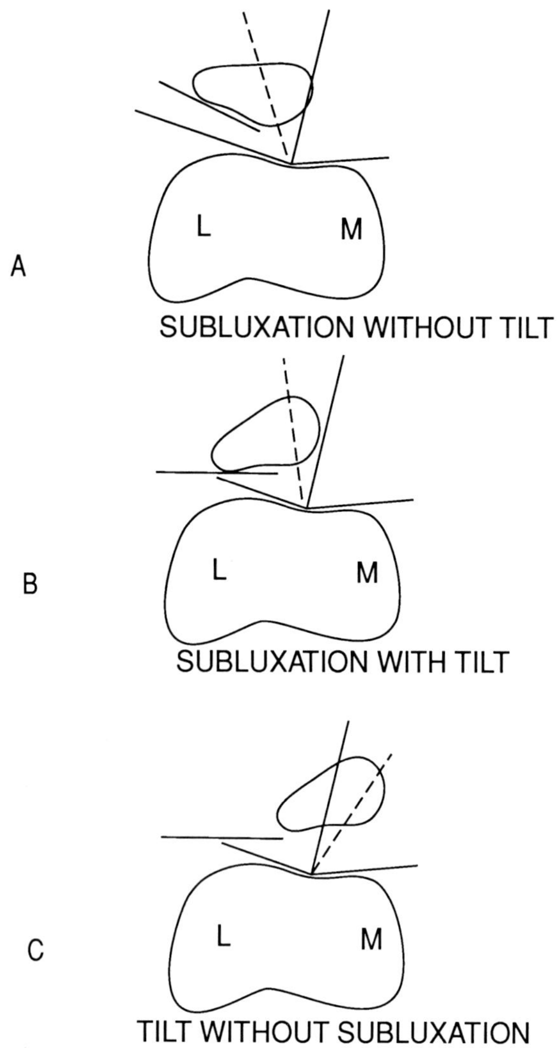

PATELLA I

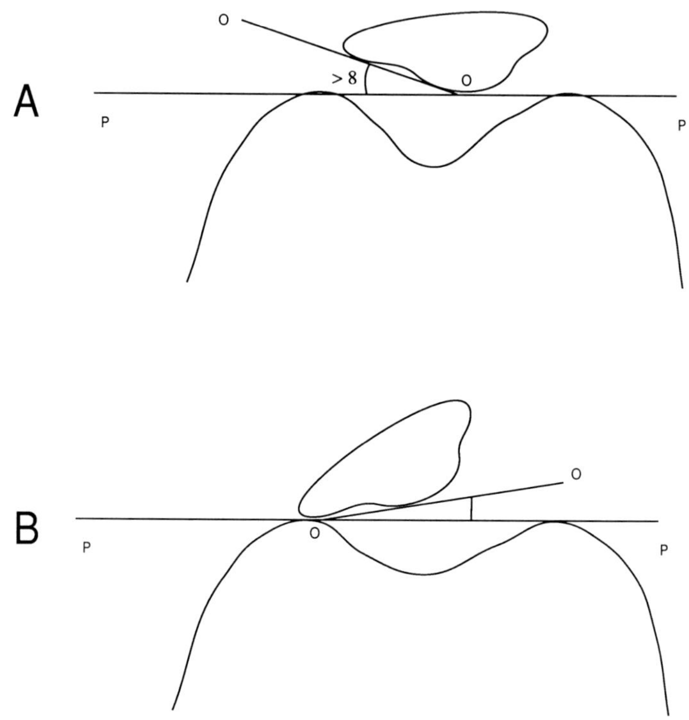

PATELLA II

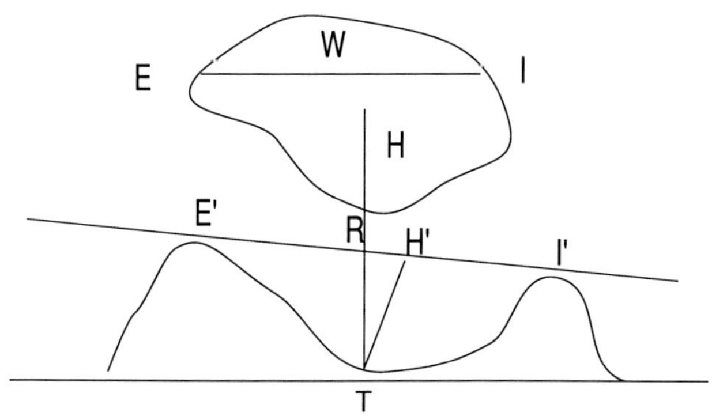

PATELLA III

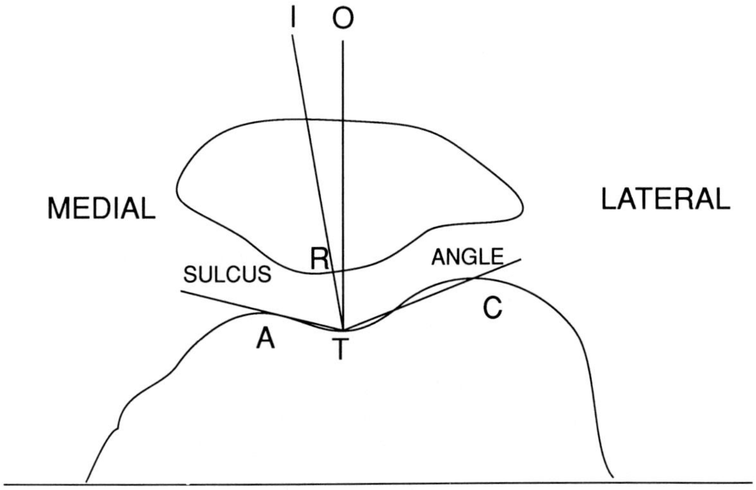

* T is placed at the lowest point of the articular ridge of the patella

PATELLA IV

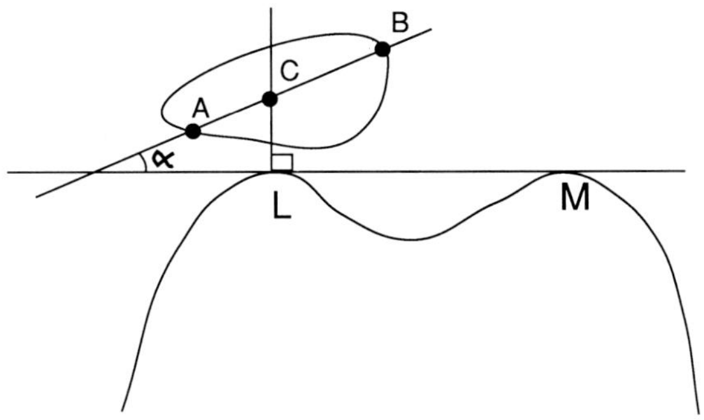

PATELLA V

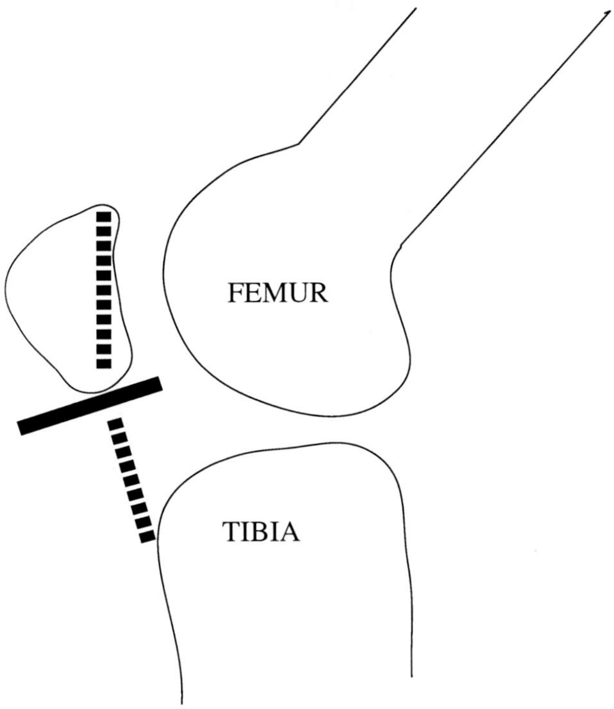

PATELLA VI

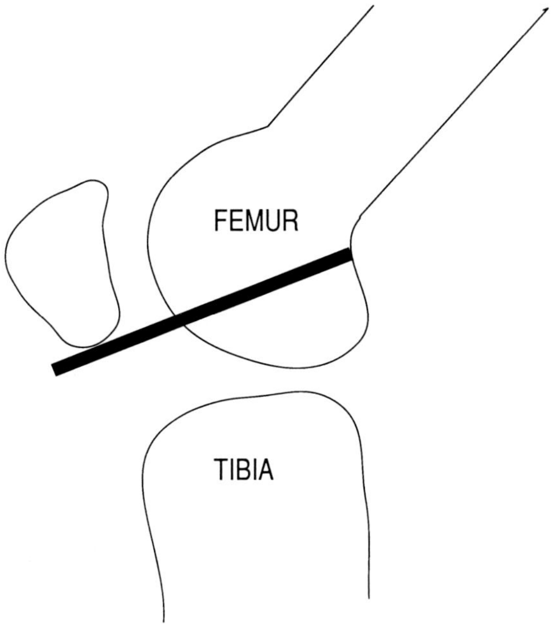

PATELLA VII

CASE 73

Differential Diagnosis of Anterior Knee Pain and Patellofemoral Disease

HISTORY: A 48-year-old man presented with chronic lateral knee pain and recent anterior knee trauma sustained in a motor vehicle accident. What is the MRI diagnosis? (Fig. 73-1: axial proton-density MR image at the level of the midpatella.)

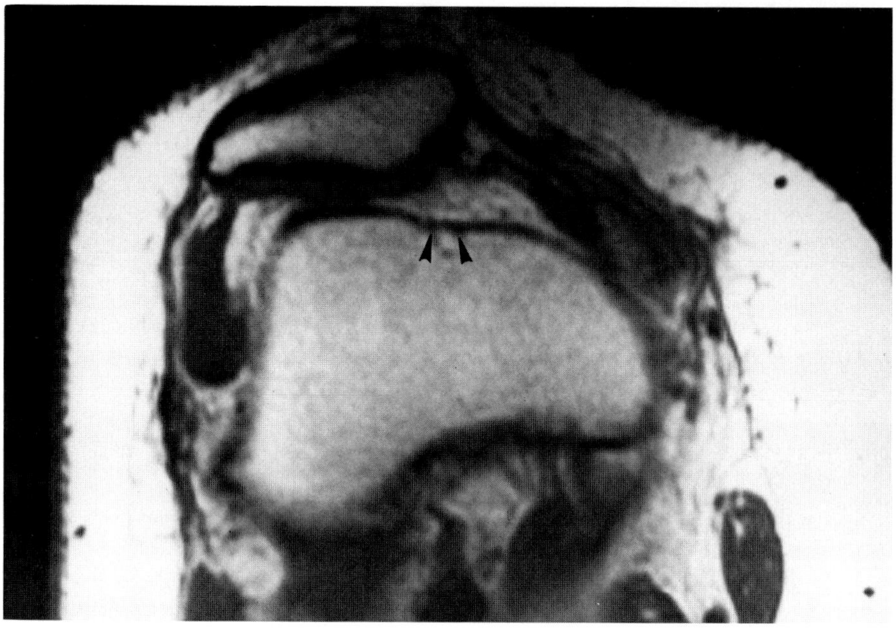

FIGURE 73-1

DISCUSSION

TROCHLEAR DEPTH/LATERAL FEMORAL RIDGE HYPOPLASIA: Weiberg has defined numerous patellofemoral configurations or subtypes. The type 3 configuration is one in which the lateral femoral component of the patellofemoral joint is diminutive in size. The trochlear groove between the femoral ridges (arrowheads in Fig. 73-1) of the knee is therefore shallow, and the patient is prone to recurrent patellar lateral subluxation or instability. The trochlear facet angle in the Patella III diagram is demarcated by *E'TI*. When this angle is greater than 145°, it is abnormal and suggests patellofemoral dysplasia.

Similarly, trochlear depth may be calculated from a ratio of a line drawn between the two peaks of the femur (*E'TI*) divided by the depth, demarcated by line *RT*. Another measure of sulcus retentiveness is the sulcus angle. A shallow sulcus angle and small lateral femoral ridge are shown in the Patella IV diagram. This ratio may have implications with regard to sulcus retentiveness, with a normal range between 4.2 and 6.5. Dynamic MRI may be used to confirm the presence of subluxation in association with instability and dysplasia. Serial axial fast scan images with varying degrees of flexion may be displayed in rapid sequence on a video tape as a cine loop.

CONGRUENCE ANGLE: A more useful and accurate measure of patellofemoral dysplasia may be obtained by measuring the congruence angle, as shown in the Patella III diagram. This is ascertained by bisecting the sulcus *ATC* with a reference line *B0*. Then a second line, *TI*, is projected from the sulcus (*T*) to the lowest point on the articular ridge of the patella (*I*). The congruence angle, *T0I*, is negative if *I* is medial to reference line *TO* and positive if it is lateral to reference line *T0*. Therefore, the *TOI* angle is expressed in positive or negative degrees or increments. Normal congruence angles are a subject of debate. They tend to lie between +6° and −6°. An angle of +16° is abnormal at the 95th percentile, and virtually all patients with an angle greater than +20° have symptoms secondary to patellofemoral dysplasia. A loose association exists between abnormalities in the sulcus trochlear angle and Insall–Salvati index (a measurement of patellar height). The normal trochlear sulcus angle approximates 140° and the normal Insall–Salvati index approximates <1.2.

LATERAL DISPLACEMENT: The trochlear groove and depth are extremely shallow in this case. The lateral femoral ridge is virtually flat, a configuration that predisposes to recurrent patellar subluxation. The patella is laterally displaced or overhangs the lateral femoral ridge. If a perpendicular line is drawn along the lateral femoral ridge, the degree of displacement is measured by approximating the amount of patella lying lateral to this perpendicular line.

The degree of lateral patella disruption or dysplasia should be determined with an axial view taken with 15° of knee flexion. The correlation of displacement severity with chondromalacia is only rough. This is illustrated in the accompanying diagram. The degree of lateral patellar displacement can be calculated by a percentage. A perpendicular is dropped (line *CL* in the Patella V diagram). The ratio of patella lateral to this line divided by that medial to it is the degree of displacement. A patella may sublux with tilt, without tilt, or it may tilt without subluxation (see Patella I diagram).

DIAGNOSIS: The patient has patellar subluxation due to lateral femoral ridge hypoplasia with a mild patellar tilt, as abnormal congruence angle, and a shallow trochlear depth.

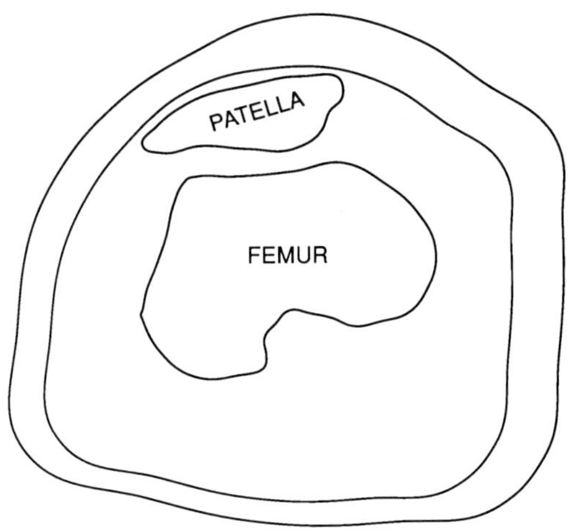

FIGURE 73-2

CASE 74

Differential Diagnosis of Anterior Knee Pain

HISTORY: A 42-year-old woman presented with chronic anterior knee pain for 2 years that was recently exacerbated by a fall and now associated with knee swelling. (Fig. 74-1: sagittal, and Fig. 74-2: axial proton-density MR images.)

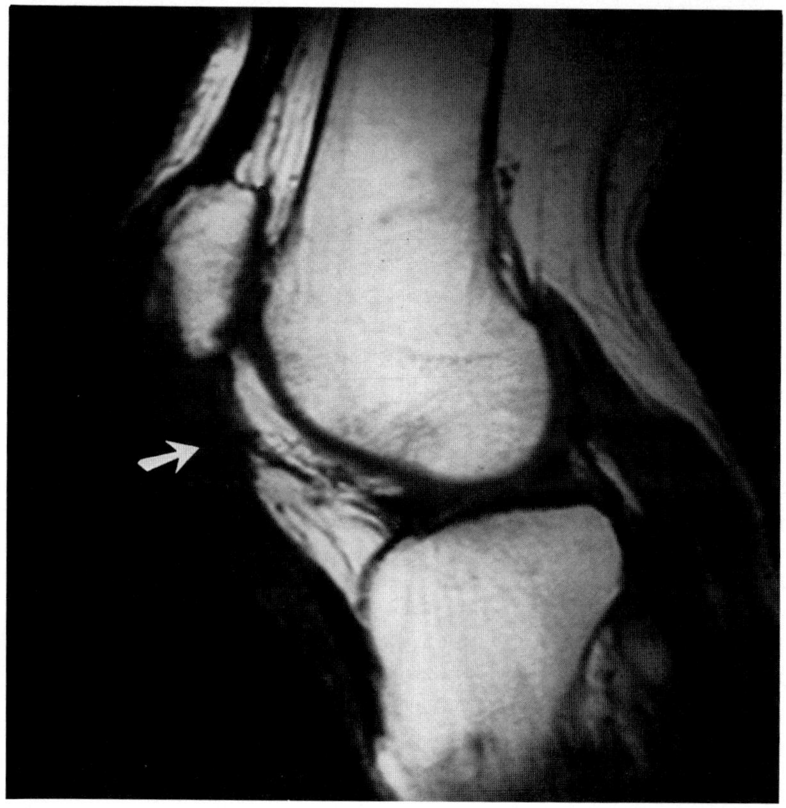

FIGURE 74-1

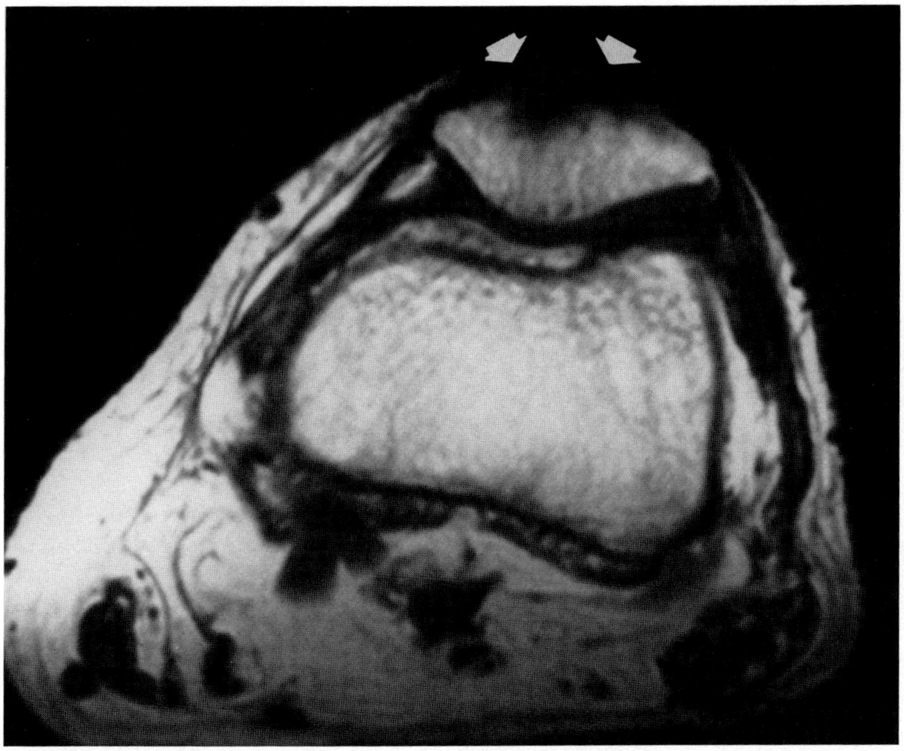

FIGURE 74-2

DISCUSSION: The sagittal midplane image of the knee was taken with the knee in 20° to 30° of flexion. The patellar height is positioned in a more proximal craniad distribution. There are four methods of determining patellar height; however, the most widely utilized is that of Insall–Salvati. At 20° to 30° of flexion, the ratio of the patellar: tendon length to that of the greatest diagonal length of the patella is calculated. The normal upper limit is 1.2. (The Insall–Salvati index is higher in women and tends to be closer to 1.2 in women and 1.0 in men.) The relationship of patellar alta is increased with both patellar instability and chondromalacia in many series; however, the relationship to patellar subluxation is stronger than the relationship to chondromalacia alone. Alta often implies the presence of patellar instability in more extended ranges of knee motion so the patella has nominal bony constraint at these angles. If one utilizes the Patella VI diagram and measures the tendon length to patellar length ratio, one sees that it exceeds 1.2 in this patient.

In addition to the anatomic alteration of patellar alta, arrows on the MR images demarcate the presence of intermediate signal intensity anterior to the infrapatellar tendon and engulfing it in both projections. The extent of this process, the patient history, and the large anterior patellar erosions seen in the axial projection (arrows in Fig. 74-2) support an aggressive etiology to this process.

DIAGNOSIS: The patient has patellar osteomyelitis with patellar alta.

CASE 75

Differential Diagnosis of Cystic and Noncystic Masses of the Knee

HISTORY: Patients with the same lesion of varying size underwent radiologic evaluation. (Fig. 75-1: sagittal fast scan gradient-echo MR image [patient 1]. The remaining images apply to patient 2. Fig. 75-2: sagittal proton-density MR image. Fig. 75-3: axial multiecho, multiformat (two-on-one) proton-density MR images. Fig. 75-4: contiguous multiformat (four-on-one) T2-weighted MR images. Fig. 75-5: magnified axial T2-weighted image.)

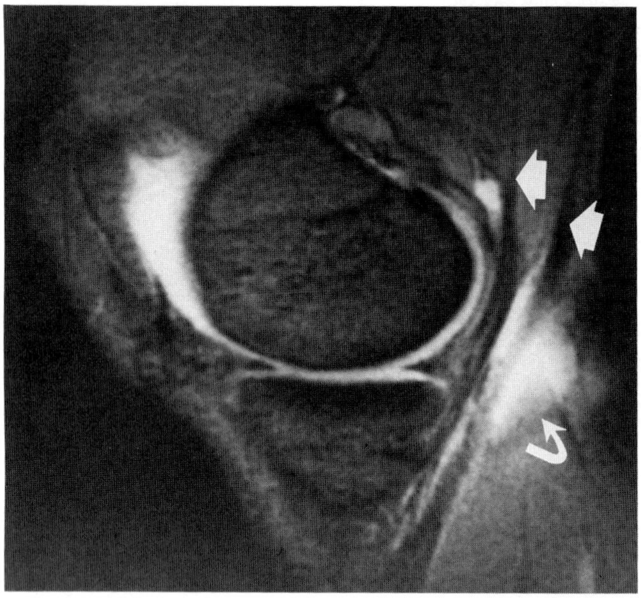

FIGURE 75-1

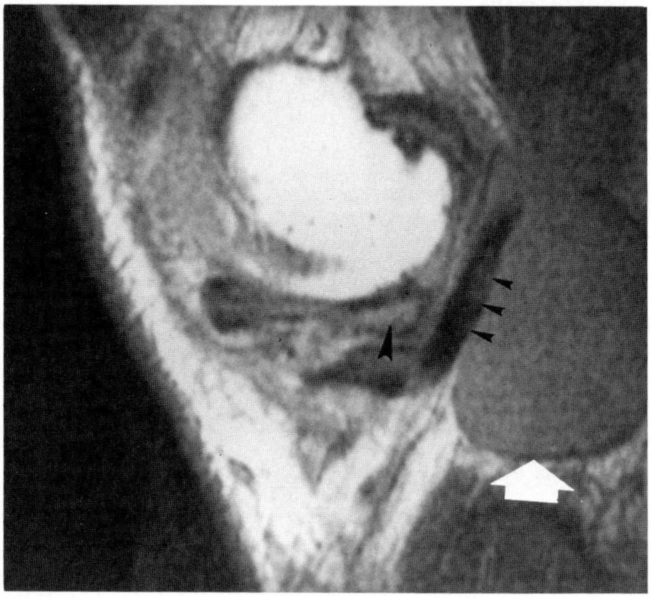

FIGURE 75-2

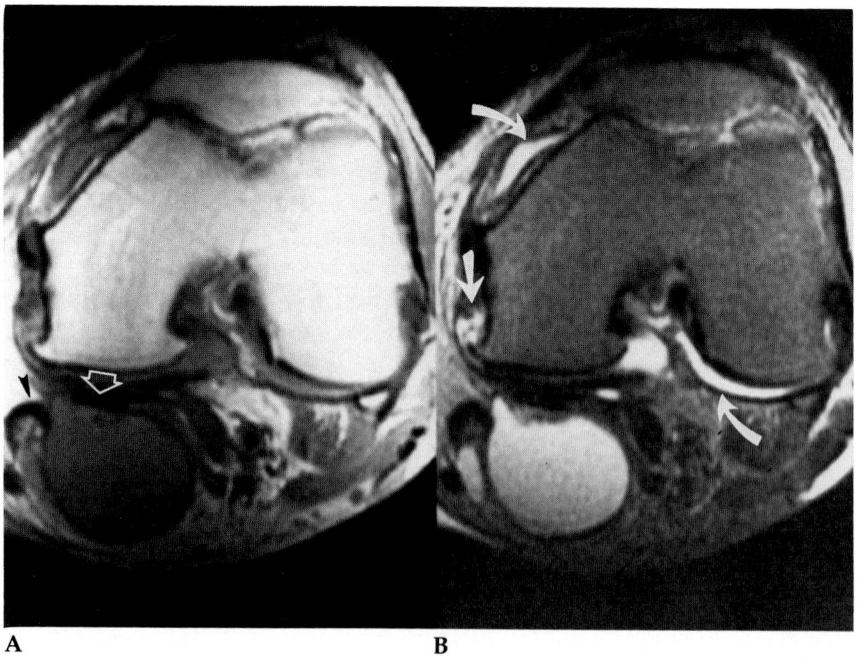

A B

FIGURE 75-3

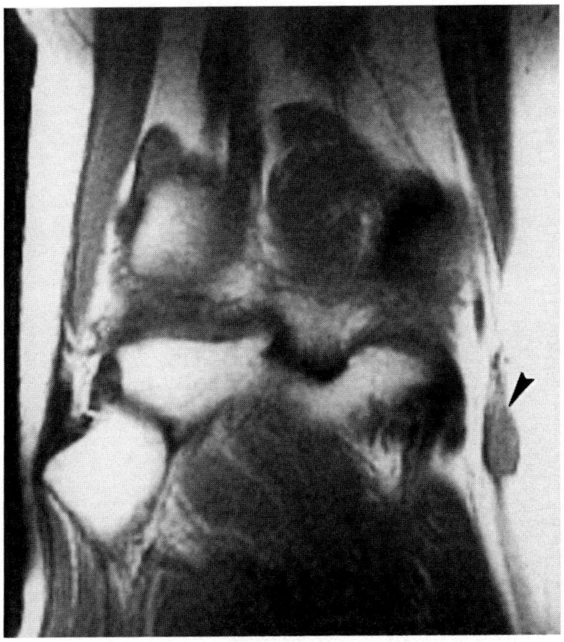

FIGURE 82-4

DISCUSSION: Masses along the medial joint line, as in patient 1 (Fig. 82-1), can be narrowed down to three or four entities, provided their signal is cystic or of water signal intensity on all pulse sequences. These entities include ganglia, bursitis or bursal enlargement, and meniscal cyst. Ganglia communicate with the joint space but not with the menisci and invariably align themselves with tendons. Meniscal cysts communicate with the menisci and are associated with meniscal tear. Bursal enlargements or popliteal cysts, when positioned medially, usually arise from the gastrocnemius–semimembranosus bursa. A posterior location predominates in such cases.

A round, hypointense mass of water signal intensity (curved arrow in Fig. 82-1*B*) ensheaths the linear hypointense pes anserine (semitendinosus, gracilis, and sartorius) tendon complex. This mass projects exactly along the course of the anserine complex, not above or below it, as do most Baker's cysts. The lesion tenderness supports an inflammatory condition rather than a remote posttraumatic etiology.

The second set of images, from patient 2, again show pes anserine bursitis. Along a bundle of the pes is an area of homogeneous, intermediate signal intensity (arrowhead in Fig. 82-4) on spin-echo imaging that becomes hyperintense on the fast scan sequence (triple arrowheads in Fig. 82-3). The differential diagnosis includes ganglion formation, pes anserinus, and bursitis. A small, thin bursa runs among and between the tendinous anatomy in this region. With bursitis, the aspirate from this lesion would be clear and waterlike; however, with ganglion, the material would appear gelatinous.

DIAGNOSIS: Two examples of pes anserine bursitis are illustrated.

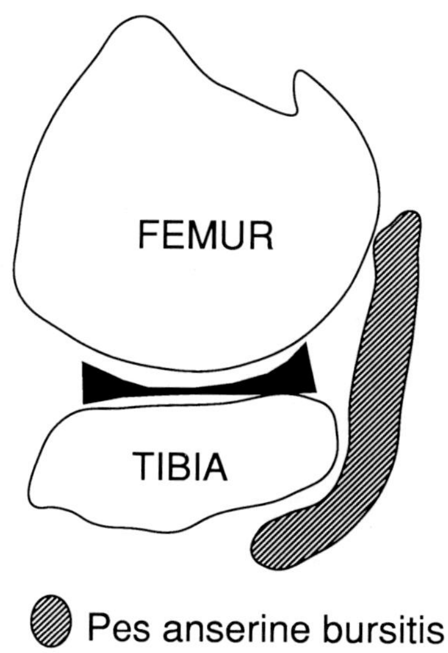

FIGURE 82-5

CASE 83

Differential Diagnosis of Knee Swelling or Mass

HISTORY: A 22-year-old woman reported swelling on the lateral side of the knee. The medial joint line was nontender. What is the MRI diagnosis? (Fig. 83-1: coronal proton-density image, TR/TE 1,000/20 msec. Fig. 83-2: multiformat (four-on-one) sagittal T1-weighted images.)

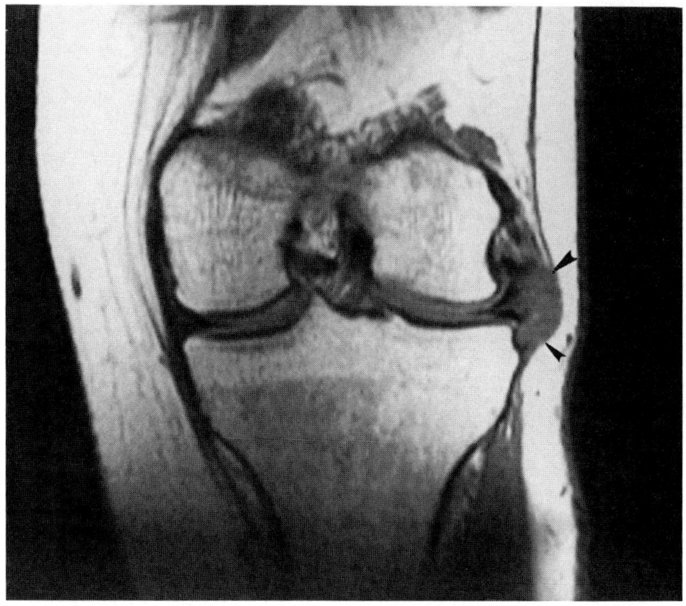

FIGURE 83-1

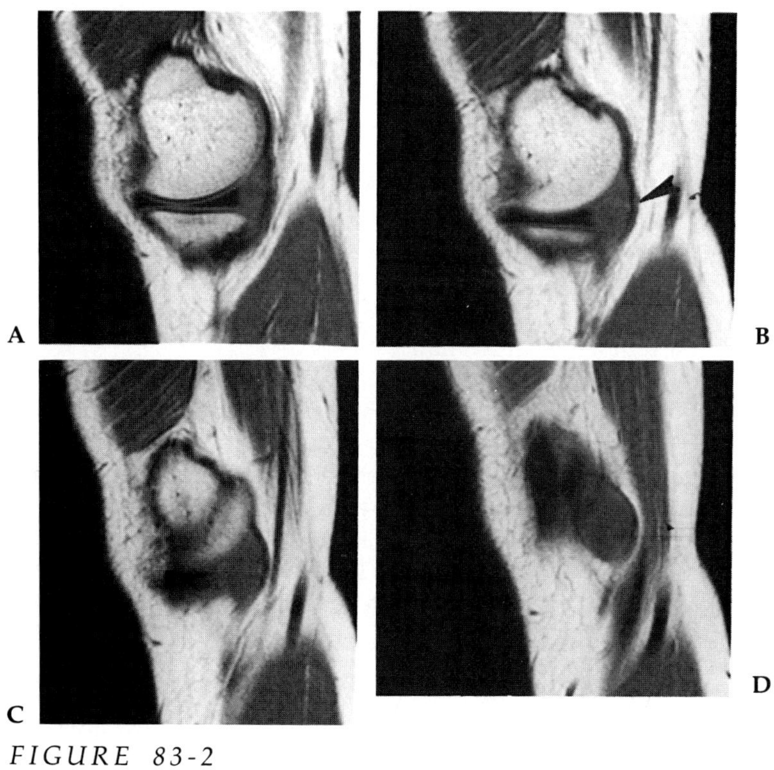

FIGURE 83-2

DISCUSSION: Meniscal cysts are of intermediate signal intensity on T1-weighted imaging, owing to their proteinaceous or gelatinous contents, and of high signal intensity on fast scan or T2-weighted imaging. They are characteristically located at the joint line and are more often lateral than medial (4:1 ratio). A definable connection to the joint and often the meniscus may be present, as in this case. Prominent intermediate intrameniscal signal intensity is apparent within the normally black triangle of the meniscus just deep to the mass (arrowheads in Fig. 83-1). If the cyst is excised but the underlying tear is not addressed, recurrence rates approximate 90%. The lesions are round or ovoid and smooth walled.

Lateral cysts tend to be smaller and are contained by the capsule and iliotibial band, usually in the midplane near the joint line. They may dissect between the iliotibial band and fibular collateral ligament and subsequently into the Hoffa fat space. Medial cysts, while less often producing pain, tend to be larger with more posterior extension, since they often occur behind the medial collateral ligament and are unrestricted. Popliteal cyst is then simulated. An example of such a cyst is illustrated in Figure 83-2*B* (arrowhead). Just behind the hypointense triangular meniscus is a homogeneous intermediate signal mass. Communication with the posteromedial capsular interface suggests either a meniscal cyst or a ganglion. The location is far more typical of meniscal cyst.

DIAGNOSIS: The patient has a lateral meniscal cyst with a horizontal meniscal tear, and a medial meniscal cyst.

CASE 84

Differential Diagnosis of Soft Tissue Masses about the Knee

HISTORY: A 74-year-old man was referred for evaluation of a posterior knee mass and knee pain, with a suspected diagnosis of popliteal cyst. Is this a popliteal or gastrocnemius–semimembranosis bursal cyst? (Fig. 84-1: axial T1-weighted image at the level of the tibial plateau.)

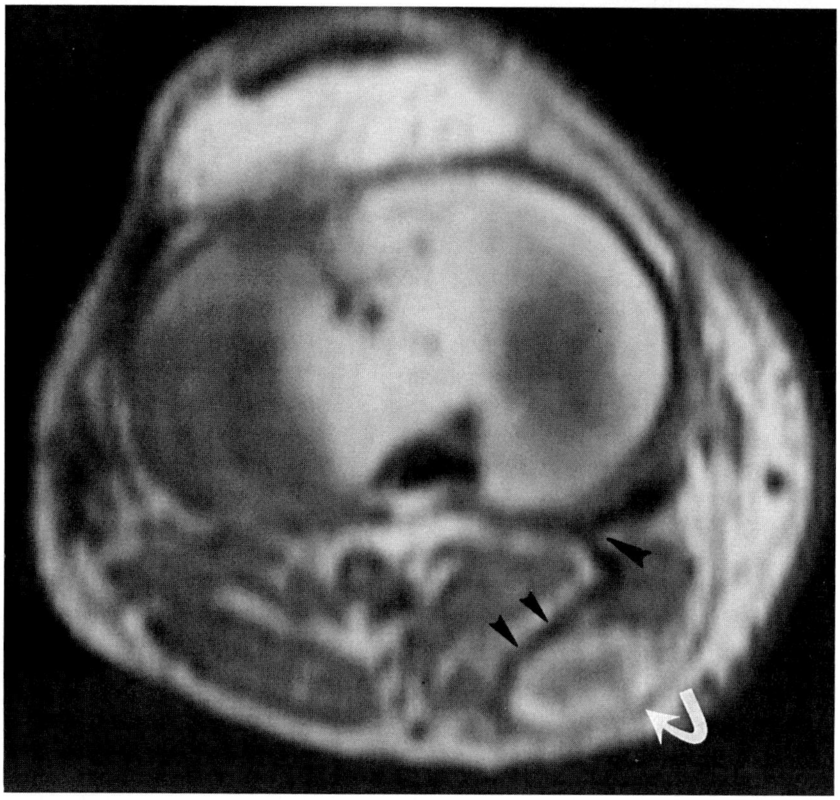

FIGURE 84-1

DISCUSSION: More than 95% of popliteal cysts occur in the posteromedial compartment of the knee, arising from the posterolateral horn of the gastrocnemius–semimembranosus bursa. The bursal reflection, apparent as a thin black line between the hypointense tendons, is barely visualized in the axial projection (large arrowhead) and is identified in Figure 84-2.

Anatomically, a hyperintense mass with a center of intermediate signal intensity lies within the medial head of the gastrocnemius muscle (paired arrowheads). The findings are typical of the subacute phase of hematoma formation (curved white arrow) with peripheral hyperintensity due to red cell lysis and methemoglobin formation. A joint effusion was also present (not shown). The evolution of hematomas elsewhere in the body is not nearly as consistent, as it occurs in a closed compartment such as the intracranial space. In fact, the preferential field-dependent T2 shortening effects of intracellular deoxyhemoglobin and methemoglobin are minimized elsewhere in the body, owing to more rapid diffusion of red cells into the surrounding normal tissues and higher or faster rates of red blood cell lysis. Simple bursal cysts are hypointense, not hyperintense, on T1-weighted images.

DIAGNOSIS: The patient has a subacute gastrocnemius muscle hematoma.

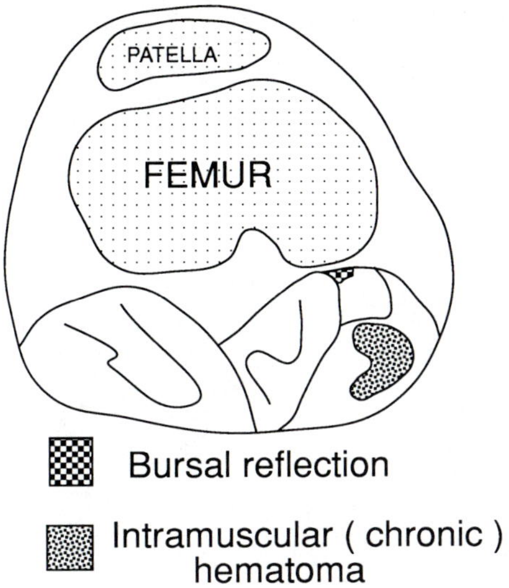

FIGURE 84-2

CASE 85

Differential Diagnosis of Soft Tissue Masses about the Knee

HISTORY: A 39-year-old man presented with lower extremity pain. What is the MRI differential diagnosis? (Fig. 85-1: sagittal T2-weighted image. Fig. 85-2: axial T1-weighted image at the level of the tibial plateau.)

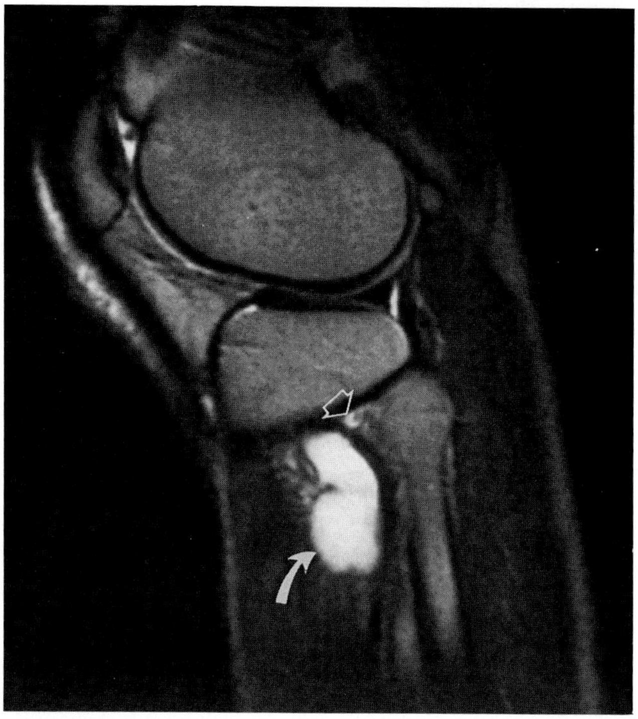

FIGURE 85-1

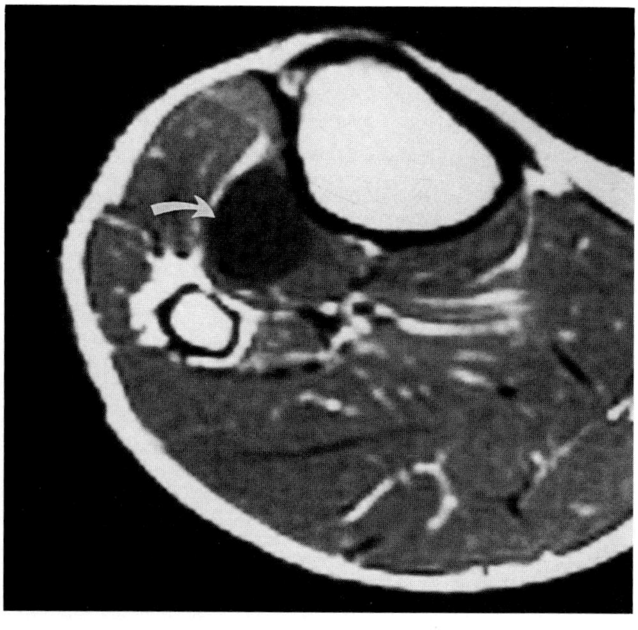

FIGURE 85-2

DISCUSSION: A homogeneous mass is apparent that is hypointense on T1-weighted imaging and hyperintense on T2-weighted imaging (curved white arrow, both images). The waterlike signal is compatible with a cystic lesion. The differential diagnosis is limited to bursitis, ganglion, and cystic soft tissue neoplasm. The latter is excluded by the lesion homogeneity, lack of hyperintense edema around the lesion periphery on T2-weighted imaging, and sharp margination.

Although a bursa does exist between the tibia and fibula, this lesion is positioned in the interosseous space between the tibia and fibula. Bursitis almost always produces a mass effect in a direct lateral orientation relative to the joint space and fibular head. A tail-like communication with the joint capsule is suggested in the sagittal projection (open arrow in Fig. 85-1). The findings are typical of ganglion formation. Ganglia result from myxoid softening of tissues surrounding tendons or the joint spaces.

DIAGNOSIS: The patient has an interosseous tibiofibular space ganglion.

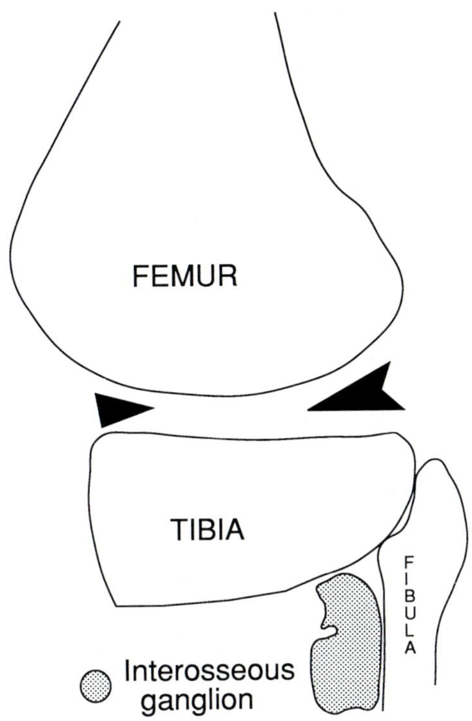

FIGURE 85-3

CASE 86

Differential Diagnosis of Masses and Tumorlike Lesions of and about the Knee

HISTORY: A 32-year-old woman was evaluated for knee pain. Is the process benign or malignant? What is the differential diagnosis? (Fig. 86-1: sagittal multiformat proton-density, and Fig. 86-2: T2-weighted MR images.)

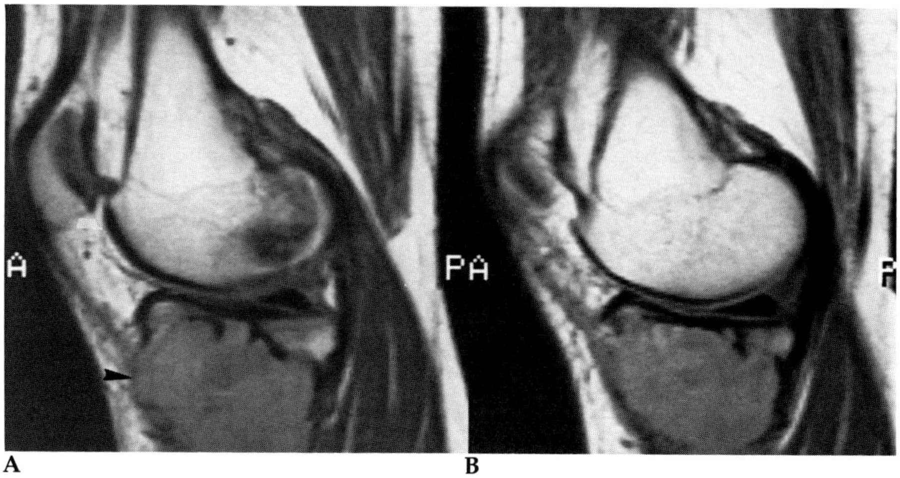

A B
FIGURE 86-1

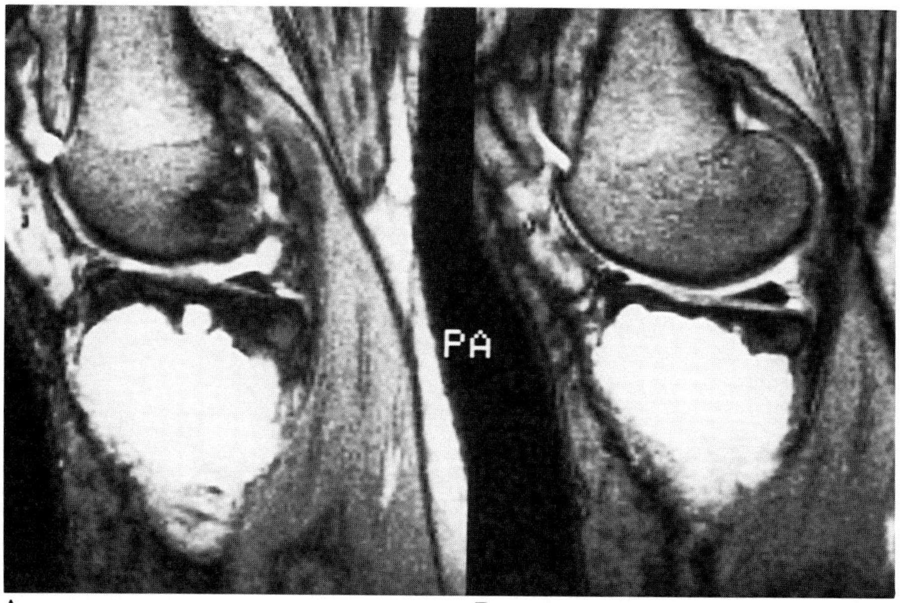

A B
FIGURE 86-2

DISCUSSION: A lesion with a homogeneous signal intensity of water, hypointense on T1-weighted imaging and hyperintense on T2-weighted imaging, is seen in a metaepiphyseal location and extends virtually to the subchondral end of the tibia. The lesion bows and displaces the tibial cortical margin anteriorly (arrowhead in Fig. 86-1*A*); however, no soft tissue component is identified. Septation within the lesion is scant.

The differential diagnosis of a lesion in the end of a bone include chondroblastoma, benign or malignant giant cell tumor, intraosseous ganglion, subchondral arthropathic cyst, Brodie's abscess (particularly from coccidioidomycosis), and pigmented villonodular synovitis. Cystic or clear cell variants of chondrosarcoma may (rarely) occur in bone epiphyses as a result of dedifferentiation from chondroblastoma. The fact that this lesion is well circumscribed and cystic makes the diagnosis of pigmented villonodular synovitis unlikely. The large size rules out intraosseous ganglion and Brodie's abscess. Absence of edema is unusual in Brodie's abscess or its look-alike, osteoid osteoma. The differential diagnosis is thus narrowed to giant cell tumor, chondroblastoma, or chondrosarcomatous dedifferentiation from chondroblastoma. Closed epiphyses, patient age (the average age of patients with giant cell tumors is 32, the average age of patients with chondroblastoma is 10), and lesion homogeneity favor the diagnosis of giant cell tumor. Giant cell tumors, both on MRI and on conventional radiography, have their epicenter in the metaphyses and subsequently engulf or involve the epiphyses.

Giant cell tumor is a lesion with variable aggression, and prognosis after excision is extremely variable. Malignant giant cell tumor tends to occur in older patients. Perilesional edema on MRI connotes a worse prognosis and may also be seen in a similar lesion, dedifferentiated (from chondroblastoma) cystic chondrosarcoma. Giant cell tumor may dedifferentiate into osteogenic sarcoma or fibrosarcoma and may arise secondarily from Paget's disease. The knee is the most common site affected. Hemorrhagic bright signal on T1-weighted imaging is unusual in giant cell tumor and suggests the diagnosis of aneurysmal bone cyst. In fact, aneurysmal bone cyst is frequently confused with or misdiagnosed histologically as a giant cell tumor. Enchondromas have hyperintense inhomogeneous signal on MRI and do not occur at bone ends.

The MRI features of giant cell tumor may be summarized as follows:

1. waterlike signal intensity (hypointense on T1-weighted images, hyperintense on T2-weighted images) rather than hemorrhagic signal intensity,
2. well circumscribed,
3. central or eccentric,
4. metaphyseal with epiphyseal involvement,
5. homogeneous or septated,
6. no soft tissue component,
7. no daughter cysts, and
8. minimal perilesional edema unless malignant.

DIAGNOSIS: The patient has a giant cell tumor.

CASE 87

Differential Diagnosis of Masses and Tumorlike Lesions of and about the Knee

HISTORY: A 62-year-old woman was evaluated for medial thigh pain and the sensation of a mass. What is the differential diagnosis? (Fig. 87-1: coronal T1-weighted image, and Fig. 87-2: coronal T2-weighted image, 0.5T.) Case was provided courtesy of Providence Hospital Radiology Department, Cincinnati, Ohio.

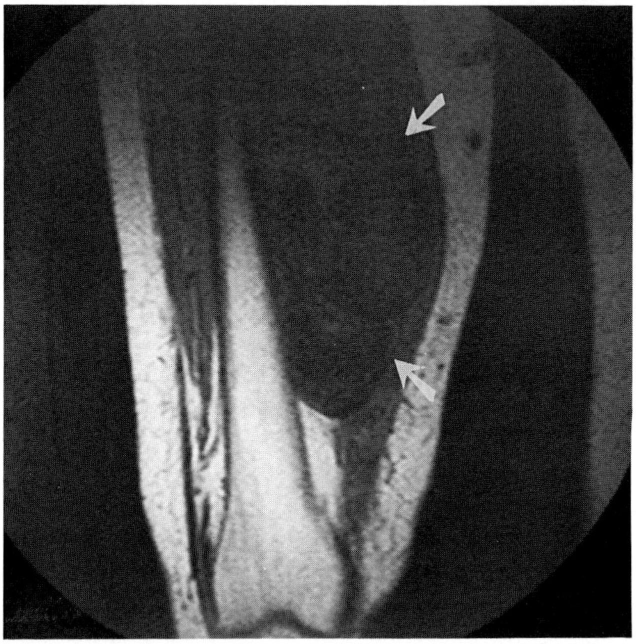

FIGURE 87-1

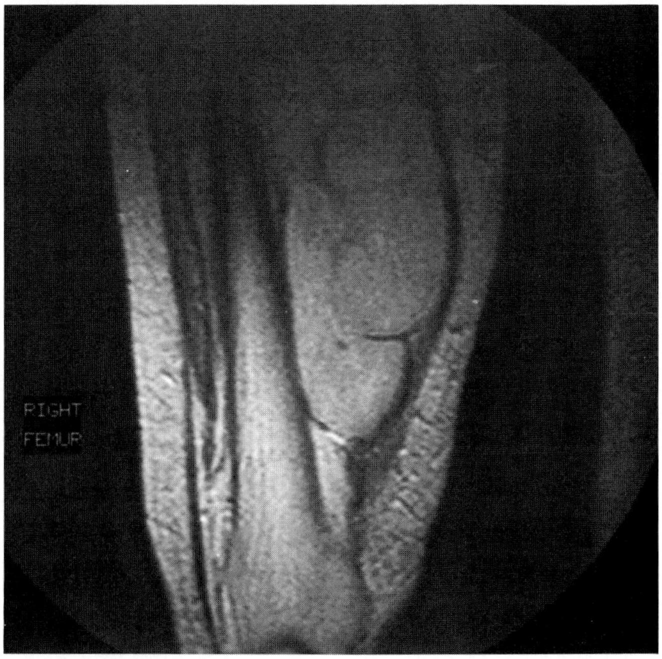

FIGURE 87-2

DISCUSSION: A mass is present in the medial thigh (arrows in Fig. 87-1) with homogeneous, water signal intensity that appears hypointense on T1-weighted imaging and hyperintense on T2-weighted imaging. Multiple septations or loculations within the mass are best seen on T2-weighted images. The vastus medialis muscle is displaced medially; therefore, this lesion lies deep within the medial compartment of the thigh.

The cystic nature of this mass, the absence of surrounding edema, and the absence of bone or soft tissue infiltration suggest a nonneoplastic etiology. The signal intensity is inconsistent with hemorrhage. The location and size are inconsistent with a sebaceous cyst. Other cystic masses of the thigh or soft tissues include hygroma, abscess, seroma, and lymphocele. Hygromas presenting in later life and having such massive size would be unusual. An abscess should be associated with fever, pain, tenderness, and more muscular or soft tissue edema that is hyperintense on T2-weighted imaging. Abscesses are not usually so homogeneous. With the patient's history of trauma, the differential diagnosis is narrowed to seroma and lymphocele.

Lymphoceles often occur in the abdomen or pelvis, particularly after ureteric or abdominal surgery, since lymphatics are numerous in these areas. Therefore, seroma is the most likely diagnosis. The signal of seroma is identical to that of cysts, hygromas, and urinomas.

DIAGNOSIS: The patient has a seroma.

CASE 88

Differential Diagnosis of Masses and Tumorlike Lesions of and about the Knee

HISTORY: A 47-year-old man presented with anteromedial pain in the posteromedial calf 16.0 cm below the knee, of 2 years' duration. What is the MRI diagnosis? For comparison, images from a second patient are shown. Is the lesion recent or old? (Fig. 88-1: sagittal proton-density (*A,C*) and T2-weighted (*B,D*) images. Fig. 88-2: axial proton-density (*A,C*) and T2-weighted (*B,D*) images. Fig. 88-3: AP radiograph. Fig. 88-4: lateral radiograph. The remaining images pertain to patient 2. Fig. 88-5: sagittal proton-density, and Fig. 88-6: T2-weighted images.)

A B C D

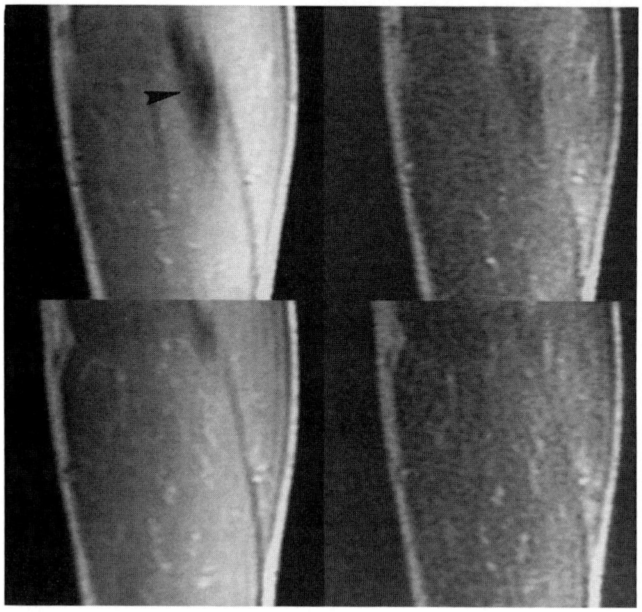

FIGURE 88-1

A B C D

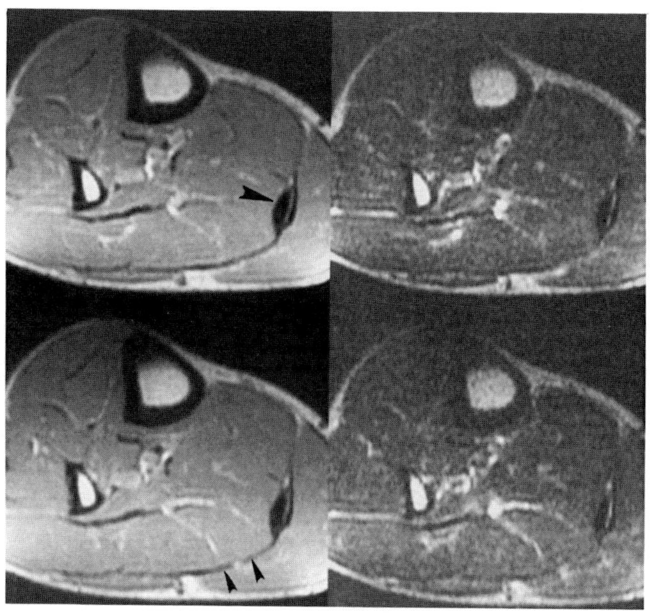

FIGURE 88-2

DIAGNOSIS: The patient has a low-grade cystic chondrosarcoma.

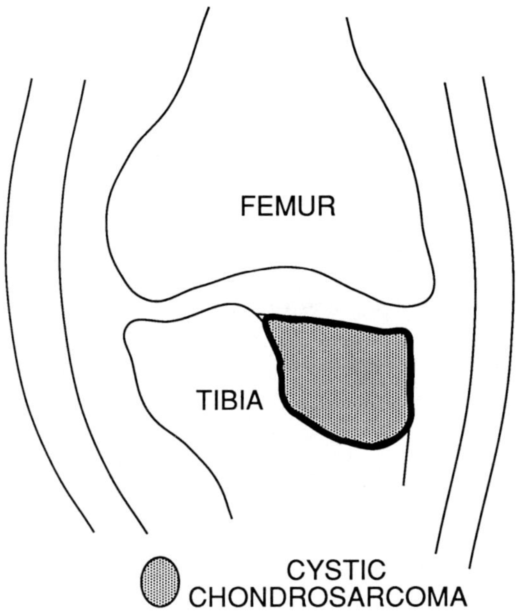

FIGURE 91-4

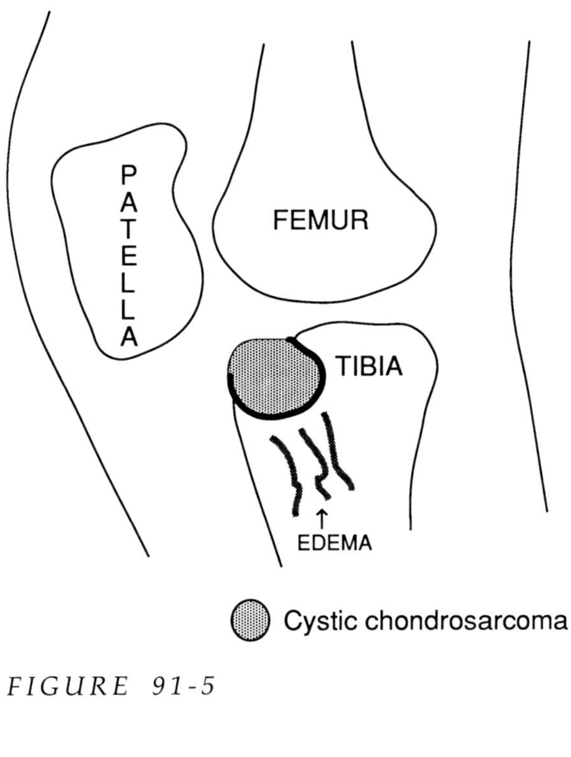

FIGURE 91-5

CASE 92

Differential Diagnosis of Masses and Tumorlike Lesions of and about the Knee

HISTORY: An 11-year-old girl presented with difficulty ambulating and severe tenderness of the anterior calf 48 hours after sustaining an injury in a soccer game. She described tingling and numbness in the dorsolateral distal extremity. (Fig. 92-1: axial multiecho proton-density (*A*) and T2-weighted (*B*) MR images, TR/TE 2,000/20, 80 msec.)

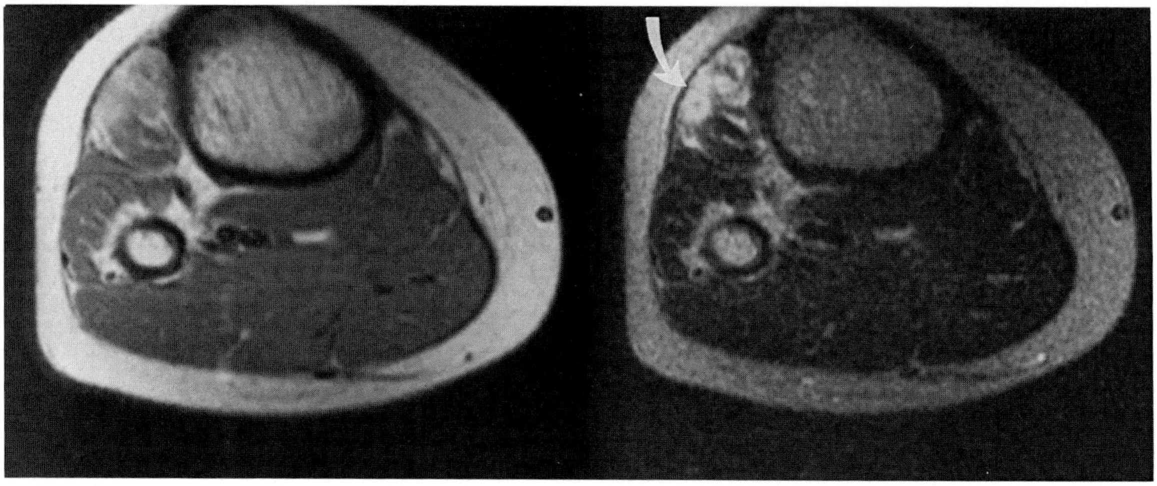

FIGURE 92-1

DISCUSSION: Foci of increased signal intensity on the axial projections (curved white arrow in *B*) are seen in the anterior compartment muscles (tibialis anterior and extensor hallucis longus). The injury is recent (48 hours old).

The swelling is due to hematoma formation. At 48 hours, a hematoma in the brain would be hypointense on T2-weighted images owing to the T2 shortening effect of the deoxyhemoglobin and methemoglobin in intact red cells. In the body, preferential T2 susceptibility effects are inconsistent, even at high field strengths. Although they may exist, they are more difficult to detect and may not be seen at all. This may relate to the diffusion of red cells into the adjacent soft tissues and the onset of rapid hemolysis that often follows direct soft tissue trauma. Such rapid diffusion and abrupt red cell injury may not occur in the protected intracranial fossa. Therefore, low or intermediate signal intensity on T1 weighting and hyperintense signal on T2 weighting should not sway one from the diagnosis of acute hematoma formation. The fact that this process is confined to one major muscle group would not support a neoplastic etiology.

DIAGNOSIS: The patient has an acute hematoma of the tibialis anterior muscle and compartment syndrome.

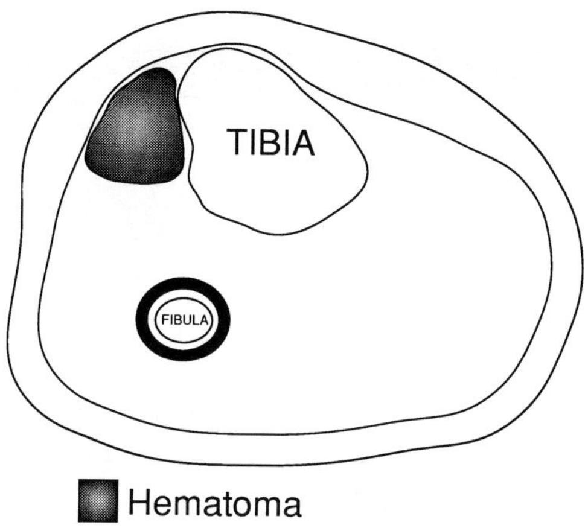

FIGURE 92-2

CASE 93

Differential Diagnosis of Bone Neoplasm

HISTORY: Two patients with knee pain underwent radiologic evaluation. The findings are pathognomonic. What are the diagnoses? (Patient 1—Fig. 93-1: conventional lateral radiography. Fig. 93-2: sagittal T1-weighted, Fig. 93-3: proton-density (*A*) and T2-weighted (*B*), and Fig. 93-4: magnified sagittal T2-weighted images. Patient 2—Fig. 93-5: conventional lateral radiograph. Fig. 93-6: sagittal multiecho proton-density (*A*) and T2-weighted (*B*) images.)

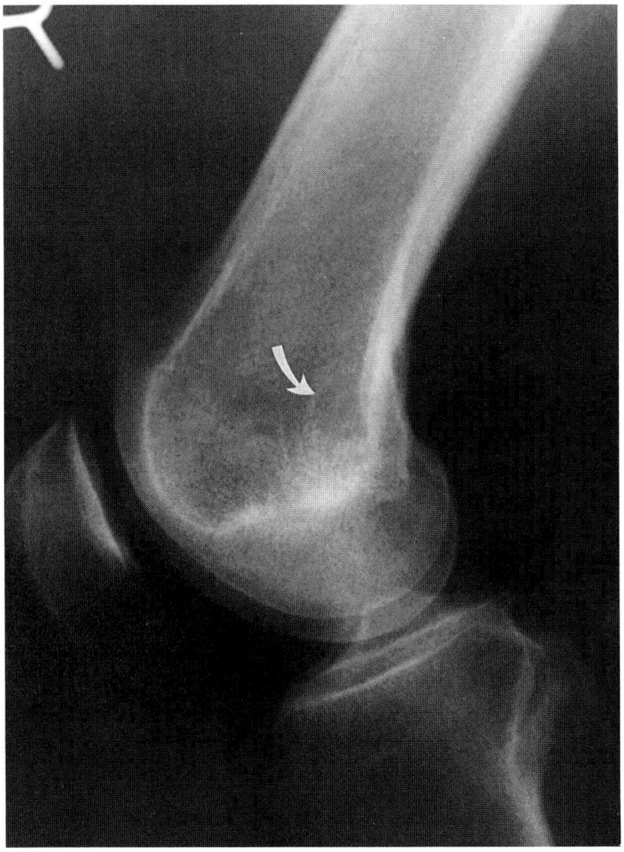

FIGURE 93-1

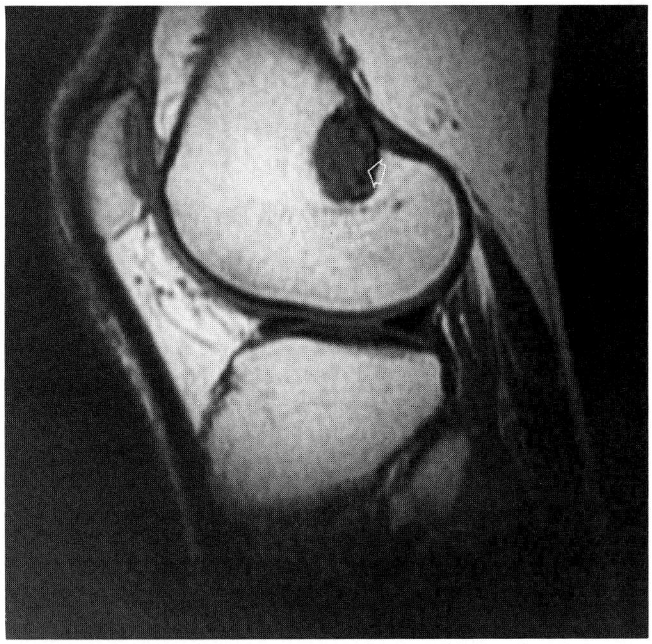

FIGURE 93-2

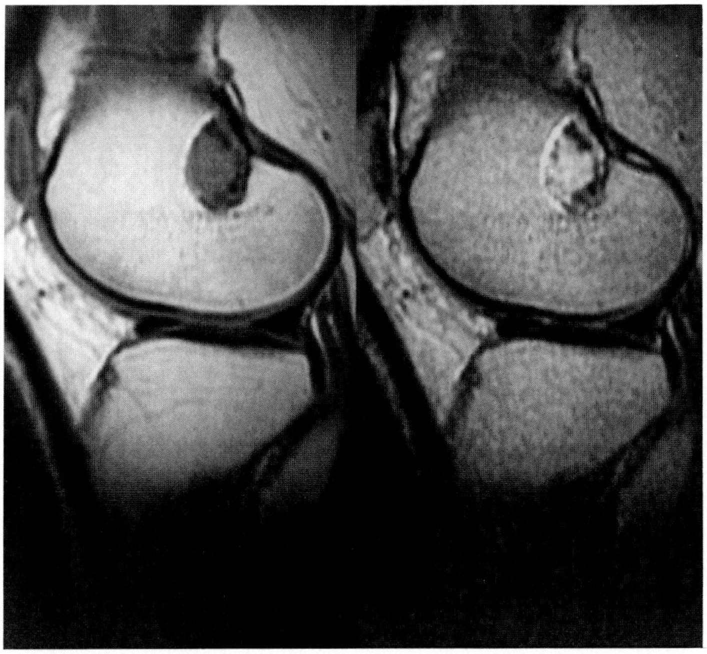

FIGURE 93-3

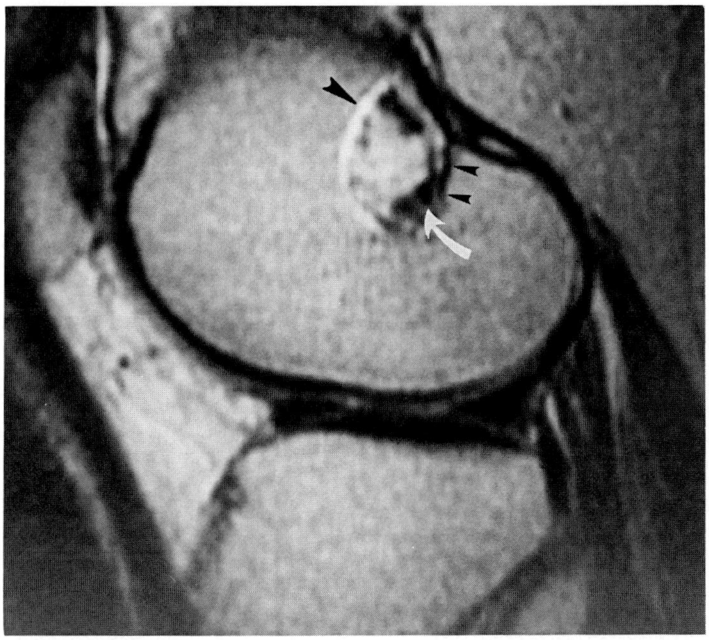

FIGURE 93-4

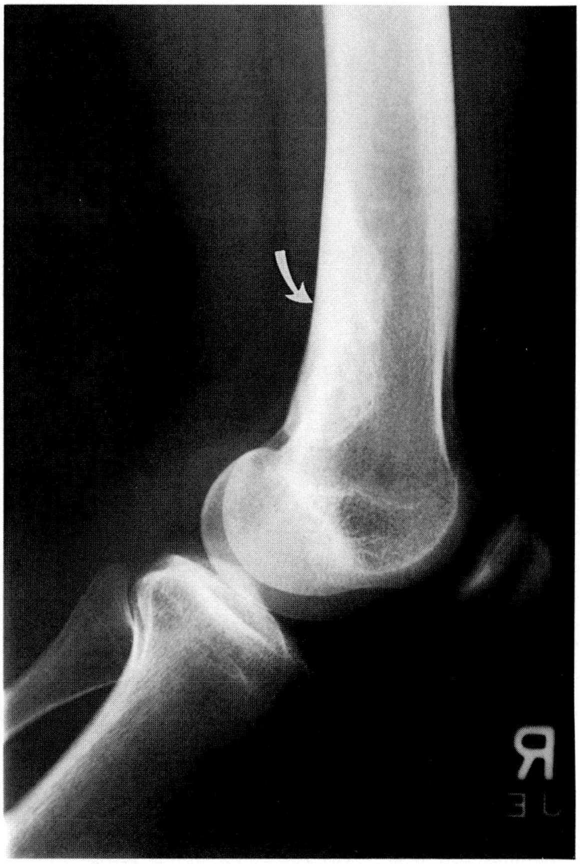

FIGURE 93-5

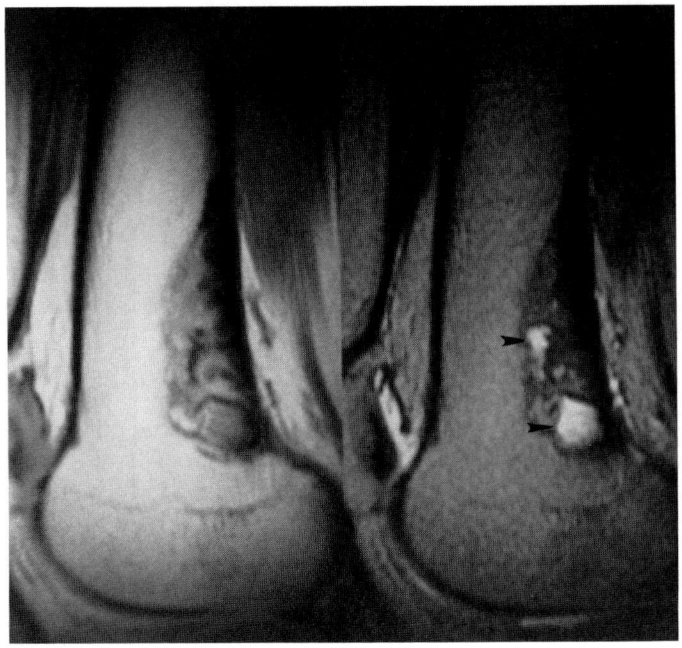

FIGURE 93-6

DISCUSSION: The lesion in patient 1 is well circumscribed, hypointense on T1 weighting, and hyperintense on T2 weighting, with its margin remaining hypointense. On the lateral radiograph the lesion is barely visible, with faint marginal sclerosis (curved arrow in Fig. 93-1). On MRI it exhibits no perilesional edema, and there is no evidence of soft tissue mass or periosteal signal change. A posteromedial femoral location and the findings just described are typical of fibrous metaphyseal cortical defect. The central cystic component of this lesion is hypointense on T1-weighted imaging and hyperintense on T2-weighted imaging. A hypointense fibrous rim (white arrow in Fig. 93-4) is common to fibrous medullary defects. This rim may be demonstrable on T1-weighted images (open arrow in Fig. 93-2). Since a water-containing lesion lies within and is surrounded by medullary fat, a chemical shift or pixel shift artifact results in a black interface (paired arrowheads in Fig. 93-4) and a white interface (large arrowhead in Fig. 93-4).

There are several MRI appearances to this lesion. The early cystic type consists of hypointense signal on T1 weighting, hyperintense signal on T2 weighting, with a hypointense well-marginated rim around the lesion periphery. The xanthomatous type consists of hyperintense signal on both T1- and T2-weighted images. Both of these subtypes result in lytic lesions on conventional radiography. Types 3 and 4 present with lesion sclerosis on conventional radiography. These are the healed type and the mixed type. The healed type results in hypointense signal on all pulse sequences, most pronounced on T2-weighted images. The mixed type consists of partial healing with mixed areas of cyst formation or hyperintense signal and occasional xanthomatous elements on T1-weighted imaging. With this lesion we have conventional radiographic sclerosis and mixed signal intensity with hypointense T1 and hyperintense T2 cystic areas. The fifth subtype we have observed consists of a heavily fibrous lesion with little in the way of xanthomatous (bright T1) or water-containing (bright T2) elements. Histologically, we have called this the fibrous type, owing to its histology and hypointense signal on both T1- and T2-weighted images in the face of a lytic lesion, not a sclerotic lesion on conventional radiology.

A critical criterion for nonossifying fibroma is the absence of hypointense T1 or hyperintense T2 edema around the lesion. A spectrum of fibrous bone defects exist. Normally, a small circular area of rarefaction exists in the metaphyseal cortex of children's long bones that disappears spontaneously. When the lesion is seen as a small hypointense or lytic area less than 2 cm in diameter, it is considered a fibrous cortical defect. Some have used the term *fibrous endosteal defect* to describe the lesion that has attained 2.0 to 4.0 cm in size. A size of 4.0 or more is considered a fibrous medullary defect or nonossifying fibroma. It is believed to be the sequela of a fibrous cortical defect that has persisted, grown, and drifted into the diametaphysis. Approximately 70% of these lesions occur between 10 and 15 years of age. The lesions are often clinically solid, and contrast enhancement on MRI is faint to nonexistent at the lesion periphery, without evidence of central enhancement.

In patient 2, an eccentric, well-marginated lesion in the posteromedial femur contains cystic areas that are hypointense on T1 weighting and hyperintense on T2 weighting (arrowheads in Fig. 93-6*B*). The radiograph shows an area of sclerosis (curved arrow in Fig. 96-5) corresponding to the healed mixed type of nonossifying fibroma.

DIAGNOSIS: Patient 1 has a nonossifying fibroma or fibrous medullary defect of the cystic type. Patient 2 has a nonossifying fibroma of the mixed type.

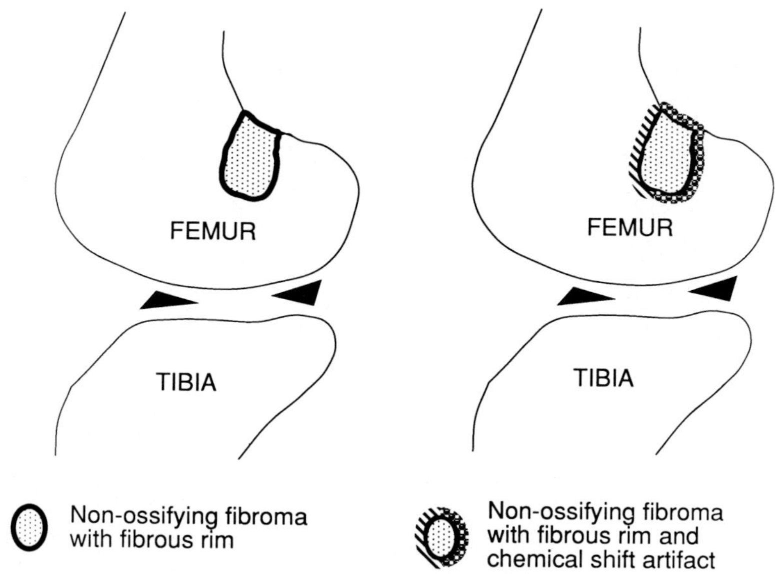

FIGURE 93-7

CASE 94

Differential Diagnosis of Masses and Tumorlike Lesions of and about the Knee

HISTORY: An 8-year-old child with knee pain of 3 weeks' duration and known prior septic arthritis, diagnosed 6 months earlier, underwent radiologic evaluation. What is the MRI diagnosis? (Fig. 94-1: conventional anteroposterior radiograph. Figs. 94-2 and 94-3: coronal T1-weighted MR images, TR/TE 600/20 msec, 20-cm FOV, 5.0-mm sections, 1 excitation, 128 × 256 pixel matrix.)

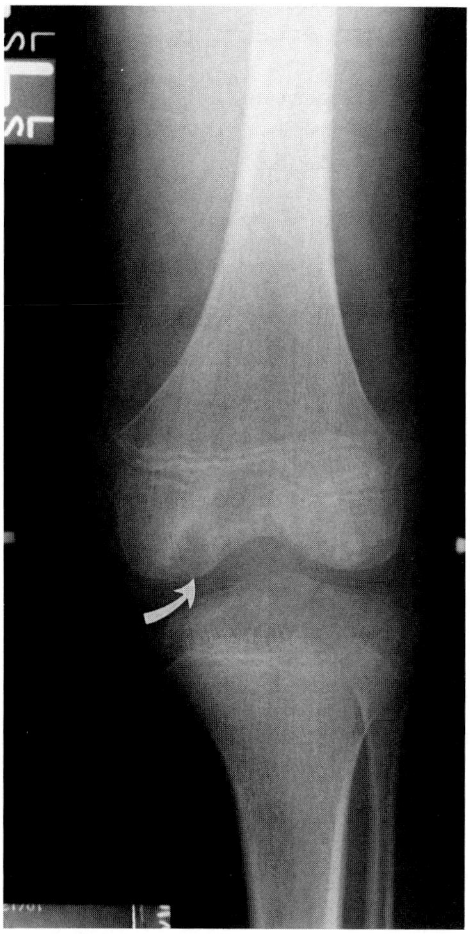

FIGURE 94-1

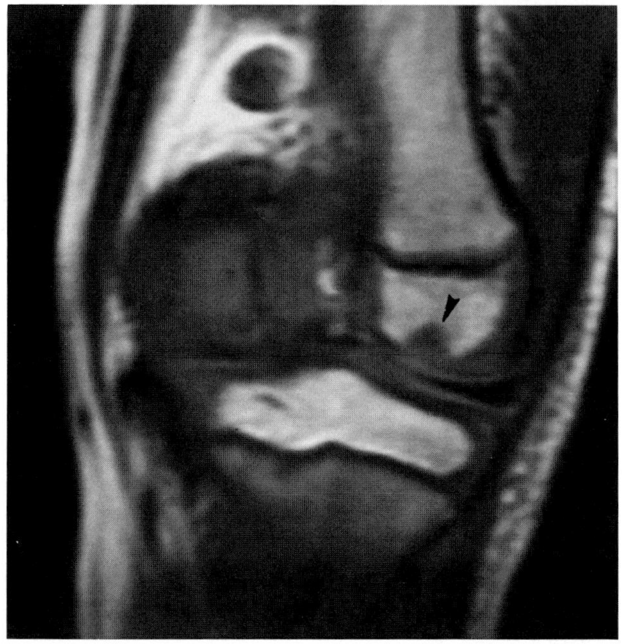

FIGURE 94-2

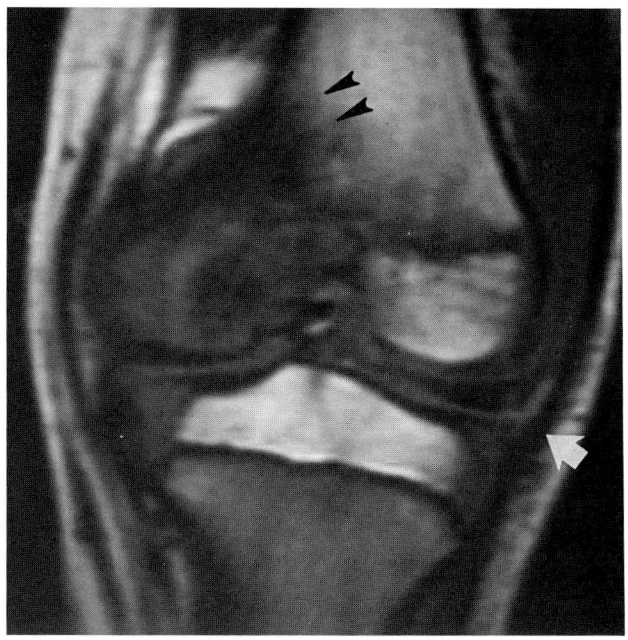

FIGURE 94-3

DISCUSSION: The AP radiograph shows areas of bone lucency (curved arrow in Fig. 94-1) and irregularity, particularly along the medial subarticular femoral condyle. The normal marrow signal in an 8-year-old child should be relatively bright on T1-weighted imaging.

At birth the marrow is normally isointense or gray, due to the domination of red over yellow marrow. Immediately after birth, yellow marrow begins to appear in the terminal phalanges and progresses centrally. The epiphyses and apophyses are often hyperintense with yellow marrow very early in life. Poorly defined metaphyseal and epiphyseal foci of decreased signal intensity are noted in the femur and tibia medially. On the lateral side, demarcated by the hypointense iliotibial band (arrow in Fig. 94-1) a smaller area of subarticular signal hypointensity is present (arrowhead in Fig. 94-2). This is an extremely rare example of septic arthritis with secondary osteomyelitis.

The signal hypointensity of medullary bone on T1-weighted images is related to bone edema. This edema is often pronounced and extensive. Unlike a condition that may simulate osteomyelitis on bone scintigraphy, transient osteoporosis or reflex sympathetic dystrophy has a more subtle but extensive hypointensity. Signal alteration or isointensity in the normally hypointense bone cortex supports an aggressive process. The areas of low signal intensity in the medial femoral condyle involve the epiphysis and cross over the epiphyseal plate to the metaphysis (paired arrowheads in Fig. 94-3).

No extremity MRI examination should be interpreted without the benefit of conventional radiographs.

DIAGNOSIS: The patient has osteomyelitis of the femur, arising from prior septic arthritis.

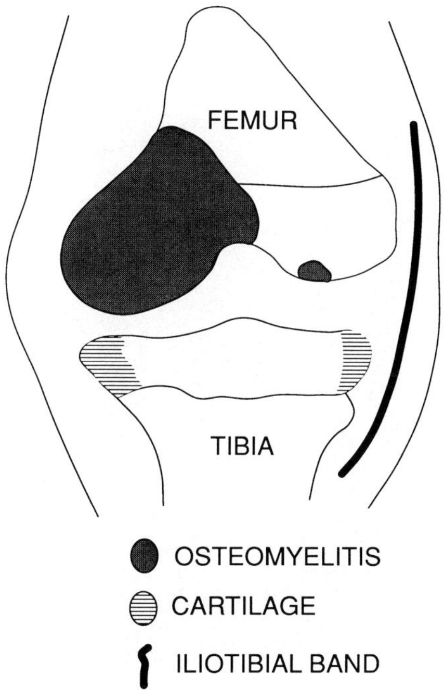

FIGURE 94-4

CASE 95

Differential Diagnosis of Masses and Tumorlike Lesions of and about the Knee

HISTORY: Two children, aged 9 and 12 years, with severe anterior knee pain underwent radiologic evaluation. What is the differential diagnosis in each case? (Patient 1—Figs. 95-1 and 95-2: lateral and anteroposterior plain radiographs. Fig. 95-3: sagittal multiformat contiguous T1-weighted images. Fig. 95-4: axial proton-density (*A*) and T2-weighted (*B*) images. Patient 2—Fig. 95-5: anteroposterior radiograph. Fig. 95-6: axial T1-weighted MR image. Fig. 95-7: sagittal multiformat adjacent T1-weighted images.)

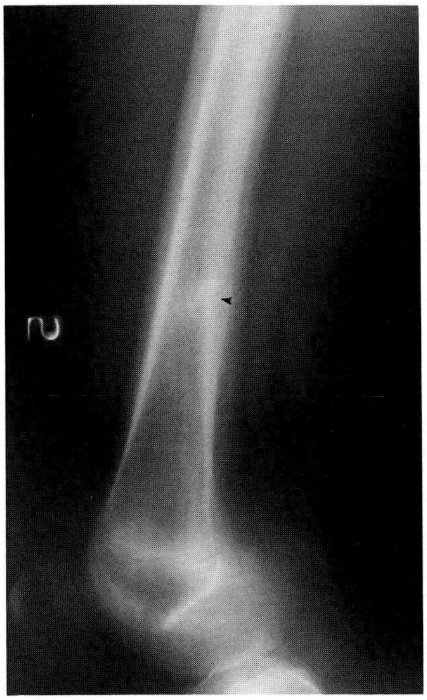

FIGURE 95-1

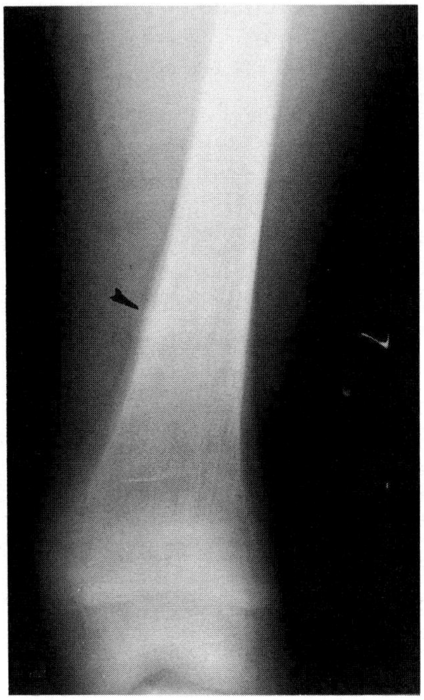

FIGURE 95-2

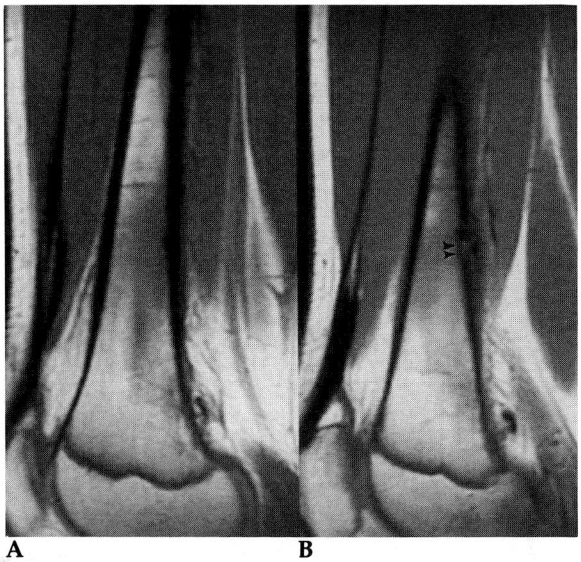

A B

FIGURE 95-3

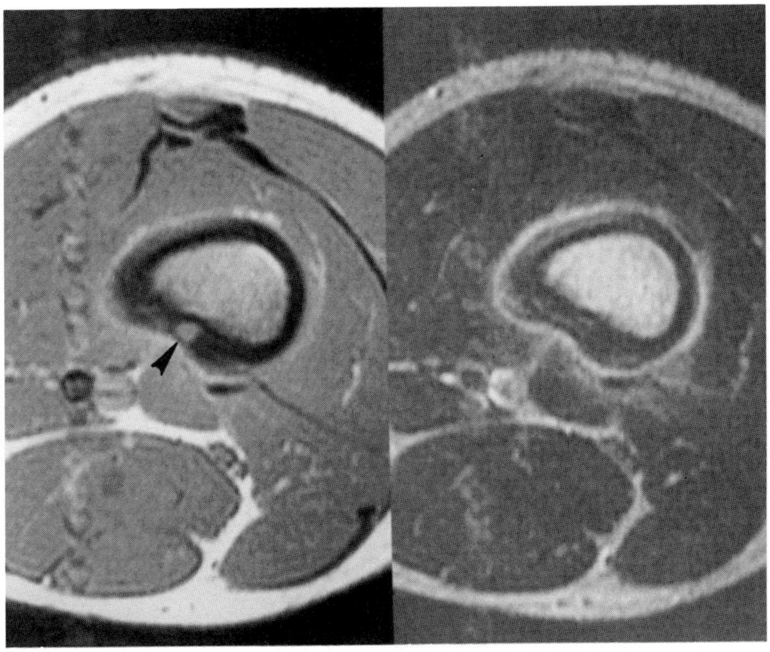

A B
FIGURE 95-4

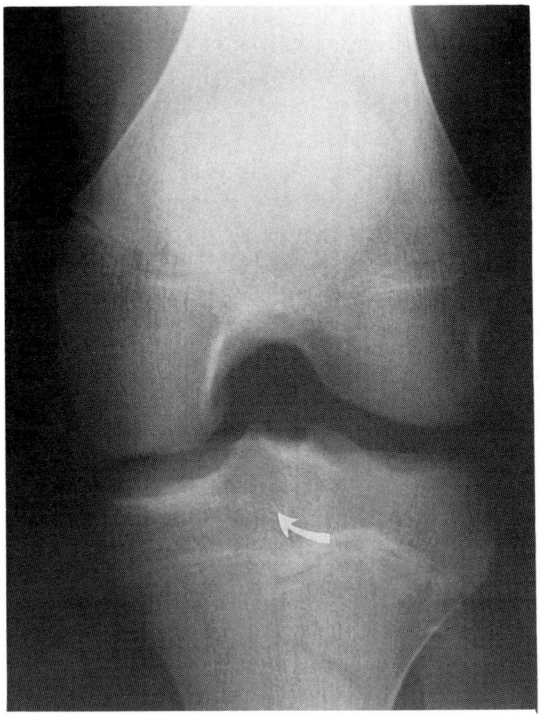

FIGURE 95-5

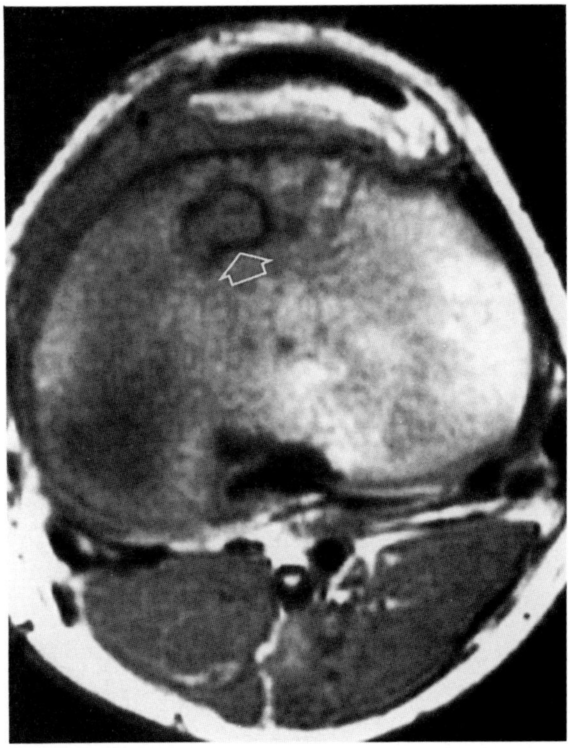

FIGURE 95-6

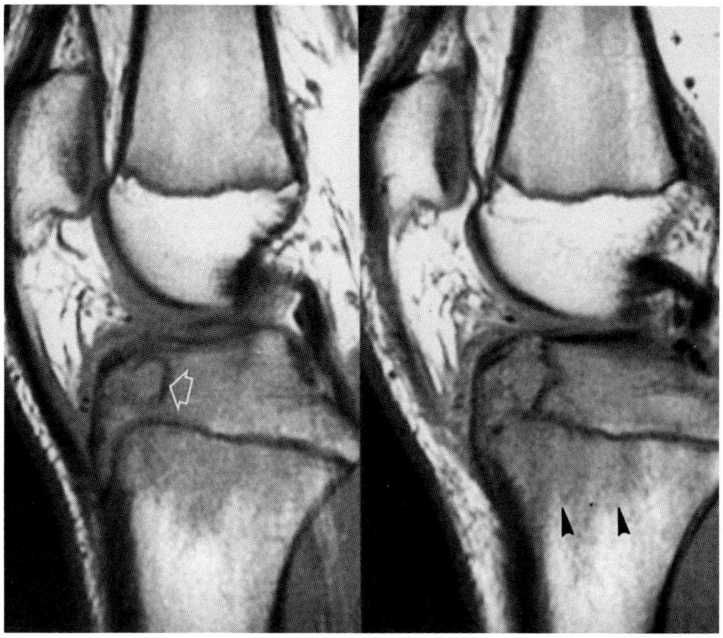

A B

FIGURE 95-7

DISCUSSION: The conventional radiographs in patient 1 show an intracortical focal tibial lucency that is best seen on the lateral view (arrowhead in Fig. 95-1); the surrounding bone and periosteal reaction is appreciated on the frontal view (arrowhead in Fig. 95-2). The lesion nidus is visible on the axial MR images as a round area of intermediate signal intensity (arrowhead in Fig. 95-4*A*), and on the sagittal view (paired arrowheads in Fig. 95-3*B*). Cortical thickening or reaction is demonstrated on MRI as a widened black or hypointense band, best evaluated on sagittal projections.

The differential diagnosis is limited because of the patient's young age, the clinical history of pain, and the lesion's intracortical location. Osteoid osteoma is the only reasonable diagnosis, with Brodie's abscess and cortical metastasis statistically unlikely.

Osteoid osteomas on MR have presented with two basic signal intensity patterns:

1. Intermediate to slightly hyperintense signal on T1 weighting that becomes quite hyperintense on T2-weighted images and is surrounded by a black rim. This type has the appearance of a target.
2. Intermediate T1 signal with intermediate T2 signal that is only faintly visible on T2 weighting. A surrounding black rim may be present in this type and may be so thick as to obliterate the central gray nidus.

The variable appearance of the lesion center may relate to the degree of calcification present. More mature lesions show more extensive calcification. The hypointense edema present in osteoid osteoma is variable but may be so extensive, severe, and irregular that malignancy is simulated.

In patient 2, sclerosis of the distal femur on the conventional radiograph obscures a subcortical lucency (curved white arrow in Fig. 95-5). On MRI irregular areas of T1 signal hypointensity are extensive and represent edema (arrowheads in Fig. 95-7*B*). The axial and sagittal projections reveal a round area of hypointense signal (open arrows in Figs. 95-6, 95-7*A*) with a hypointense rim. The differential diagnosis includes osteoid osteoma, osteomyelitis, osteogenic sarcoma, metastasis and intraosseus ganglion.

Location at a bone end is unusual in osteogenic sarcoma; however, the degree of edema is disturbing. Brodie's abscess or cystic foci of osteomyelitis are not common at bone ends except in certain fungal osteomyelitic processes like coccidioidomycosis. This patient is not from the southwestern United States. Intraosseous ganglion is a cystic lesion at the bone ends that does not communicate with the joint space and is more hypointense on T1 weighting and hyperintense on T2 weighting than the lesions shown here. It should not be associated with such extensive edema. Metastatic disease is impossible to exclude; however, the patient's age, the lack of a primary neoplasm, and the location at a bone end make this diagnosis unlikely. The "nidus" appearance of this lesion axially suggests the correct diagnosis of osteoid osteoma.

Osteoid osteoma is a benign neoplasm occurring before age 25. It has a 2:1 male–female predilection. Over 50% occur in the femur or tibia. Lesions in the spine usually involve the neural arch. Giant osteoid osteomas (osteoblastomas) are over 2.0 cm in size and are less painful, enabling them to reach large volumes without detection. Intramedullary, intracortical, and subperiosteal locations may occur with intramedullary lesions producing nominal edema or bone reaction. Lesions of the hip deep to the capsule in particular produce almost no bone reaction (T1 hypointensity) and are frequently calcified and hypo- or isointense on T1- and T2-weighted imaging.

DIAGNOSIS: Both patients have osteoid osteomas.

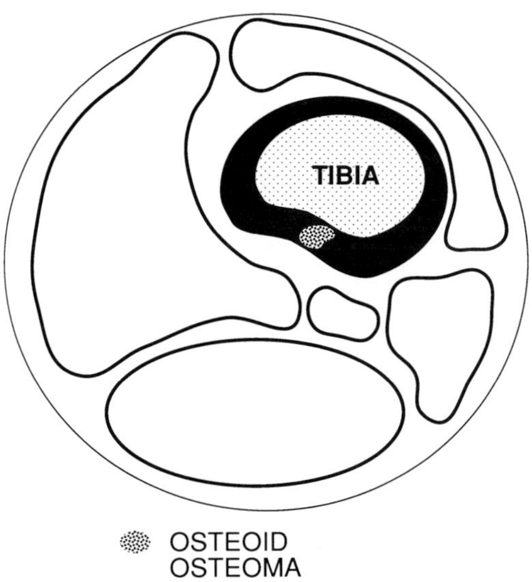

FIGURE 95-8

CASE 96

Differential Diagnosis of Masses and Tumorlike Lesions of and about the Knee

HISTORY: A 16-year-old girl was evaluated for posterior knee pain exacerbated by high school soccer games. Is the process benign or malignant? (Fig. 96-1: conventional lateral radiograph. Fig. 96-2: axial multiformat (two-on-one) T1-weighted images.)

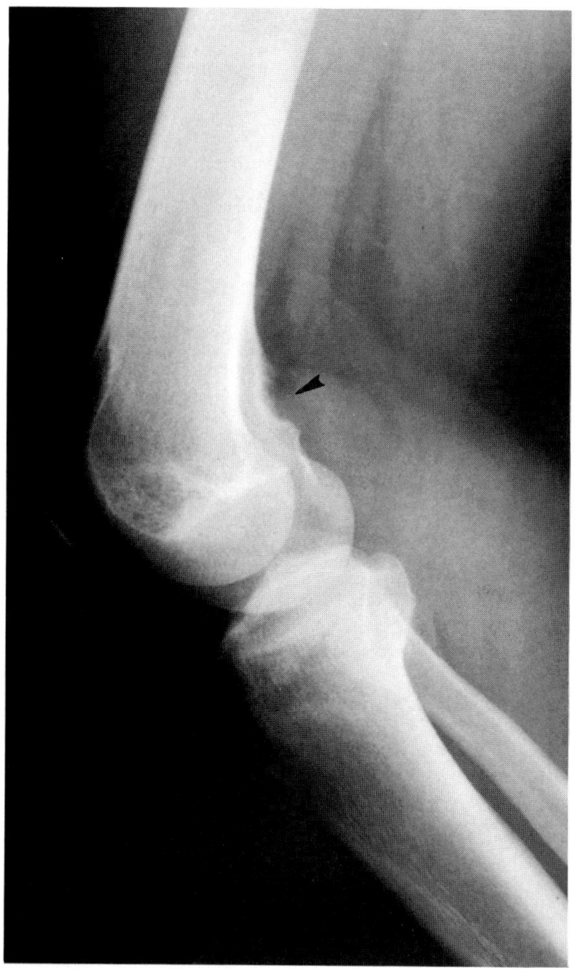

FIGURE 96-1

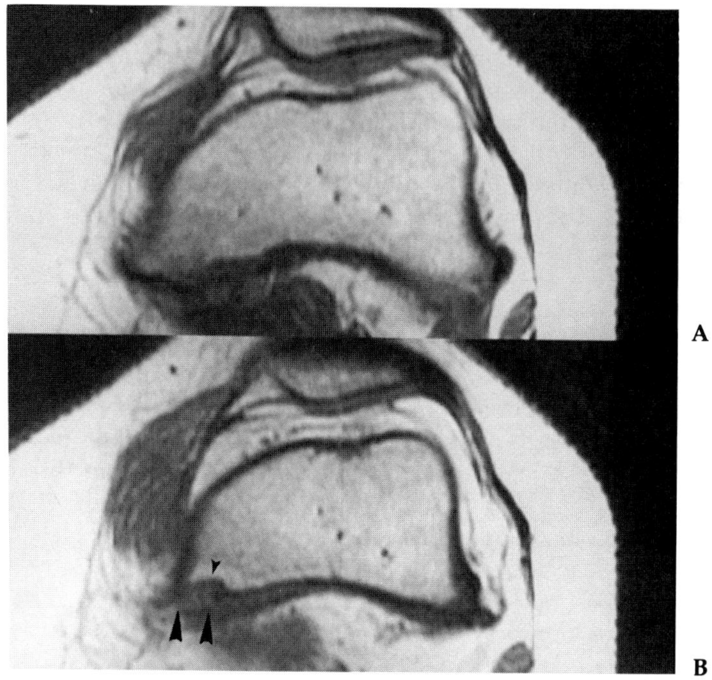

FIGURE 96-2

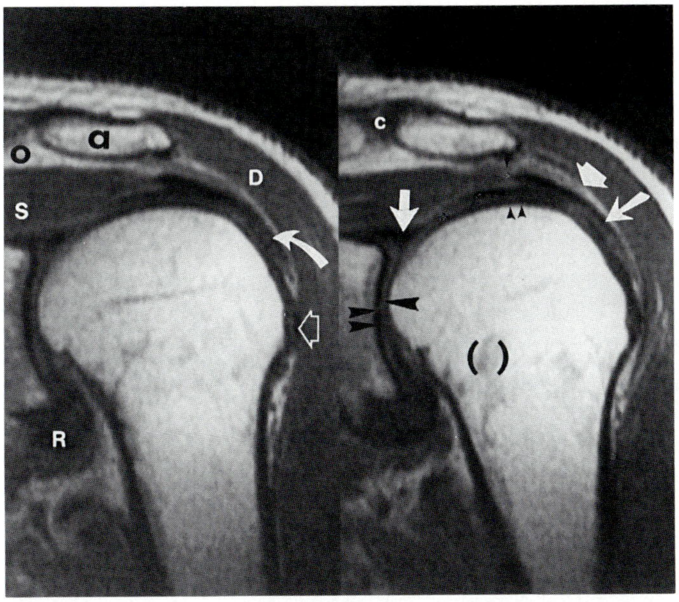

A B

FIGURE 1-2

DISCUSSION: No normal supraspinatous muscle is visualized on any of these sections. Severely atrophic and irregularly atrophied muscle fibers (single arrowhead in Fig. 1-2*B*) occupy the subacromial space. No anatomic linear hypointense rotator cuff is visualized. Instead, relatively homogeneous foci of intermediate signal intensity obliterate the subacromial fat interface and extend laterally into the subdeltoid fat space. T2-weighted images are not required with such dramatic findings as these, documenting complete musculotendinous cuff interruption and retraction. That this is a late phase of impingement is implied by the fact that the humerus lies directly underneath the clavicle. Narrowing of the acromiohumeral distance is considered a late finding of impingement. Other manifestations and presentations of musculotendinous cuff atrophy are presented in case 13.

Figure 1-2: c, acromioclavicular joint/capsule; a, acromion; o, subacromial fat; D, deltoid muscle, short white arrow, deltoid fat line; s, supraspinatus muscle; oblique white arrow, supraspinatus tendon; curved white arrow (*A*), conjoined (infra- and supraspinatus) tendon; open arrow (*A*), teres minor superior insertion; R, axillary recess; single black arrowhead (*B*), glenoid cartilaginous labrum/interface; paired black arrowheads (*B*), glenoid cortical bone; three horizontal white dashes (*B*), suprahumeral capsular interface (capsular reflection); single horizontal white dash (*B*), suprahumeral hyaline cartilage; parentheses enclose islands of red marrow.

DIAGNOSIS: The images show grade 3 impingement syndrome with complete rotator cuff transection and musculotendinous retraction and atrophy.

CASE 2

Differential Diagnosis of Acute Shoulder Pain

HISTORY: A 43-year-old man fell with an outstretched arm. The following day he noted pain on movement and inability to abduct or externally rotate the right shoulder. What is the MRI diagnosis? (Fig. 2-1: coronal multiformat, multiecho contiguous proton-density (*A,B*) and T2-weighted (*C,D*) images.)

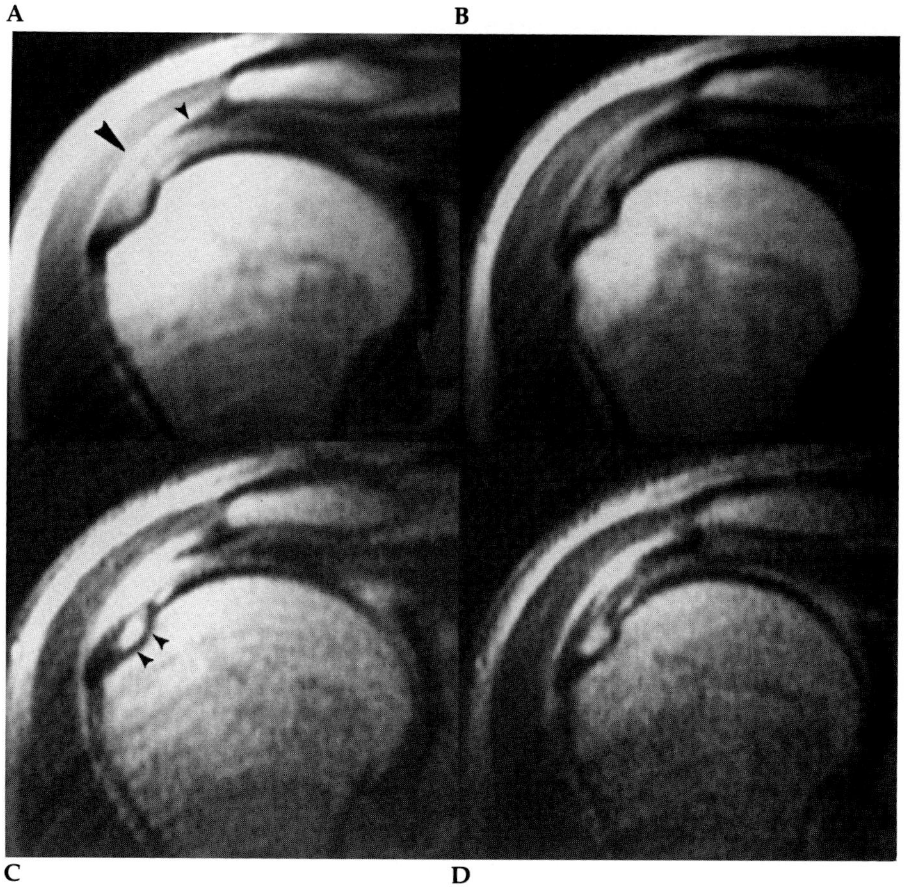

FIGURE 2-1

DISCUSSION: The coronal T1-weighted image is used to detect anatomic abnormalities and confirm rotator cuff contiguity. Most sequences include sagittal and coronal oblique T1-weighted images oriented parallel and perpendicular to the supraspinatus muscle (see Fig. 2-2). Superior image quality is afforded by the inherently superior signal-to-noise ratio (S/N) characteristics of single-echo imaging. Fields of view of 16 to 18 cm are employed, with a section thickness of 5 mm and a 192 by 256 pixel matrix. Multiecho coronal oblique proton-density and T2-weighted images are routinely employed, and T1-weighted, proton-density, and T2-weighted images are compared at each anatomic location to distinguish signal changes from fat, fluid, and blood. The field of view may have to be increased by 2.0 cm in some instances, and the matrix should be altered to 128 × 256. Section thickness should remain at 5.0 mm with a 1-mm gap. To reduce motion-related and coherent noise artifacts, two techniques should be used:

1. Position the surface coil superolaterally rather than directly anterior to the humeral head.
2. Use craniocaudal and mediolateral saturation pulses.

The T2-weighted images show discontiguity of the hypointense cuff, which is replaced by increased signal intensity in the critical zone distribution (paired arrowheads in *A*). The critical zone is defined as the avascular area, approximately 1.0 to 2.0 cm adjacent to the distal cuff insertion, that is prone to rupture. The proton-density image confirms that signal intensity in the area of anatomic cuff discontiguity on T2-weighted images is replaced by fluidlike signal that extends into the adjacent subdeltoid bursa (large arrowhead in *B*) and thickens the bursa on T2-weighted imaging. The small arrowhead in *B* identifies the proximal margin of the acromiohumeral ligament, not the proximal rotator cuff tendon.

DIAGNOSIS: The patient has a full-thickness rotator cuff tendon tear in the critical zone.

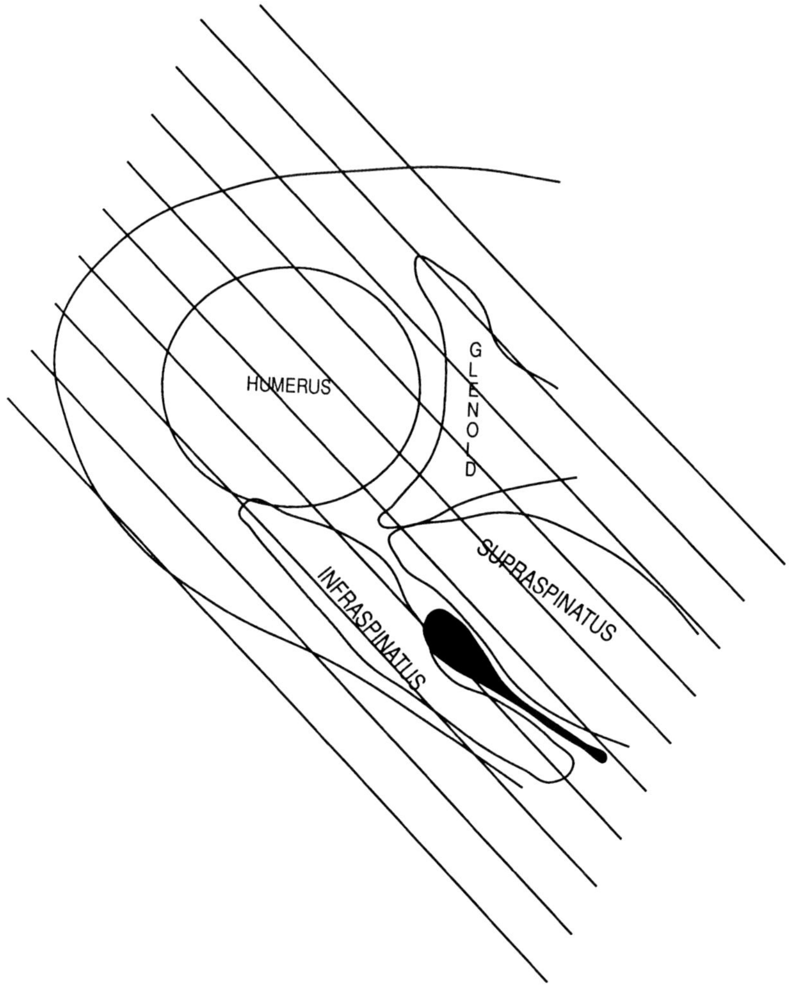

FIGURE 2-2

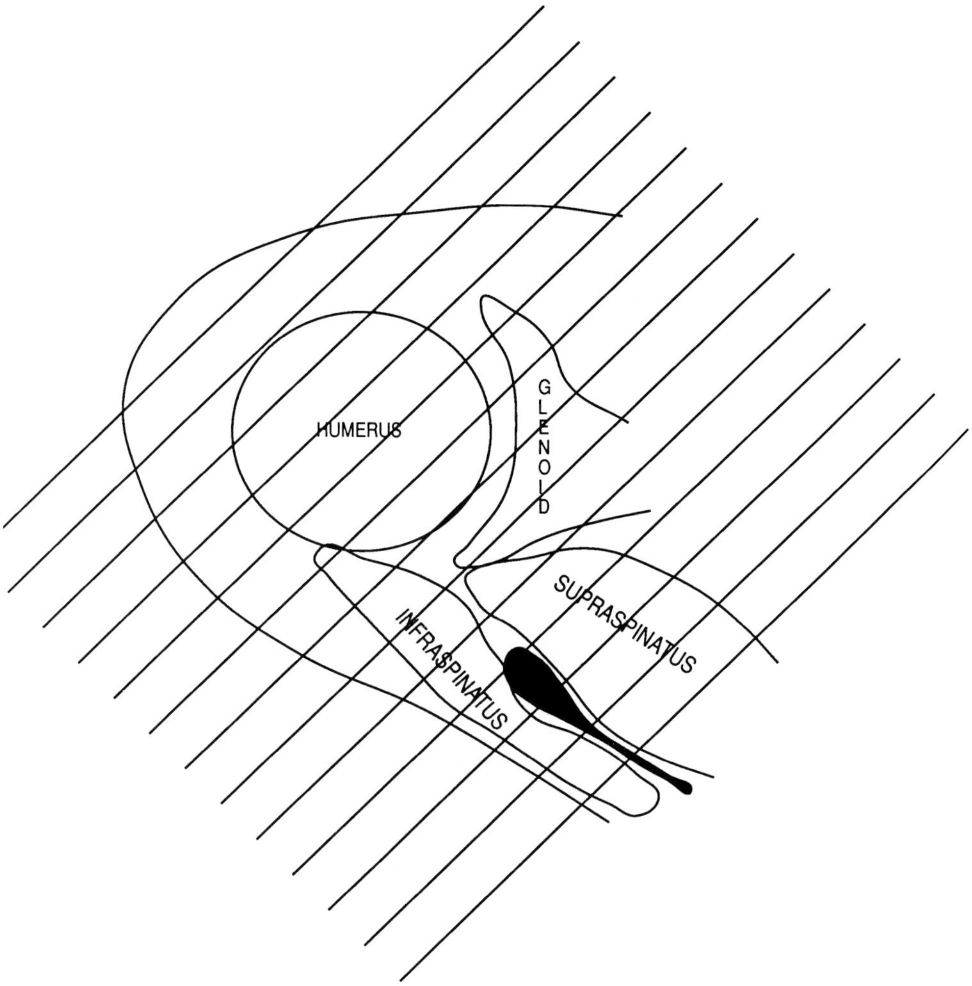

FIGURE 2-3

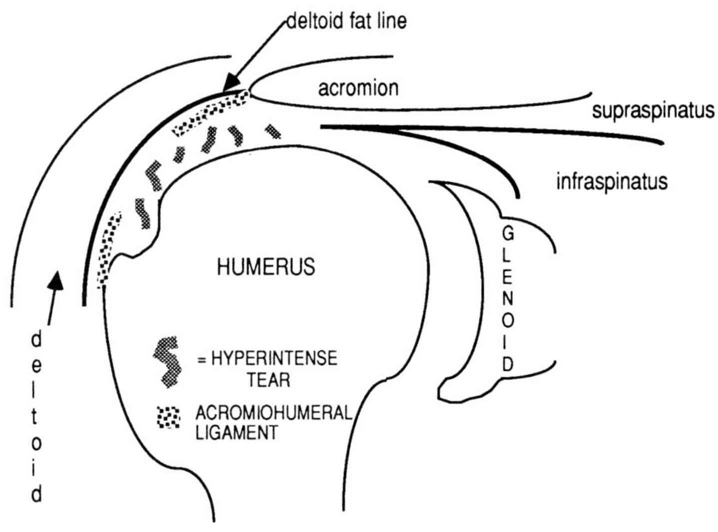

FIGURE 2-4

CASE 3

Differential Diagnosis of Chronic Shoulder Pain

HISTORY: A 44-year-old man presented with inability to abduct his arm more than 15° away from his body. What is the MRI diagnosis? (Fig. 3-1: coronal multiecho proton-density (*A*) and T2-weighted images of the left shoulder.)

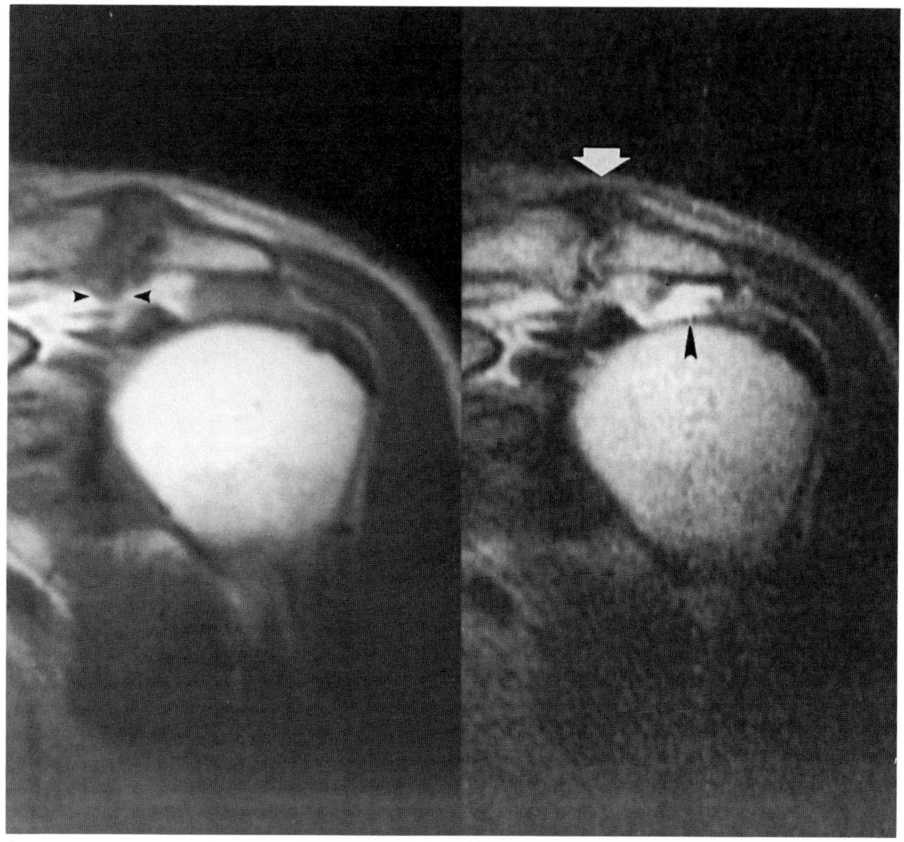

A **B**

FIGURE 3-1

DISCUSSION: Exuberant intermediate signal intensity pannus formation (white arrow in *B*) and eburnation affect both the acromion and the clavicular side of the joint space. Cortical and medullary bone spur formation (small arrowheads in *A*) extend caudally to efface the subacromial fat. The musculotendinous anatomy is difficult to identify. No tendon is visualized, and only a hypointense mass on the T2-weighted image is appreciated superomedial to the humeral head and directly beneath the acromioclavicular joint. This mass represents the retracted, curled-up tendon. Structures not seen on these images but also hypointense and located in this region are the superior labrum (triangular in shape), and the origin of the long head of the biceps from the glenoid superior tubercle. Distal to this region is an area of intermediate signal intensity on proton-density images and high signal intensity on T2-weighted imaging, representing fluid where the tendon should have been (arrowhead in *B*). These findings are compatible with a grade III impingement syndrome, which consists of the following criteria on MRI: (1) a mass effect on the subacromial arch arising from the acromioclavicular joint, due to bony spur, pannus formation, granulation tissue, bone malalignment, subluxation, fracture, or cyst formation; (2) retraction or absence of the musculotendinous anatomy and rotator cuff complexes; and (3) replacement of the normal hypointense cuff signal by confluent signal hyperintensity on T2-weighted imaging.

DIAGNOSIS: The patient has a grade 3 impingement syndrome with complete rotator cuff interruption.

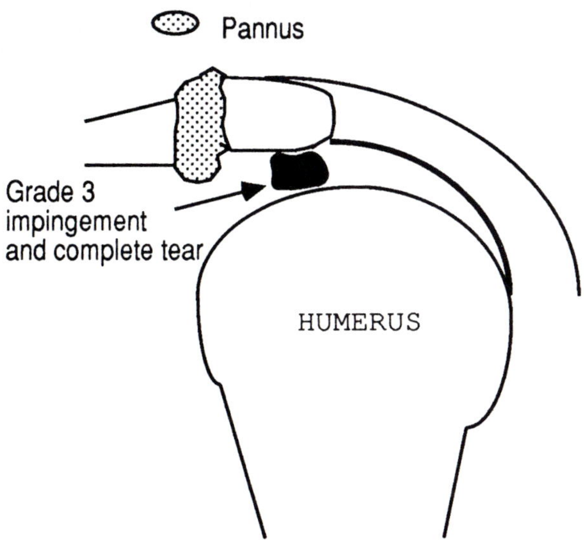

FIGURE 3-2

CASE 4

Differential Diagnosis of Acute Shoulder Pain

HISTORY: A 54-year-old man reported shoulder pain and complete loss of abduction capability. What is the MRI diagnosis? (Fig. 4-1: coronal multiecho proton-density (*A*) and T2-weighted (*B*) MR images of the left shoulder.)

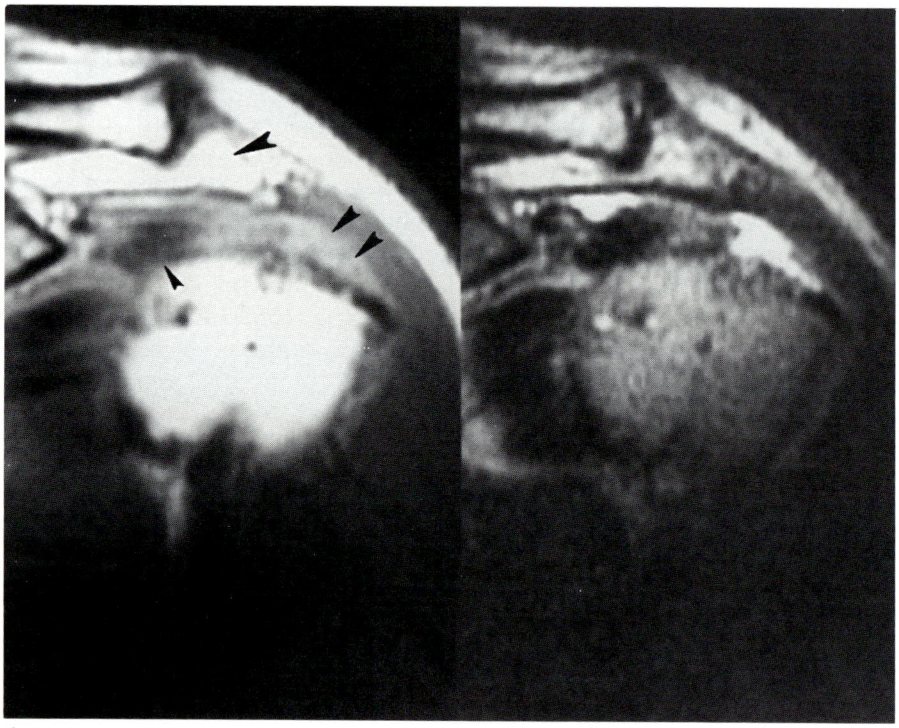

A **B**

FIGURE 4-1

DISCUSSION: As in case 3, a hypointense mass (small arrowhead in *A*) identifies the proximal supraspinatus portion of the rotator cuff. The superior glenoid labrum has been volume averaged with the cuff. The infraspinatus portion has a more posterior and lateral orientation relative to the humeral head, while the teres minor has an extreme lateral and inferior humeral attachment (see Fig. 4-2). All three attach to the greater tuberosity promontory. The subscapularis tendon crosses anterior to the humerus and inserts on the lesser tuberosity. An area of intermediate signal intensity on the proton-density image and hyperintensity on the T2-weighted image (paired arrowheads in *A*) is located where the normal critical zone attachment of the rotator cuff should be. In contradistinction to the previous case of complete rotator cuff tear, the subacromial fat space (large arrowhead in *A*) is patulous; therefore, impingement is not apparent.

DISCUSSION: A curvilinear area of hypointense signal adjacent to the most distal aspect of the rotator cuff complex insertion and overlying the greater tuberosity appears blacker on the T2-weighted image (open arrow in *B*). The conventional AP radiograph shows this area as calcification. The hypointense linear tendon is thickened and contains a focal area of bright signal (curved arrow in *B*) that does not clearly communicate with the subacromial space or interface. If such a communication were demonstrable or if a substantial change in signal in this space existed, a diagnosis of associated rotator cuff tear would be more likely. Just superior or superficial to the tendon and circumscribing it is a linear area of increased signal intensity localized to a segment of the subdeltoid bursa (straight white arrow in *B*). The tendon itself is of slightly higher signal than normal but is not transected.

DIAGNOSIS: The patient has calcific tendinitis and peritendinitis.

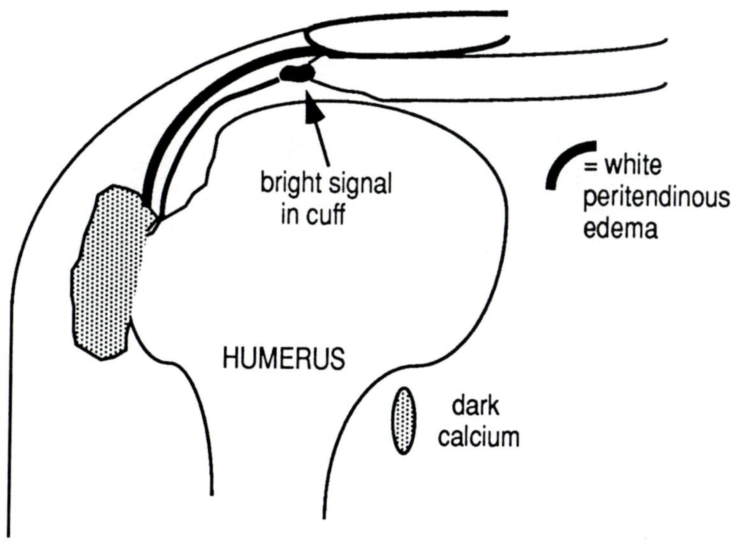

FIGURE 9-3

CASE 10

Differential Diagnosis of Chronic Shoulder Pain

HISTORY: A 35-year-old man presented with a painful right shoulder. He was unable to serve when playing tennis. Is the rotator cuff torn? (Fig. 10-1: coronal multiformat, multiecho proton-density (*A*) and T2-weighted (*B*) MR images.)

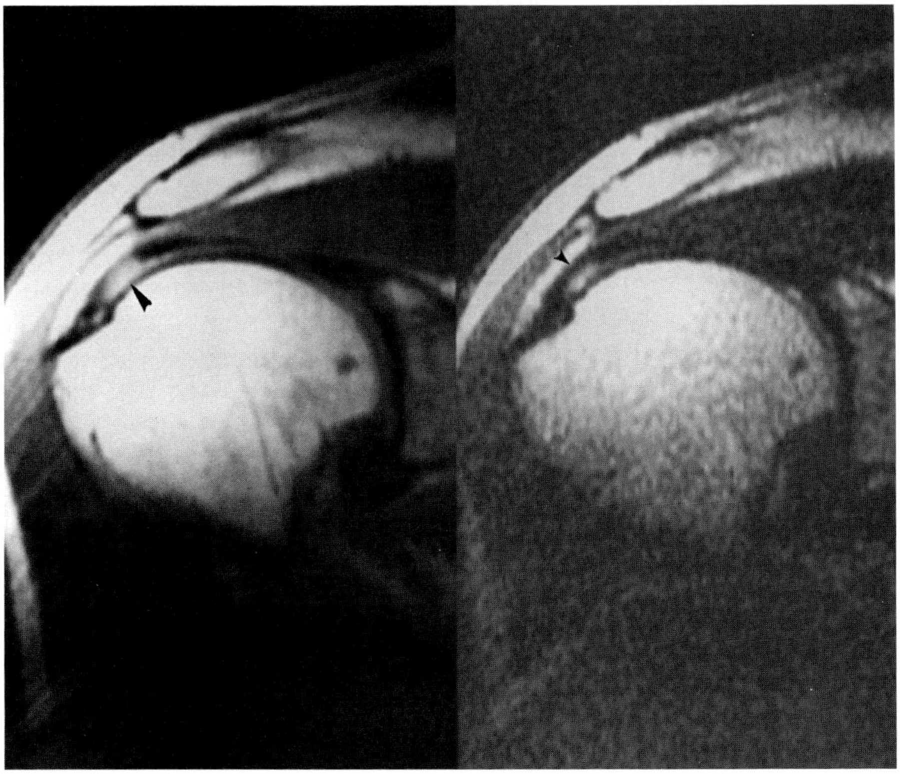

A **B**

FIGURE 10-1

DISCUSSION: The patient has a well-developed supraspinatus muscle and a large, thick, hypointense conjoint tendon consisting of the supraspinatus and infraspinatus tendons (arrowhead in *B*). Tendon discontiguity might be incorrectly deduced if only the proton-density images are inspected. Contiguity is more apparent on the T2-weighted image, further emphasizing the need for comparison of T1-weighted, proton-density, and T2-weighted coronal images at the same anatomic locations. Superficial to the tendon is a hyperintense region that becomes less bright with increased T2 weighting and therefore is incompatible with fluid. It represents the normal subdeltoid fat. However, just deep to the tendon is an area of increased signal intensity (arrowhead in *A*) that does not traverse the tendon. The absence of fluid in either the subdeltoid bursa (a potential reflection located in the subdeltoid fat space) or in the subacromial bursa (a potential reflection located in the subacromial fat space) does not support a diagnosis of partial or complete rotator cuff tear. In addition, the subacromial fat space (not shown) was visible, and the subdeltoid fat space is also visible and does not become less distinct on spin-density or T1-weighted imaging. No evidence of impingement was seen on the adjacent sections, another finding reducing the likelihood of rotator cuff tear.

In summary, other than a subtendinous and intratendinous signal increase, there are no ancillary signs to support the diagnosis of a partial tear. In such a case, at least three of the four indirect signs of rotator cuff tear should be present, including hyperintense fluid on T2-weighted imaging, and indistinctness or disappearance of the subdeltoid and subacromial fat interfaces on T1-weighted or proton-density imaging.

DIAGNOSIS: The patient has rotator cuff tendinitis.

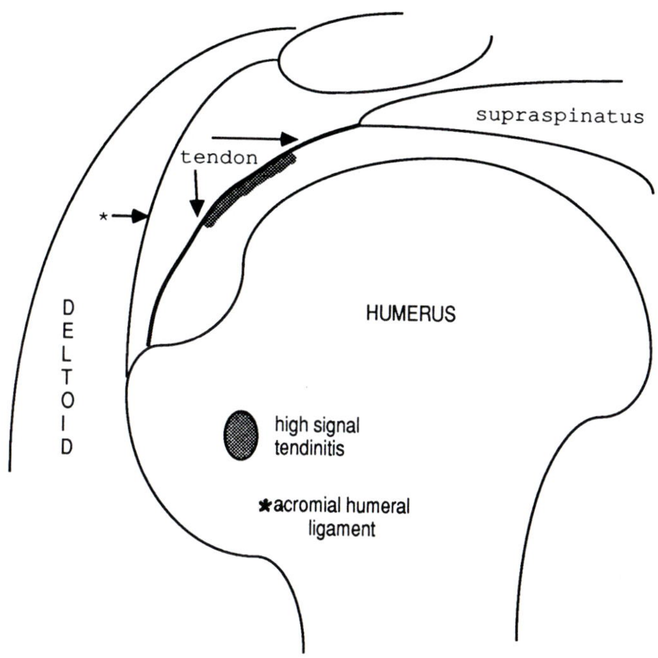

FIGURE 10-2

CASE 11

Differential Diagnosis of Shoulder Pain

HISTORY: A 52-year-old woman presented with inability to move her shoulder and a history of shoulder pain for 8 months. Identify the structures and signal areas indicated. What is the MRI diagnosis? (Fig. 11-1: coronal multiformat, multiecho proton-density (*A*) and T2-weighted (*B*) images. Fig. 11-2: sections adjacent to those shown in Fig. 11-1; 5-mm section thickness, 2-mm intersection gap.)

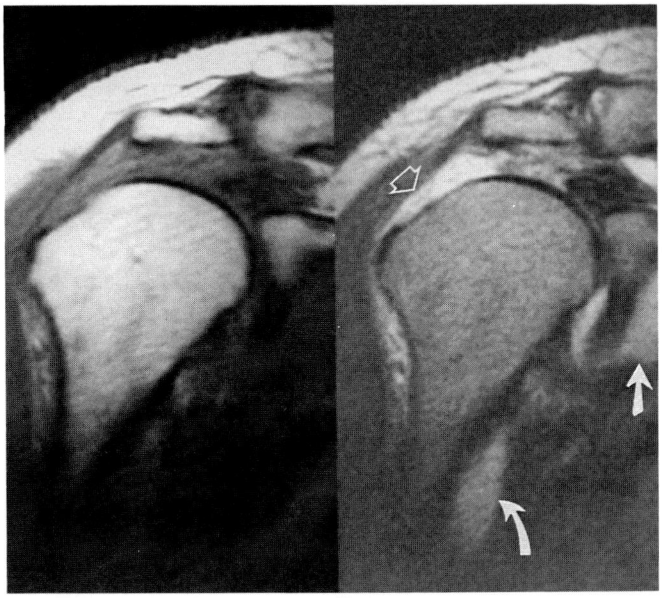

A B

FIGURE 11-1

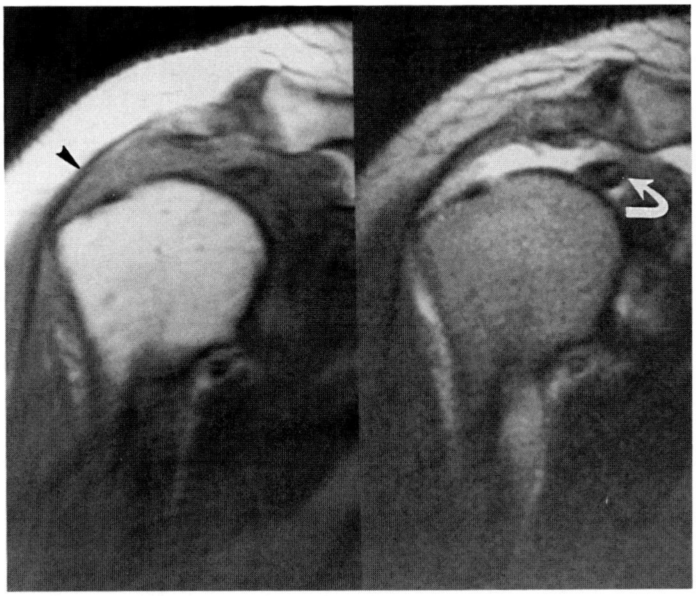

A B

FIGURE 11-2

DISCUSSION: All the signs direct and indirect of rotator cuff tear are present. The cuff is not visualized but is replaced by the signal intensity of fluid (open arrow in Fig. 11-1*B*), a direct sign of tear. Superficial to this fluid/edema interface is the hypointense acromiohumeral ligament (arrowhead in Fig. 11-2*A*), not to be confused with the rotator cuff. A joint effusion extends along the bicipital sheath (curved white arrow in Fig. 11-1*B*) and involves the subscapularis/axillary recess bursal complex (straight white arrow in Fig. 11-1*B*). The triangular or "pointed" superior glenoid labrum appears as a pseudomass (curved white arrow in Fig. 11-2*B*) and may be misconstrued as the rolled-up proximal supraspinatus tendon or as the origin of the biceps long head tendon. Occasionally the proximally ruptured supraspinatus tendon, the biceps long head tendon origin, and the superior glenoid labral tubercle are volume averaged together.

The four indirect signs of rotator cuff transection are illustrated in this case: (1) absence of the deltoid fat interface on proton-density or T1-weighted imaging, (2) hyperintense fluidlike signal in the deltoid interface distribution on T2-weighted imaging, (3) obliteration of the normal hyperintense subacromial fat on T1-weighted or proton-density imaging, and (4) fluidlike signal in the subacromial fat space distribution. Note that the distal clavicle has irregular distal margins and encroaches on the subacromial triangle, almost touching the glenoid superior tubercle.

DIAGNOSIS: The patient has impingement syndrome with complete rotator cuff tear and retraction.

CASE 12

Differential Diagnosis of Shoulder Pain

HISTORY: A middle-aged woman was unable to abduct her right shoulder. What is the MRI diagnosis? Identify the area of hypointense signal along the humeral tuberosity. (Fig. 12-1: coronal oblique multiformat contiguous T1-weighted images.)

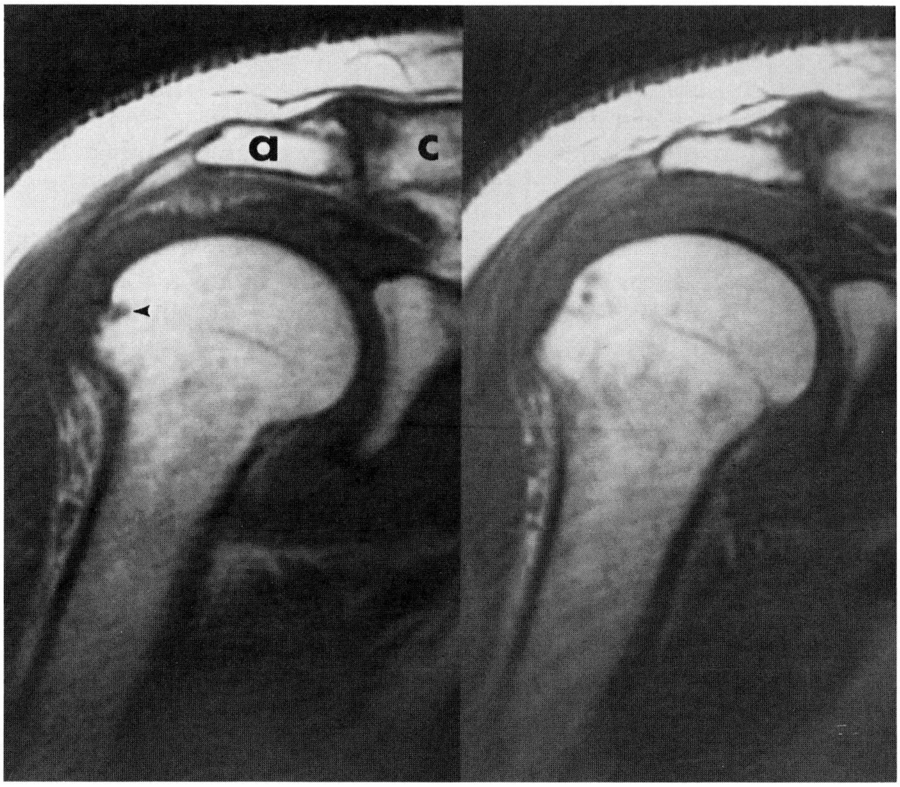

A **B**

FIGURE 12-1

DISCUSSION: The T1-weighted images should be used as an anatomic road map, particularly to identify the rotator cuff. In this case, no linear hypointense signal is demonstrable in the cuff. Instead, it is replaced by homogeneous isointense subacromial signal that has obliterated the normal subacromial fat beneath the acromion (*a*) and the clavicle (*c*). Acromioclavicular joint arthropathy is evident as foci of hypointense periarticular signal with associated pannus formation. Over 80% of rotator cuff tears are related to impingement from acromioclavicular joint arthropathy, pannus, spur formation, granulation tissue, capsular hypertrophy, or subluxation. A reactive change related to traction of the previously intact rotator cuff insertion creates the punctate hypointense signal (arrowhead in *A*).

DIAGNOSIS: The patient has an impingement syndrome with complete rotator cuff tear.

CASE 13

Differential Diagnosis of Chronic Shoulder Pain

HISTORY: A 56-year-old man presented with chronic shoulder pain and decreased strength in the left shoulder. Is a rotator cuff tear present? (Fig. 13-1: coronal T1-weighted image.)

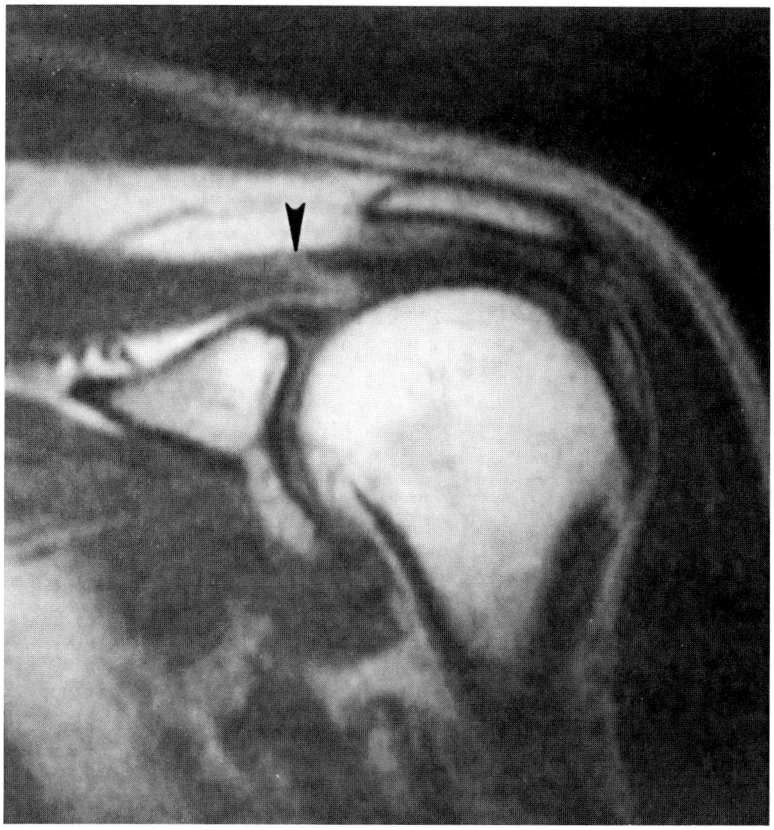

FIGURE 13-1

DISCUSSION: The normal hypointense signal of the rotator cuff complex and conjoined tendon inserting on the promontory of the greater tuberosity is replaced by intermediate signal intensity. The rotator cuff is not visible.

Just above the humeral apex between it and the acromion is an area of gray signal compatible with subacromial fluid.

The presence of upward humeral migration and atrophy of the supraspinatus muscle (arrowheads) is a poor prognostic sign and suggests that rotator cuff repair would be difficult or impossible. Supraspinatus muscle atrophy is a late finding in patients with impingement and rotator cuff complex disease. Such severe wasting can be seen in patients with prior stroke, neuromuscular dysfunction, muscular dystrophies and chronic impingement-related trauma.

DIAGNOSIS: The patient has late stage impingement with complete rotator cuff tear and supraspinatus muscle atrophy.

CASE 19

Differential Diagnosis of Frozen Shoulder

HISTORY: A 67-year-old woman who was completely unable to abduct her arm was referred for evaluation of possible adhesive capsulitis. What is the area of intermediate signal intensity indicated by the arrowheads? What is the MRI diagnosis? (Fig. 19-1: coronal oblique multiformat (two-on-one) T1-weighted images.)

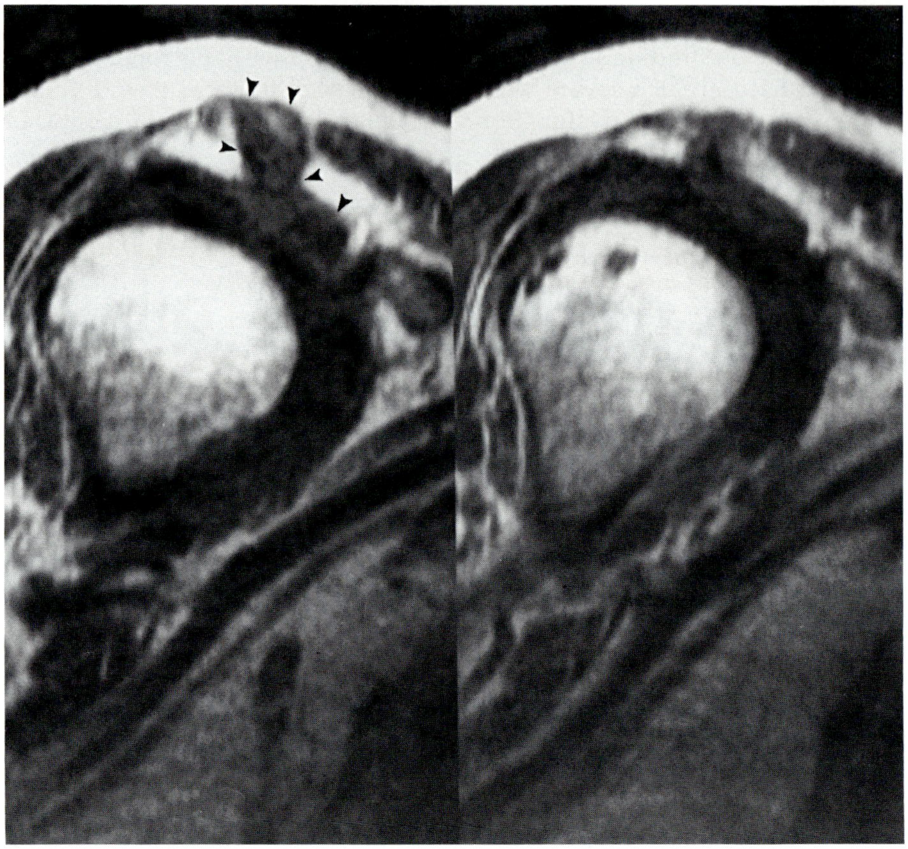

A **B**

FIGURE 19-1

DISCUSSION: Adhesive capsulitis is difficult to diagnose, and MRI is not the best imaging examination for this purpose. The diagnosis is implied on arthrography when the joint space capacity is reduced (<5 cc) on injection. In adhesive capsulitis the capsular anatomy deep to the rotator cuff appears thickened and edematous on MRI, with hyperintense T2 signal. However, that is not the diagnosis in the present case. A mass of moderate signal intensity that is higher in signal than adjacent muscle protrudes from the acromioclavicular joint space. The acromioclavicular joint itself is abnormal, exhibiting irregularity and sclerosis or hyperintensity of its margins. The mass presses down on the subadjacent musculature, completely preventing abduction. On more anterior sections (not shown), the cuff was completely transected and retracted. Resection of the mass was followed by marked clinical improvement. Pathologically, the mass consisted of granulation tissue, fibrous tissue, and pannus.

Impingement syndrome most often results from encroachment on the subacromial arch by spurs, displaced bone, pannus, fibrous tissue, or old hemorrhage. Just as the lumbar spine canal may be congenitally small, predisposing to stenosis, so too the subacromial arch may be diminutive, placing the patient at risk for shoulder impingement. We divide impingement into the following stages on MRI:

1. Simple encroachment on the underlying subacromial fat space and musculature without alteration in signal intensity.
2. Encroachment with signal hyperintensity in the musculotendinous complex, usually at the critical zone (1 cm proximal to the cuff insertion).
3. Encroachment with rotator cuff tear.
   a. Cuff and muscle diastasis/retraction.
   b. Muscle atrophy and upward migration of the humerus.

DIAGNOSIS: The patient has a grade 3b impingement syndrome secondary to giant pannus formation.

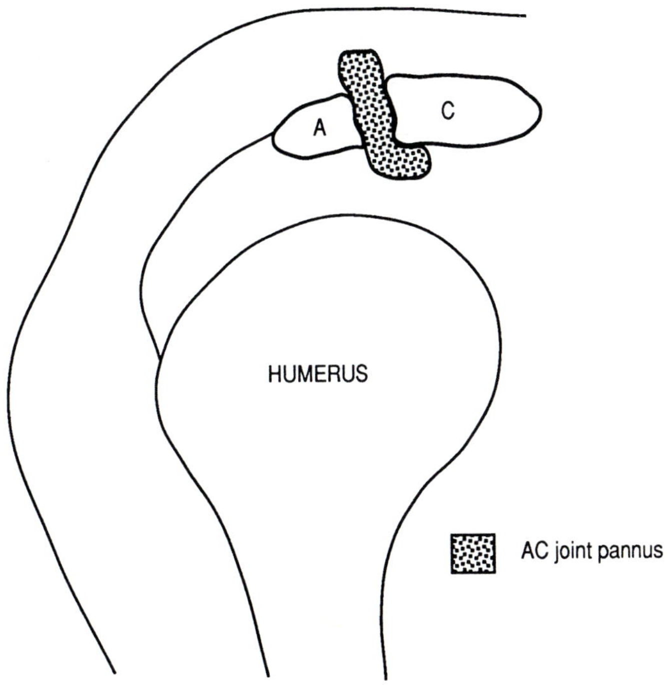

FIGURE 19-2

CASE 20

Differential Diagnosis of Chronic Shoulder Pain

HISTORY: A 65-year-old woman presented with a vague history of upper extremity pain of 3 years' duration but normal range of motion. What is the hypointense structure indicated by the curved white arrow in Figure 20-3*B*? (Fig. 20-1: conventional anteroposterior radiograph of the right shoulder. Fig. 20-2: coronal T1-weighted image. Fig. 20-3: axial multiecho proton-density (*A*) and T2-weighted image.)

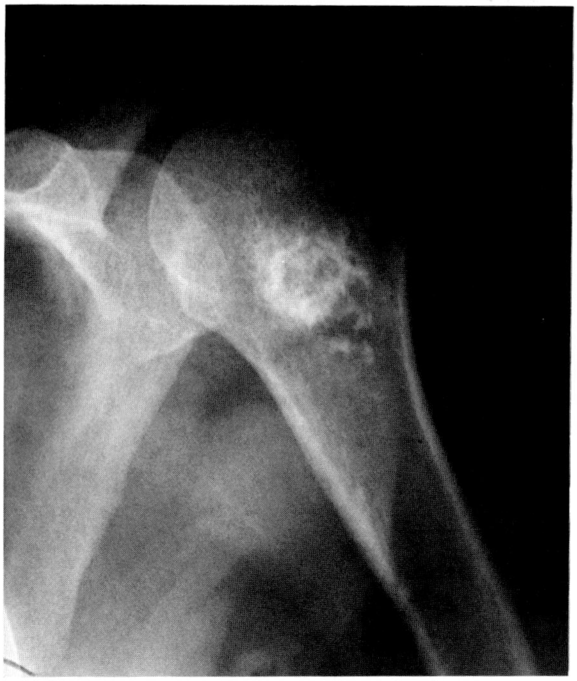

FIGURE 20-1

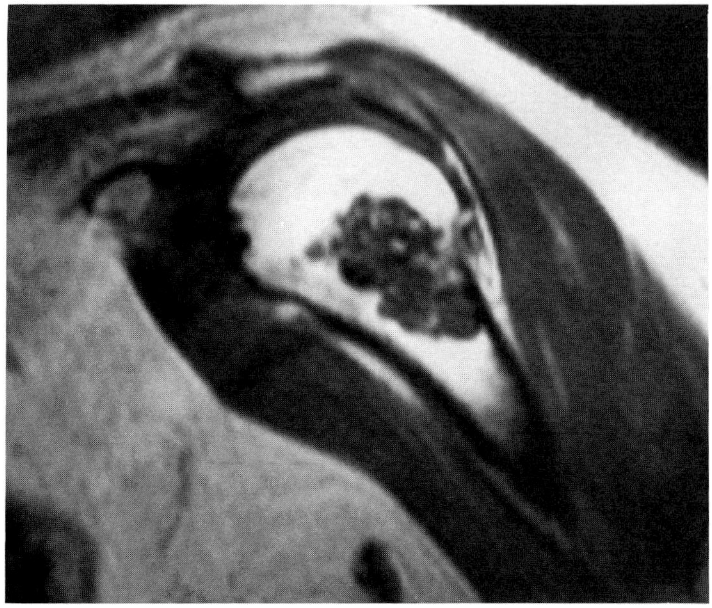

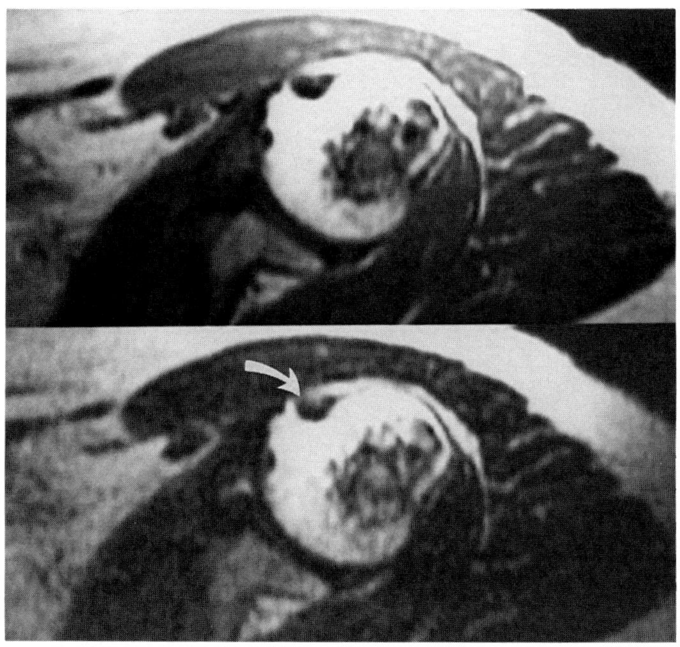

A

B

FIGURE 20-3

DISCUSSION: A hypointense multiloculated mass is visible on all pulse sequences. The mass lacks evidence of hypointense circumferential edema, does not interrupt the cortex, is multiloculated, and is hypointense on the T1-weighted imaging with only a nominal increase in signal intensity with T2 weighting. These are the MRI criteria for diagnosing a bone infarct. Typically a chondrosarcoma, which may mimic bone infarct, has much higher signal intensity on T2-weighted imaging unless calcification is present within the lesion. In fact, chondrosarcoma frequently has cystic components that are extremely hyperintense on T2-weighted imaging. Bone infarcts may exhibit marginal peripheral signal hyperintensity in the late subacute or early chronic phase, but their overall signal intensity remains relatively low. Large bone infarcts may be mildly hyperintense on the T2-weighted image acutely but revert to T2 signal hypointensity within 3 to 6 months. A malignant chondral lesion of this size would be surrounded by edema and would likely produce a soft tissue mass effect. Chondroid lesions are "hot" on scintigraphy, while bone infarcts, unless giant and acute, are not radionuclide avid. The hypointense structure (curved white arrow in Fig. 20-3*B*) is the normal biceps long head tendon (compare with case 6). It is housed in the bicipital groove and secured by the transverse humeral ligament (not seen).

Again, no extremity MRI studies should be interpreted without conventional radiographs, as the diagnosis on MRI is simple with the accompanying plain film.

DIAGNOSIS: The patient has a giant bone infarct.

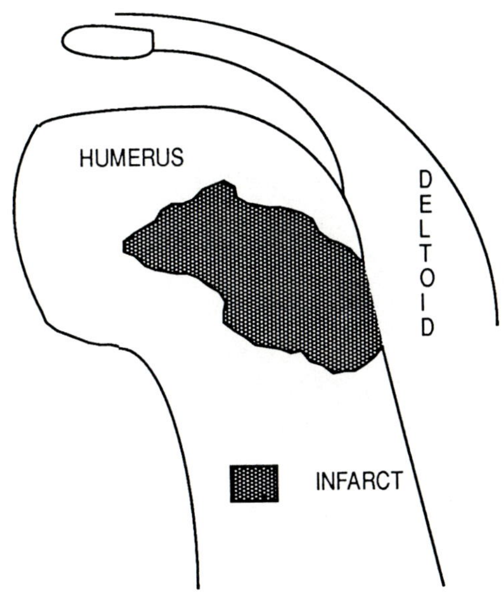

FIGURE 20-4

CASE 21

Differential Diagnosis of Chronic Shoulder Pain

HISTORY: A 68-year-old woman with chronic anemia of unknown origin presented with shoulder pain and tenderness of 3 months' duration. What is the MRI diagnosis? (Fig. 21-1: conventional anteroposterior radiograph of the left shoulder. Fig. 21-2: coronal T1-weighted MR image. Fig. 21-3: multiecho, multiformat proton-density (*A*) and T2-weighted (*B*) images.)

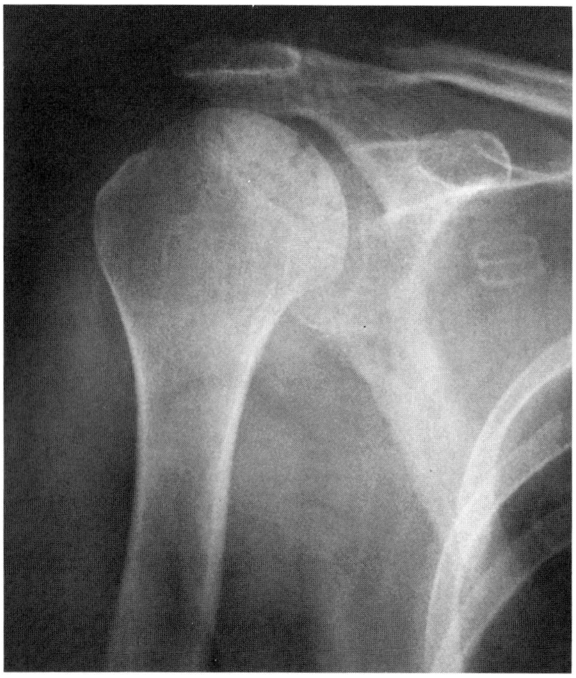

FIGURE 21-1

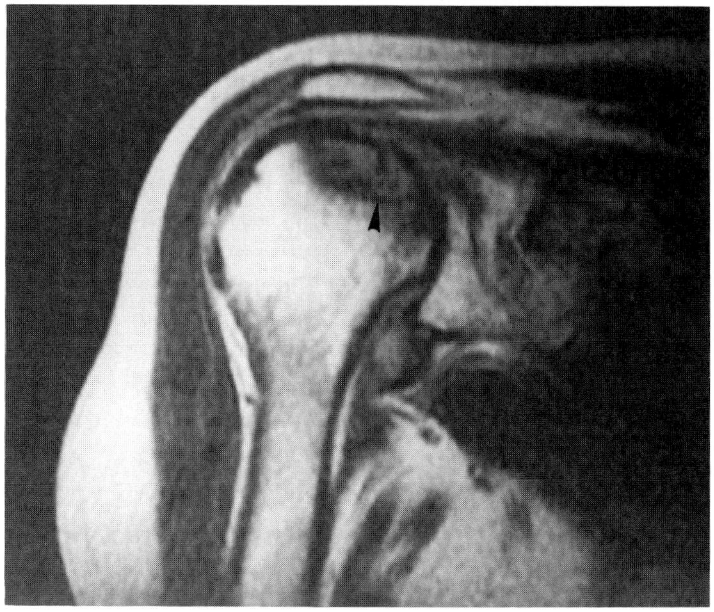

FIGURE 21-2

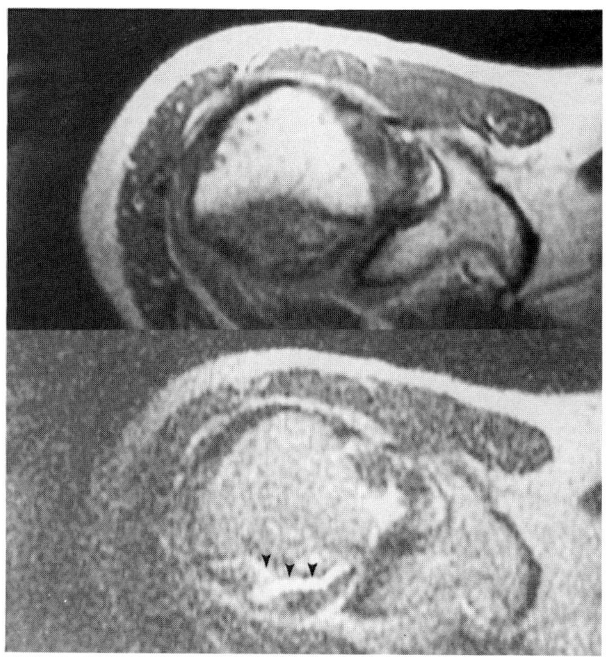

A

B

FIGURE 21-3

DISCUSSION: Although not mentioned in the history, the patient has been taking steroids for 6 months. A confluent subcapital hypointense curvilinear T1 signal is visible in the coronal projection. The AP radiograph shows sclerosis in this region, with fissural interruption of the cortex seen on this frontal projection and on the T1-weighted image as vertical lucent or hypointense lines. The findings are compatible with avascular necrosis with articular surface linear cortical fractures that have resulted in a large joint effusion (not shown). In the axial projection (Fig. 21-3), a reactive hyperintense linear interface is noted on the T2-weighted image (arrowheads in Fig. 21-3*B*). This reactive interface may be displaced from its correct location with respect to marrow fat by a chemical shift (frequency shift) artifact, so that on the T2-weighted image a thin white line lies adjacent to a thin dark line. The dark line on the T2-weighted image may also be due to the fibrous interface. A hypointense rim on the T1-weighted coronal image (arrowhead in Fig. 21-2) and the axial proton-density image is compatible with a fibrous interface.

Once bone ischemia occurs, hematopoietic cells are most sensitive, dying after 6 to 12 hours. This phase is followed by osteocytic/bone cell death at 12 to 48 hours, and the death of marrow fat cells in 2 to 5 days. Pathologically, osteonecrosis may be broken down into five phases:

Phase 1: Interruption of blood supply to red cells, osteocytes, and fat cells over a 5-day period, as described.

Phase 2: Hyperemia in surrounding bone with associated osteoporosis over a 3-week period.

Phase 3: Modulation of ischemic fat cells into fibroblasts with a hypointense reactive interface at the infarct margin on T1-weighted imaging that is hyperintense on T2-weighted imaging, as occurred in this case.

Phase 4: Widening of the reactive interface, acellularity, and sclerosis that appears hypointensity on T1-weighted imaging and less pronounced on T2-weighted imaging. This is seen posterior and superior to the reactive interface in this case.

Phase 5: Trabecular weakening with subchondral fracture beginning as linear micro- and macrofractures in a subcapital distribution and eventuating in bony collapse.

DIAGNOSIS: The patient has early phase 5 osteonecrosis with a reactive interface (phase 3) and fibrosis (phase 4).

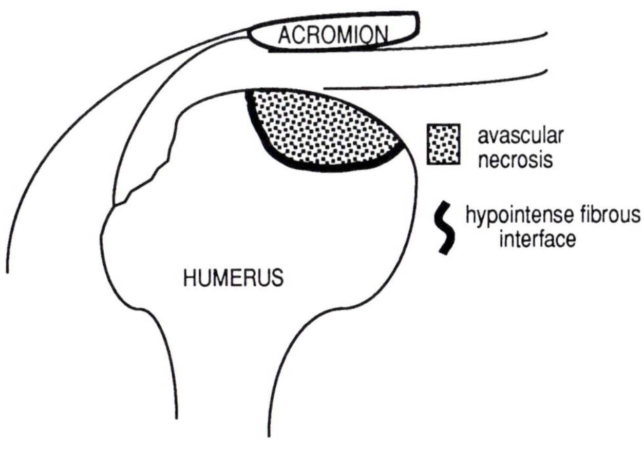

FIGURE 21-4

CASE 22

Differential Diagnosis of Chronic Shoulder Pain

HISTORY: A 57-year-old man with known lung carcinoma presented with chronic right shoulder pain. The patient reported numbness, tingling, and weakness in his upper extremities, more so on the right side, than on the left. What is the MRI diagnosis? (Fig. 22-1: conventional anteroposterior radiograph. Fig. 22-2: coronal T1-weighted MR image.)

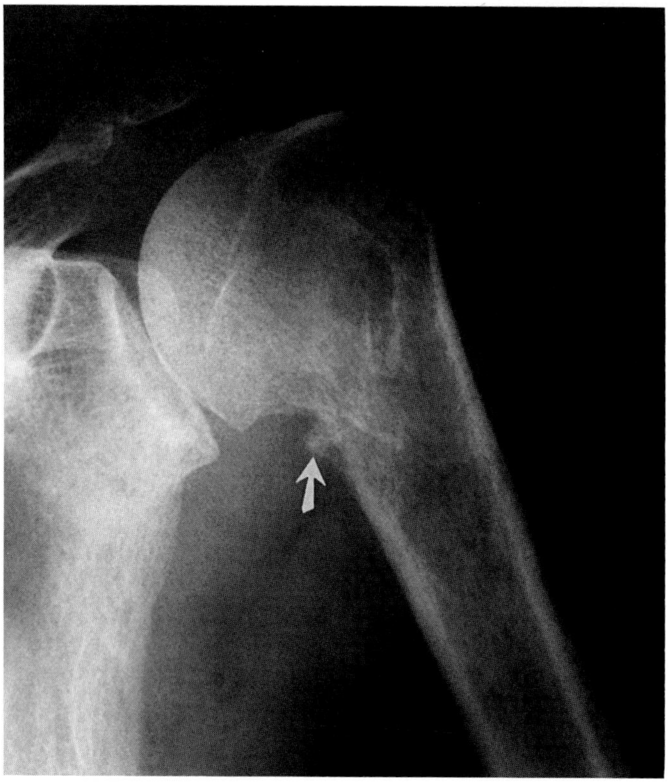

FIGURE 22-1

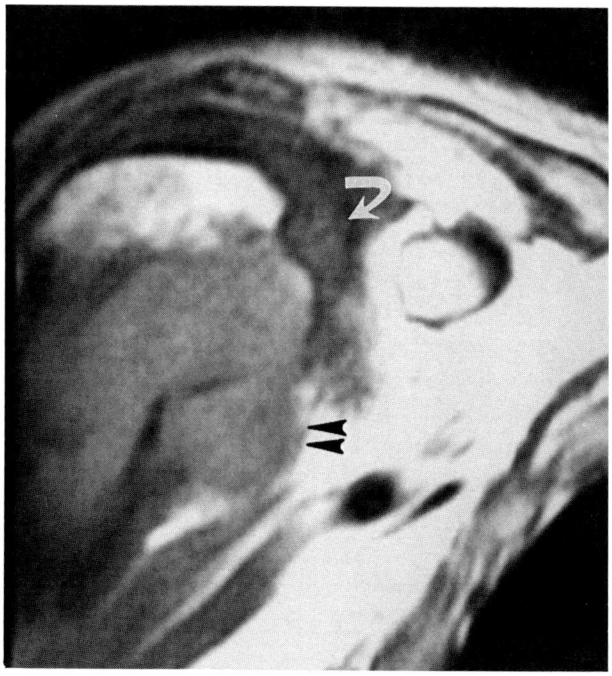

FIGURE 22-2

DISCUSSION: Normally the humeral head has a slightly mottled but hyperintense signal on T1-weighted imaging. This signal mottling is most often related to islands of hematopoietic marrow (see case 1). Areas of red marrow formation, particularly in the anemic patient and child, may be associated with such pronounced signal inhomogeneity on T1-weighted imaging that they may be mistaken for neoplasm.

In this case a globular, confluent, hypointense mass replaces the humeral head and extends out into the adjacent soft tissues. This is not a cystic lesion, since the T1 signal (paired arrowheads in Fig. 22-2) is not as hypointense as that of fluid in the joint space (curved white arrow in Fig. 22-2). The cortex is broken by the lesion, confirming its aggressive nature. The conventional radiograph shows a pathologic humeral neck fracture with mixed bone lysis and sclerosis and cortical irregularity (arrow in Fig. 22-1). However, the subtlety of the findings on plain film is disturbing, in light of the size and extent of disease appreciated on MRI. It is not unusual in the axial or appendicular skeleton to observe dramatic T1 signal alterations on MRI with normal conventional radiographs. The T2 signal of skeletal neoplasm is extremely variable. Proton-density–weighted imaging may obscure both the lesion and the gross medullary bone pathology. Short-time inversion-recovery sequences (STIR) may be useful for identifying with great sensitivity the signal hyperintensity of pathologic, neoplastic bone.

Focal bright areas are occasionally seen in bone, particularly in the spine on T1-weighted images. The T1 rule of thumb, "White is right," is reliable since malignant neoplasia with bright T1 signal is extremely rare.

DIAGNOSIS: The patient has metastatic lung carcinoma.

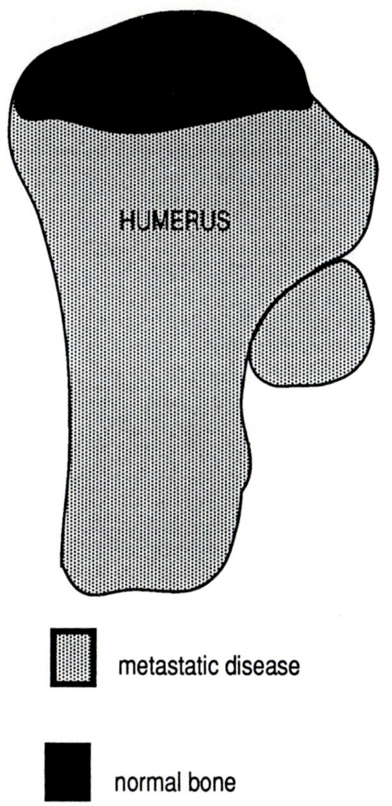

FIGURE 22-3

CASE 23

Differential Diagnosis of Chronic Shoulder Pain

HISTORY: A 68-year-old woman with a 7-year history of keratitis sicca and intermittent low-grade fever presented with deep-seated shoulder discomfort for 1 year. What is the MRI diagnosis? The history and MRI findings are pathognomonic. (Fig. 23-1: coronal multiformat (two-on-one) multiecho proton-density (*A*) and T2-weighted (*B*) MR images.)

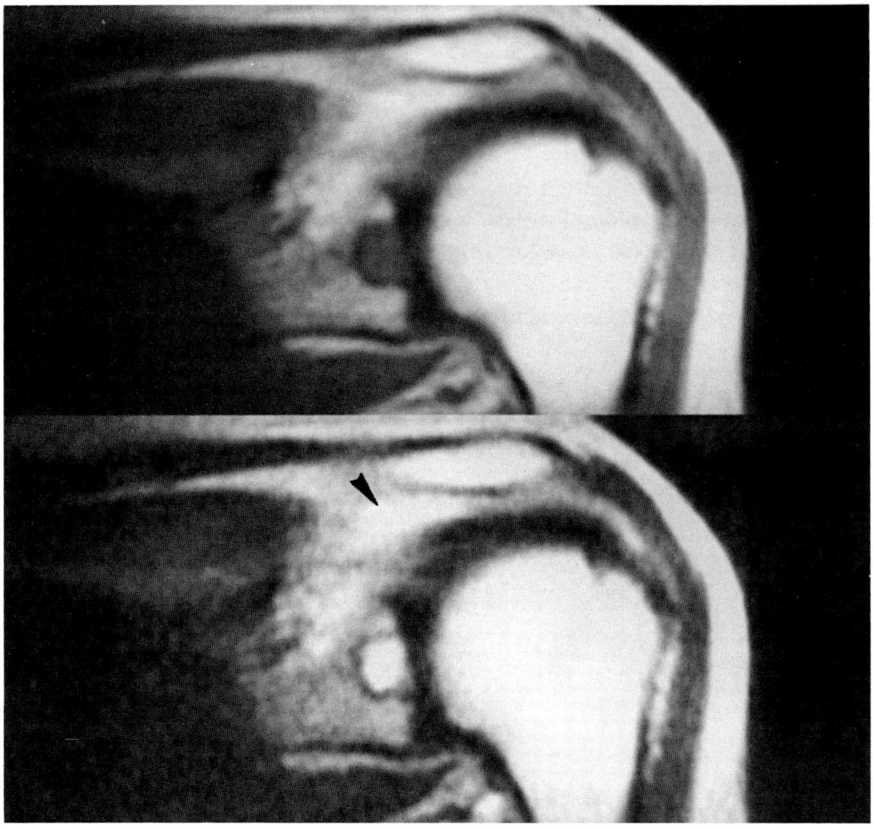

A

B

FIGURE 23-1

DISCUSSION: The MR images show a well-circumscribed subchondral focal area that is hypointense on T1 weighting and hyperintense on T2 weighting. The mass is well marginated, exhibits no edema, and is not associated with an extraskeletal soft tissue mass. The lesion is marginated by a hypointense rim representing rheumatoid granulomas. The central homogeneous portion of the lesion represents cyst formation secondary to synovial invagination and ulceration of the articular surface. Alone, this is a nonspecific finding. However, in a patient with systemic disease (fever) of long standing and associated with keratitis sicca (dry eye), the diagnosis of rheumatoid arthritis is all but certain. Other arthropathies could produce similar lesions on MRI. In addition, lesions that occur at the ends of bones, such as an intraosseous ganglion, would have the same signal intensity, but intraosseous ganglion is a much rarer lesion, typically does not occur at this location, and does not communicate with the joint space, as this lesion does. Only one side of the joint is involved, and the absence of edema and joint fluid greatly reduces the likelihood of an infectious process or Brodie's abscess. A small joint effusion exists (arrowhead in *B*). The humeral head is normal.

DIAGNOSIS: The patient has a rheumatoid granuloma-lined synovial cyst and rheumatoid arthritis.

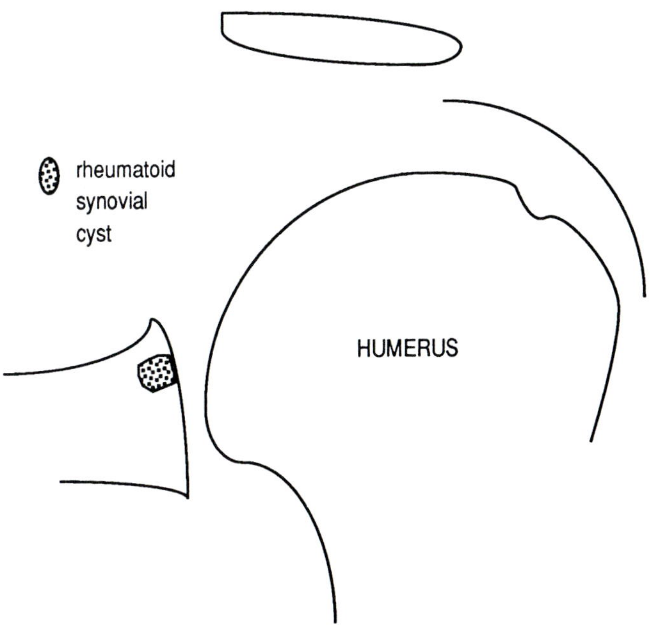

FIGURE 23-2

CASE 24

Differential Diagnosis of Shoulder Masses

HISTORY: A 10-year-old boy presented with chronic left shoulder and upper arm pain. What is the MRI diagnosis? (Fig. 24-1: frontal conventional radiograph of the left humerus in internal rotation. Fig. 24-2: coronal T1-weighted MR image. Fig. 24-3: coronal multiecho proton-density (*A*) and T2-weighted (*B*) MR images.)

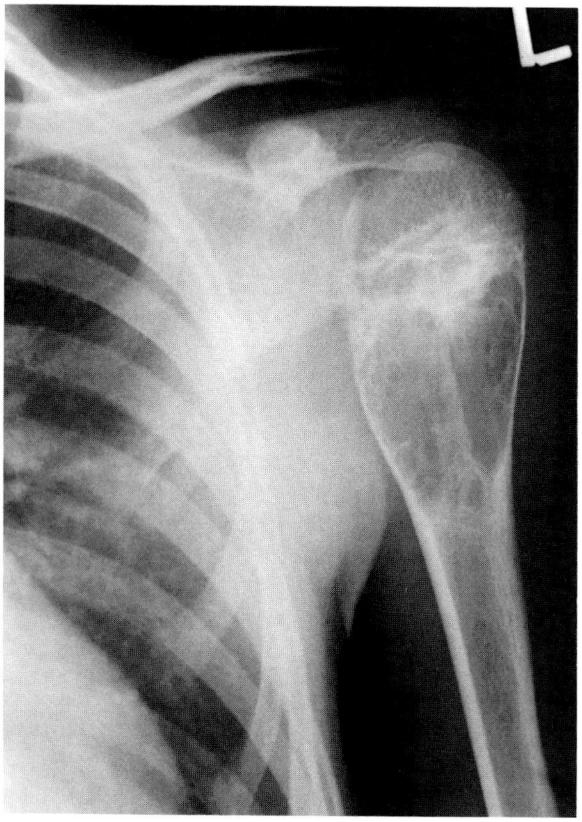

FIGURE 24-1

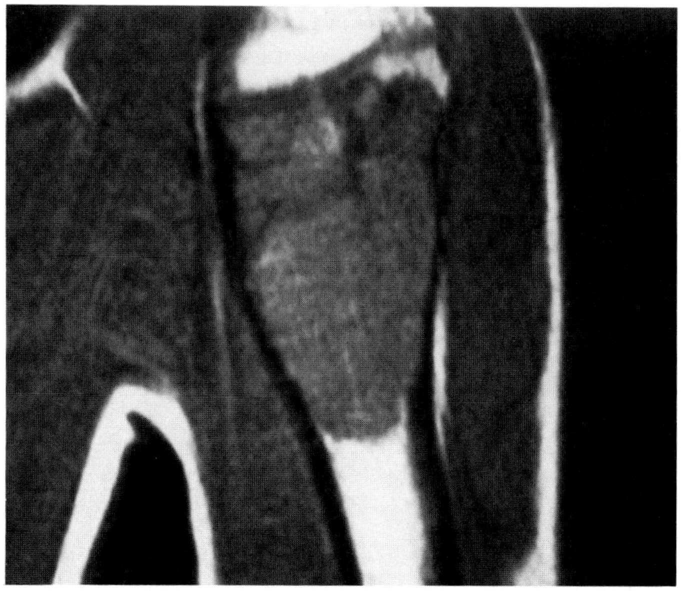

FIGURE 24-2

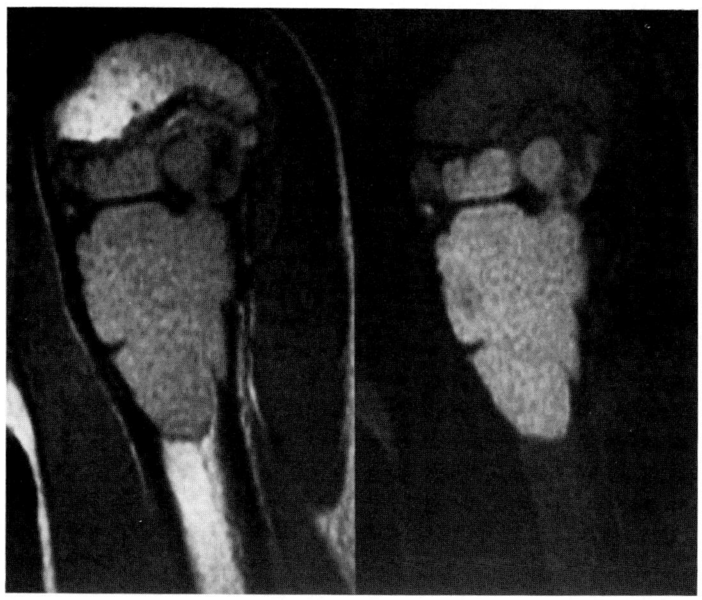

A **B**

FIGURE 24-3

DISCUSSION: A multiloculated lytic lesion is present in the proximal humerus that is well-demarcated, expansile, and devoid of matrix formation, calcification, or periosteal reaction on the conventional radiograph. The T1-weighted image shows a hypointense mass with septations extending through it. Other than the septations, the lesion is relatively homogeneous and exhibits homogeneous signal increase on the T2-weighted image, as well as homogeneity on spin-density imaging. The lesion stops directly at the unclosed epiphysis, is expansile, and is non-hemorrhagic on MRI.

The signal characteristics, sharp demarcation, absence of edema, absence of soft tissue mass, and location in the proximal humerus in a young male are characteristic of unicameral bone cyst. The proximal humerus is the most common site of this lesion, the proximal femur the second most common site. Eighty percent of these lesions occur in children aged 3 to 14 years, and males predominate in a ratio of 3:1.

Because the lesion is expansile, consideration should be given to the diagnosis of aneurysmal bone cyst. Approximately 30% of aneurysmal bone cysts have hyperintense signal on T1-weighted images due to their propensity for hemorrhage. Most aneurysmal bone cysts are secondary to other neoplasms such as chondroblastoma, osteoblastoma, chondromyxoid fibroma, giant cell tumor, and telangiectatic osteogenic sarcoma. Giant cell tumor tends to involve the epiphyses in patients whose epiphyseal plates have closed. The average age at discovery is 33 years. Chondroblastoma occurs in the epiphysis before it has closed and will often contain matrix exhibiting signal inhomogeneity on T2-weighted MRI. Osteoblastoma should exhibit some hyperdensity on conventional radiography and reactive bone formation, not present in this case. Chondromyxoid fibroma is an expansile, eccentric lesion with matrix formation that occurs in an older age group. Telangiectatic osteogenic sarcoma is a deadly, lytic, expansile variant of malignant bone neoplasm that often forms secondary cysts. It may be associated with a soft tissue mass but can have a benign appearance on conventional radiographs.

DIAGNOSIS: The patient has a unicameral bone cyst.

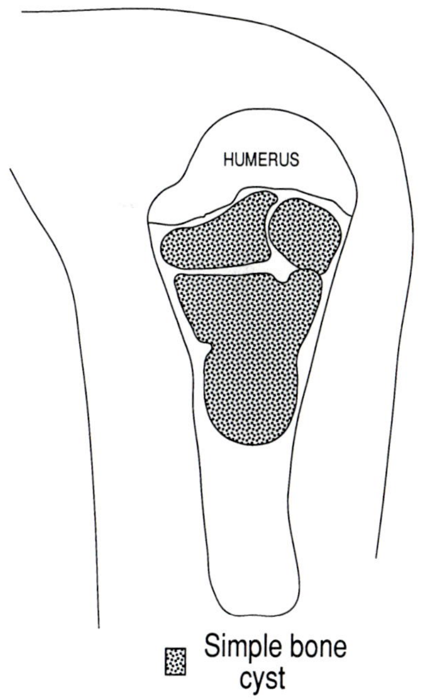

FIGURE 24-4

CASE 25

Differential Diagnosis of Shoulder Pain

HISTORY: A 23-year-old quarterback underwent radiologic evaluation for an aching sensation, decreased throwing velocity, and decreased range of motion. What is the MRI diagnosis? (Fig. 25-1: axial gradient-echo fast scan. Fig. 25-2: coronal proton-density (*A*) and T2-weighted (*B*) MR images.)

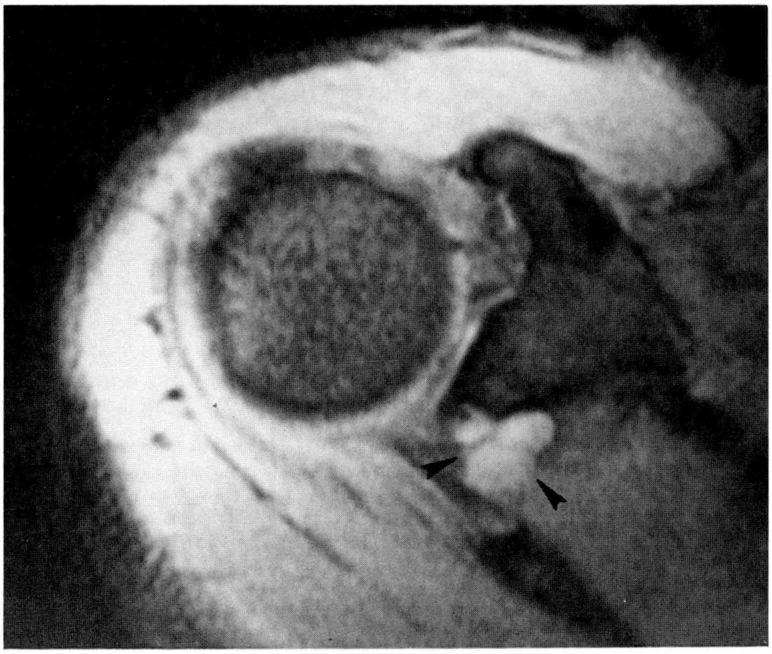

FIGURE 25-1

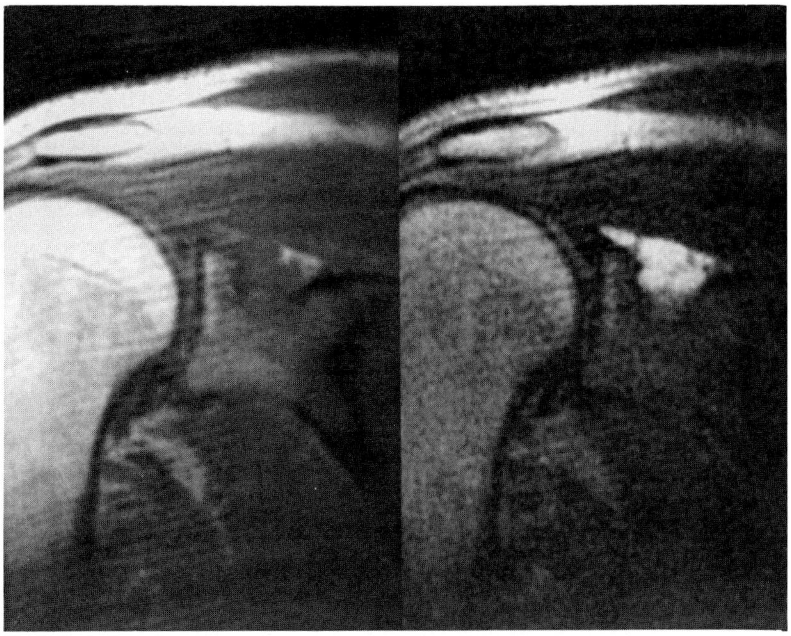

A **B**

FIGURE 25-2

DISCUSSION: Beneath the articular surface of the femoral head is a hypointense line or interface that parallels the curved femoral surface in the shape of a linear crescent (arrowheads). The findings are typical of the early phase of avascular necrosis (AVN). Based on MRI appearance, AVN can be subdivided into five basic types (see Fig. 1-2):

1. crescent type,
2. ring type,
3. homogeneous type,
4. speckled or irregular type, and
5. extended type.

After the formation of a subcapital crescent, the crescent extends to a ring. Within the hypointense ring, normal hyperintense T1 fat signal persists uninterrupted. Eventually, the ring fills in on T1-weighted images to form a homogeneous subarticular ellipse, the homogeneous type. Involvement in other areas of the femoral head with patchy signal hypointensity in and around the ring results in the speckled type. Finally, the extended type occurs when signal inhomogeneity progresses toward the intertrochanteric region, particularly along stress lines.

DIAGNOSIS: The patient has avascular necrosis of the crescent type.

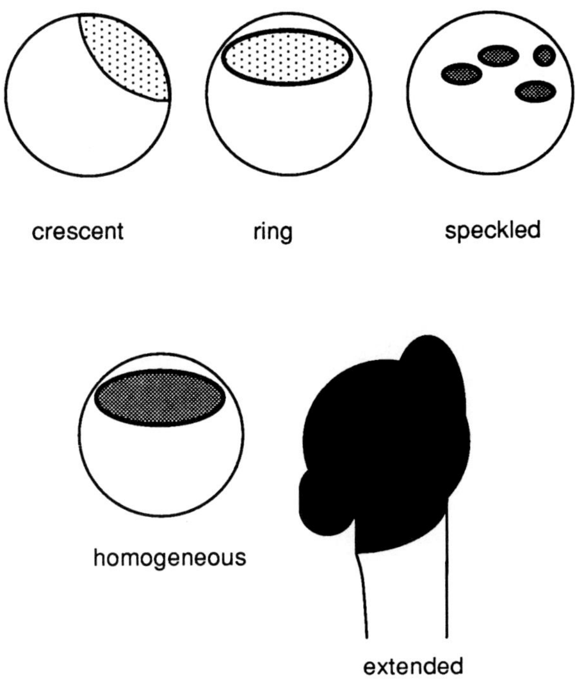

FIGURE 1-2

CASE 2

Differential Diagnosis of Hip Pain and Avascular Necrosis

HISTORY: Two presents are described in this case study. A 26-year-old man presented with chronic hip pain. He had taken steroids for 3 weeks for a questionable diagnosis of multiple sclerosis. The second patient was a 46-year-old man who had idiopathic avascular necrosis of the left hip and presented with right hip pain. What are the MRI diagnoses? (Patient 1—Fig. 2-1: conventional anteroposterior radiograph of the pelvis. Fig. 2-2: coronal, and Fig. 2-3: axial body coil T1-weighted images. Patient 2—Fig. 2-4: coronal T1-weighted MR image. Fig. 2-5: magnified T1-weighted image of the right hip.)

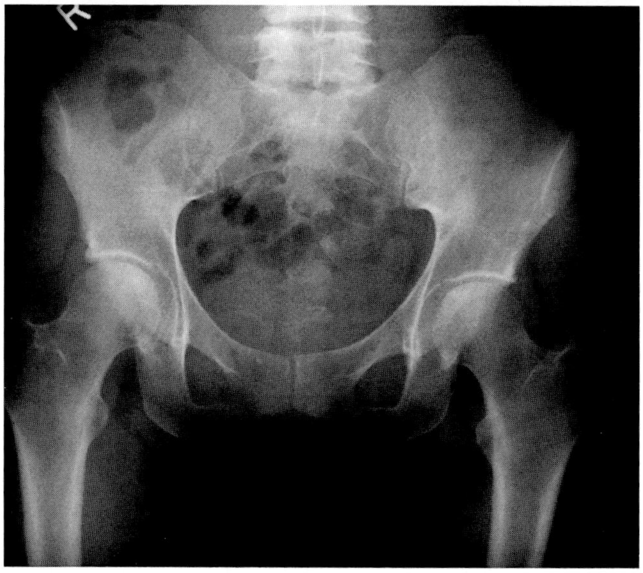

FIGURE 2-1

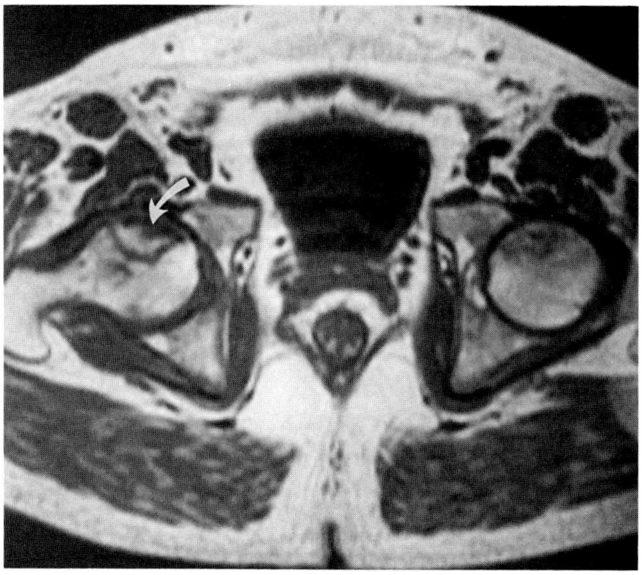

FIGURE 2-2

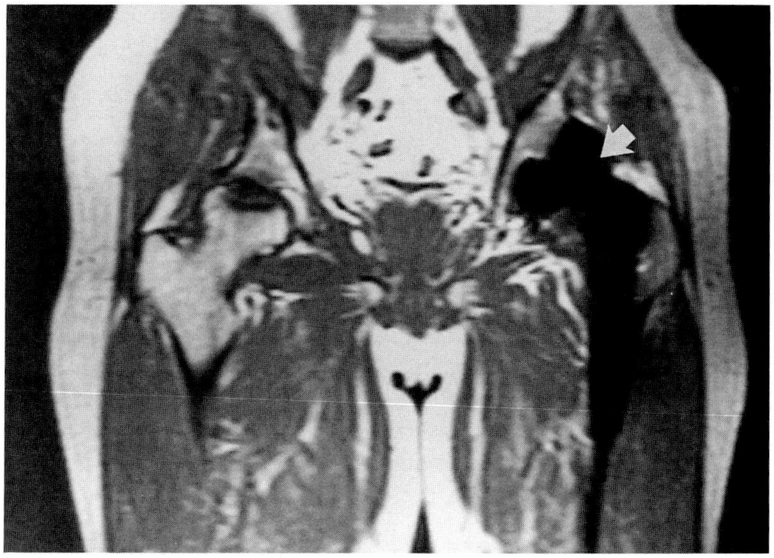

FIGURE 2-3

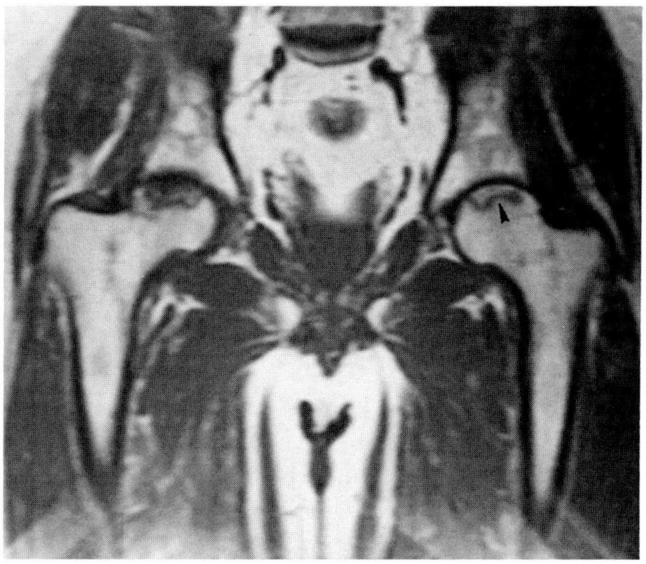

FIGURE 2-4

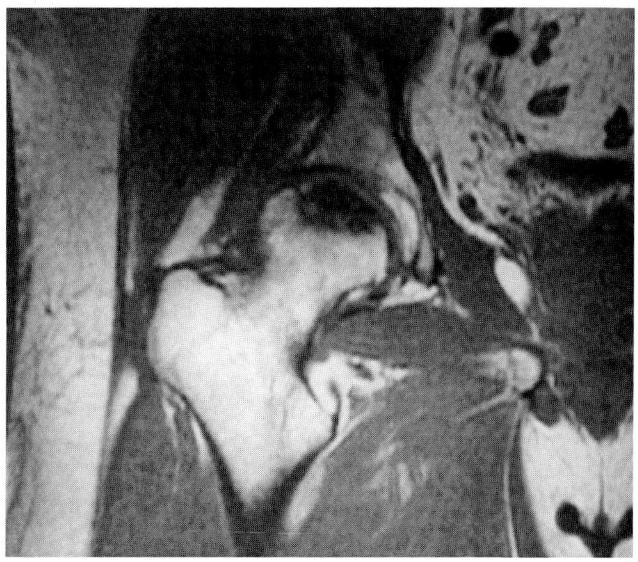

FIGURE 2-5

DISCUSSION: Five of the more common MRI phases or appearances of avascular necrosis (AVN) were described in case 1:

1. cresent type,
2. ring type,
3. homogeneous type,
4. speckled or irregular type,
5. extended type.

In patient 1 the linear foci of hypointensity have assumed a ring appearance in the coronal (arrowhead in Fig. 2-4) and axial (curved white arrow in Fig. 2-2) projections. Within this ring is an area of normal hyperintense fat signal on the left and early hypointensity beginning in the anterior aspect of the hip (curved white arrow in Fig. 2-2). The areas of patchy hypointensity in the acetabulum and the intertrochanteric hip represent islands of normal hematopoietic or red marrow. These normal areas of red marrow production should not be mistaken for neoplasm or inflammatory sites.

The pathophysiologic phases of AVN can be subdivided by temporal phenomena:

1. a. Ischemic RBC death (12 hours).
   b. Subsequent osteocytic death (24 hours).
   c. Yellow marrow death (72 hours).
2. Secondary hyperemia and osteoporosis (1 to 3 weeks).
3. Fat cell conversion to reactive fibroblasts (MRI stages 1 to 3).
4. Wide reactive interface, with acellularity and sclerosis (early MRI stage 4).
5. Subchondral fractures with loss of head height (late MRI stage 4).

MRI signal alterations in the hip cannot be detected until pathophysiologic phase 2, at 1 to 3 weeks. Therefore, the earliest phase of AVN may simply manifest as osteoporosis or as diffuse T1 hypointensity, subtle but extensive. This appearance is unusual. Other unusual appearances of early AVN are:

1. Prominence or early appearance of bright T1 yellow marrow in a young patient, so-called early red to yellow marrow conversion. (Approximately 95% of healthy subjects have some red marrow in the intertrochanteric region before age 50.)
2. Exaggeration of the linear, hypointense, vertically oriented weight-bearing trabecula.

The sensitivity of MRI in the overall detection of AVN is 93%, whereas radionuclide scintigraphy is 80% to 90% sensitive and computed tomography is 60% to 70% sensitive.

Patient 2 has undergone left hip replacement with a nonferromagnetic prosthesis that produces an area of signal void (arrow in Fig. 2-3) with little spatial distortion or obscuring of the surrounding anatomy. Almost all orthopaedic prosthetic devices can be safely scanned at high field strengths without complications of heating or torsion. Skin staples should be removed before scanning, however, as their alloy content varies, and bending or twisting may produce staple torsion in the magnet's isocenter. A subcapital ring or ellipse is visible in the right hip; this ring has now filled in and is of homogeneous signal intensity on T1-weighted imaging (Fig. 2-5).

DIAGNOSIS: Patient 1 has AVN of the ring type in the left hip, in transition to the homogeneous type in the right hip. Patient 2 has homogeneous AVN.

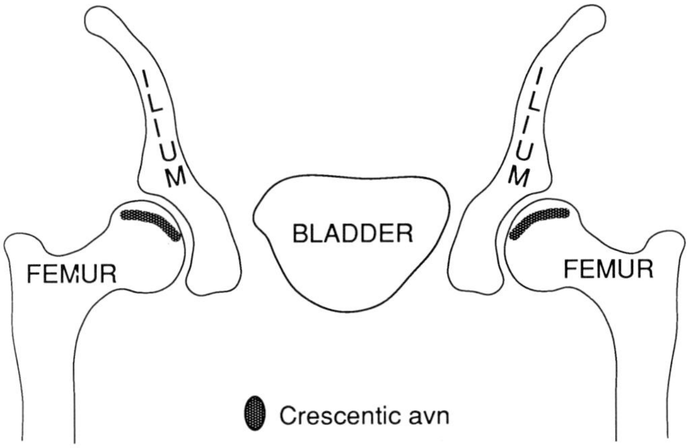

FIGURE 2-6

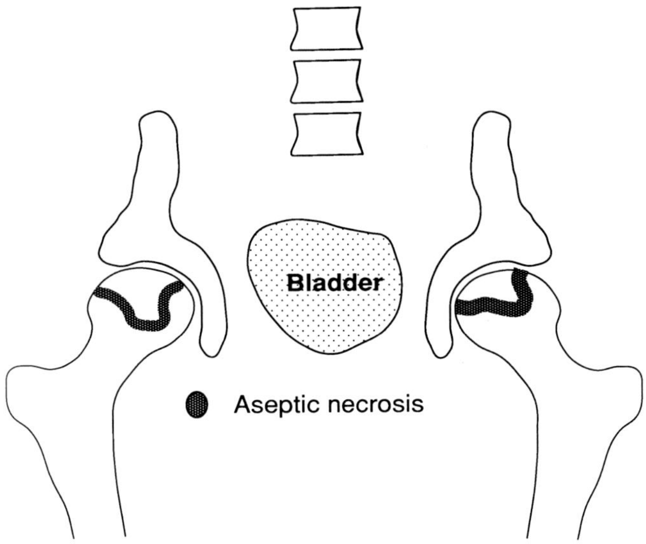

FIGURE 2-7

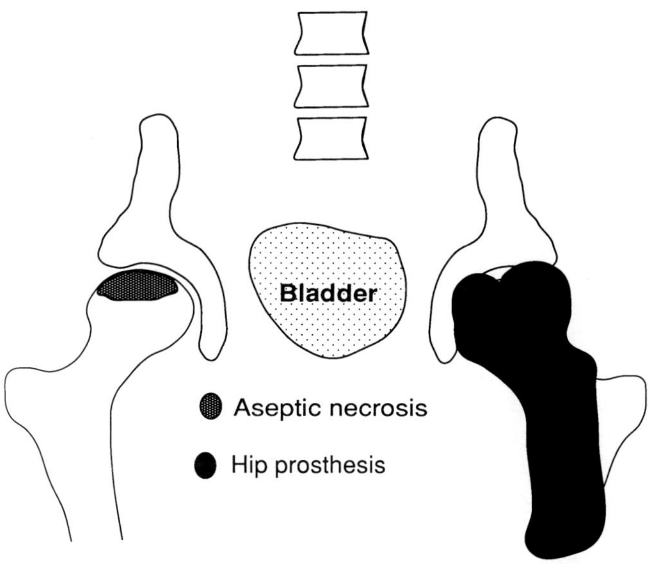

FIGURE 2-8

CASE 3

Differential Diagnosis of Hip Pain and Avascular Necrosis

HISTORY: Two 30-year-old men presented with bilateral hip pain. Did both have avascular necrosis? Explain the differences in marrow signal between the two patients. (Fig. 3-1: coronal T1-weighted image, patient 1. Fig. 3-2: coronal multiformat (two-on-one) T1-weighted images, patient 2.)

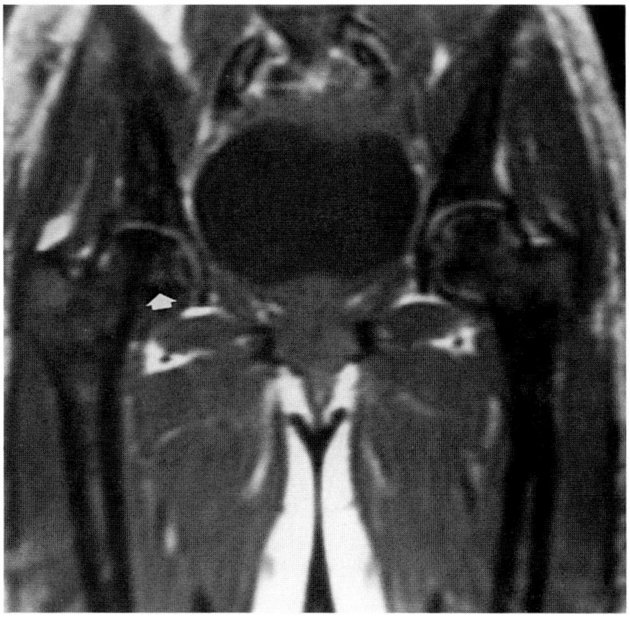

FIGURE 3-1

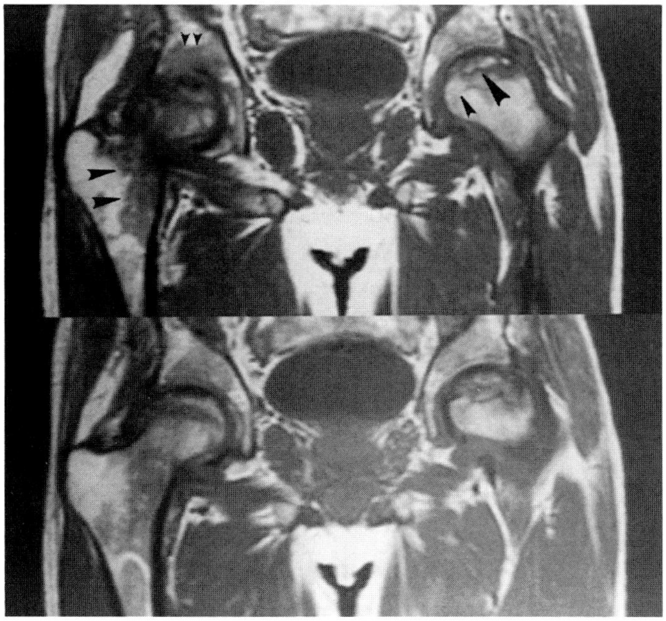

FIGURE 3-2

DISCUSSION: Distinct differences in marrow signal are noted between the two men, although they are of the same age. The marrow in patient 1 is diffusely hypointense; the hypointensity is pronounced and involves the acetabula, ilia, and lumbar spine. Diffusely dark bones may be seen in myeloid metaplasia, osteopetrosis, yellow to red marrow reconversion, osteosclerotic lymphoma, and (rarely) secondary hyperparathyroidism. In osteopetrosis, the bones are even blacker than shown here. Of the diagnostic possibilities, only sickle cell disease with red to yellow marrow reconversion is commonly associated with avascular necrosis (AVN) in a patient not taking steroids. Severe peripheral anemia is the obvious cause of RBC overproduction. Ring type AVN is barely visible (white arrow in Fig. 3-1) in both hips.

A more normal pattern of marrow intensity is seen in patient 2. Normal patchy islands of red marrow are present in the acetabula bilaterally (smallest paired arrowheads in Fig. 3-2*A*). The MR images show a normal left hip epiphysis (small arrowhead in Fig. 3-2*A*) and a subcapital crescent (large arrowhead). A more patchy distribution of signal hypointensity is seen in the right hip. A ring is barely visible, and diffuse inhomogeneity is present down to the intertrochanteric and subtrochanteric regions (medium-sized paired arrowheads in Fig. 3-2*A*).

MRI is the imaging examination of choice in early AVN. The scintigraphic appearance may be normal in 80% to 90% of cases of early AVN, and conventional radiographs may appear normal for up to 2 years. A hyperintense band may be present at the margin of AVN, circumscribing the AVN ring on T2-weighted imaging. This band may represent a chemical shift artifact or a reactive interface of hypervascularity or bone repair. Signal intensity may prove valuable in the assessment of AVN stage, lesion reversibility, and correlation with hip pain.

A staging system based on signal intensity is as follows:

A. T1 hyperintensity, T2 hypointensity (fatlike).
B. T1 hyperintensity, T2 hyperintensity (bloodlike).
C. T1 hyperintensity, T2 hyperintensity (waterlike).
D. T1 hypointensity, T2 hypointensity (fibrous-like).

Later stages are associated with more severe symptoms, poorer response to core decompression, and later radiographic stage. A commonly used plain film classification system, modified by Cruess, follows:

I. Normal radiograph.
II. Areas of bone sclerosis and lysis.
III. Subchondral sclerotic crescent.
IV. Femoral head collapse.
V. Arthritis with erosions and acetabular involvement.

All patients with suspected AVN should have both hips imaged and examined simultaneously.

DIAGNOSIS: Patient 1 has sickle cell disease with ring-type AVN. Patient 2 has the speckled and extended pattern of AVN.

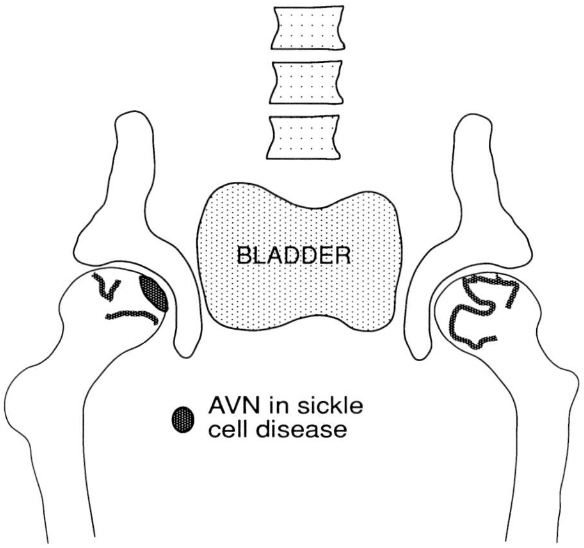

FIGURE 3-3

CASE 4

Differential Diagnosis of Hip Pain and Avascular Necrosis

HISTORY: A young boy presented with chronic left hip pain. He walked with a limp and had had decreased range of motion for 6 months. What is the MRI diagnosis? (Fig. 4-1: coronal body coil T1-weighted image. Fig. 4-2: axial multiecho proton-density (*A*) and T2-weighted (*B*) images. Fig. 4-3: for comparison, conventional anteroposterior radiograph from another patient.)

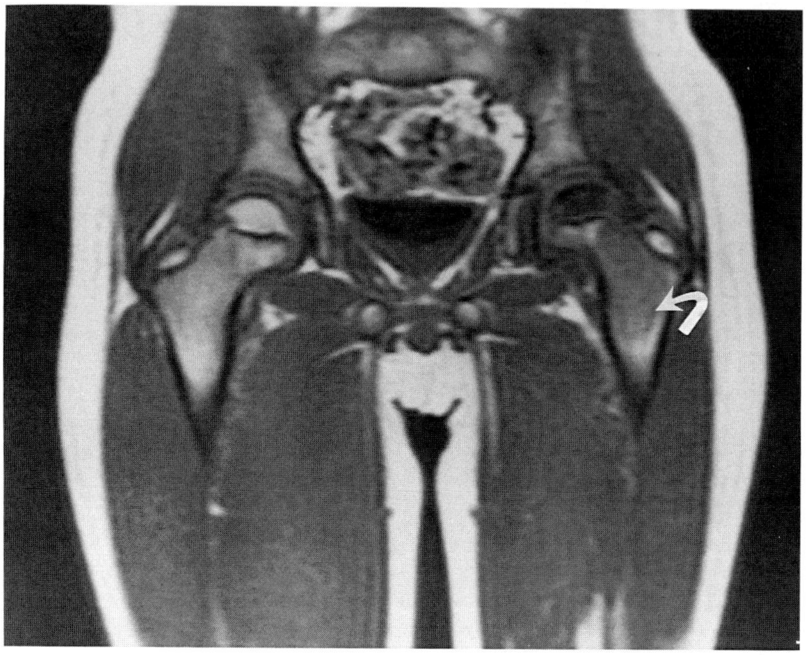

FIGURE 4-1

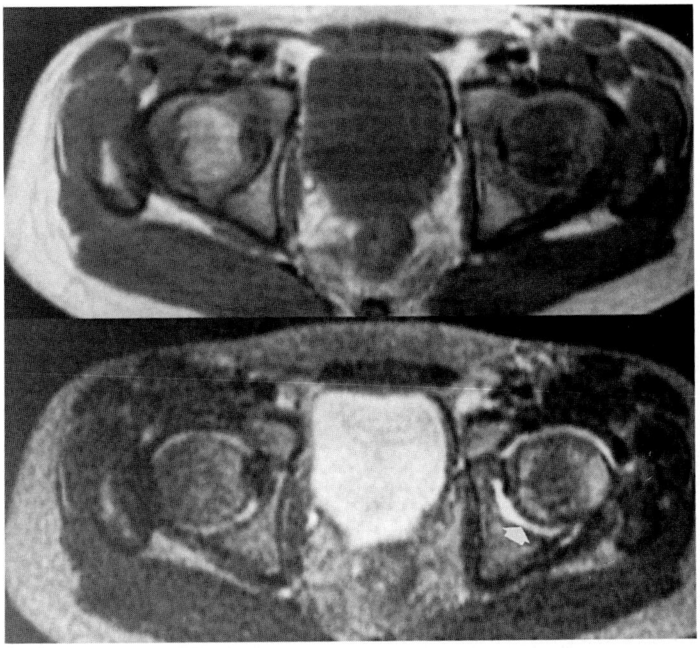

FIGURE 4-2

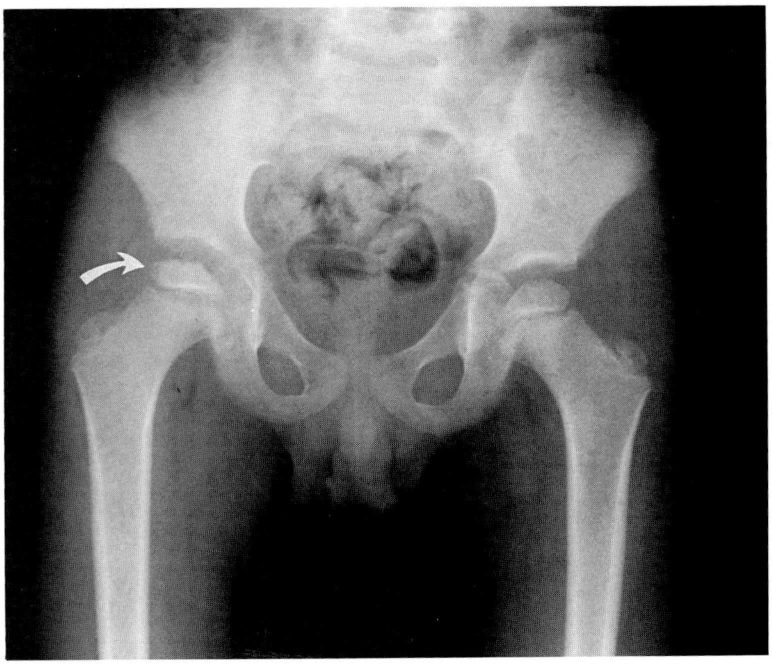

FIGURE 4-3

DISCUSSION: Like adults with avascular necrosis (AVN), children with Legg–Calvé–Perthes disease have low T1 signal in the crescent, ring, homogeneous, speckled, or extended patterns. Joint effusion (white arrow in Fig. 4-2*B*) is common on MRI in association with this entity and is important to recognize, since it may exacerbate ischemia by producing joint tamponade, but elevating intravascular and intracapsular pressures, or by compressing the retinacular vessels.

Early in the course of Legg–Calvé–Perthes disease the MR signal hypointensity may revert to normal, a phenomenon related to transient edema and observed on MRI in transient osteoporosis, stress fractures, osteomyelitis, and sickle cell crisis. Edema in the child may be quite extensive, extending into the intertrochanteric and subtrochanteric regions in many cases (curved arrow in Fig. 4-1). The edema is distinguished from areas of true necrosis or AVN by its less pronounced hypointensity on T1-weighted imaging.

Legg–Calvé–Perthes disease peaks in the 4- to 8-year-old age group, likely related to high rates of skeletal metabolism and a vascular supply that has difficulty keeping pace. Transient hip effusions due to minor trauma and congenital predisposition to increased joint pressure may contribute to the vascular tamponade and bone ischemia. The earliest MRI changes are those of simple edema. Eventually the femoral epiphysis becomes small relative to the normal side. Fragmentation, flattening, and cyst formation are common sequelae.

Of great utility in MRI is the ability of this modality to demonstrate hyaline cartilage, which permits assessment of containment of the femoral head. Containment in the acetabular fossa is a major determinant of the need for surgery versus conservative therapy.

Two methods of assessing containment are available:

1. The *acetabular head index* is calculated by dividing the width of the acetabulum by the width of the femoral head and multiplying by 100.
2. The *acetabular head quotient* is calculated by dividing the acetabular head indices of the abnormal and normal sides and multiplying by 100.

If containment is not achieved, and if the disease progresses, a small, irregularly shaped femoral head may result (curved arrow in Fig. 4-3).

DIAGNOSIS: The patient has Legg–Calvé–Perthes disease.

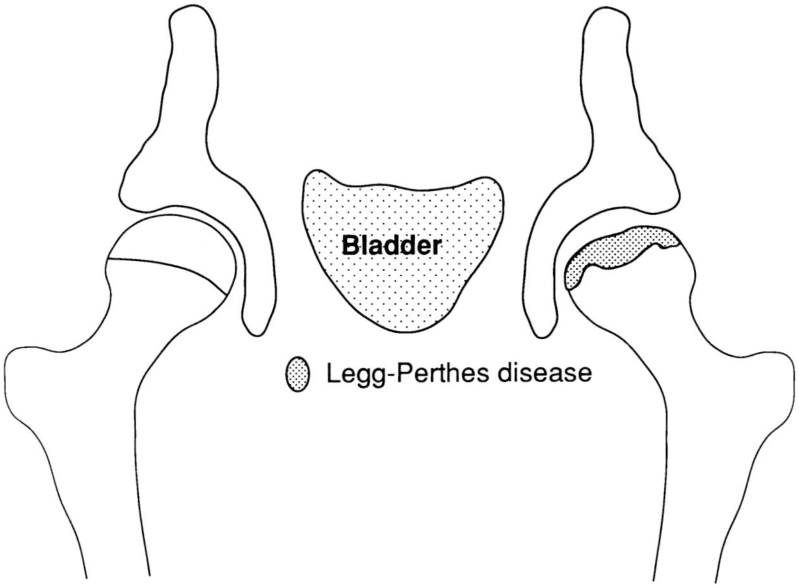

FIGURE 4-4

CASE 5

Differential Diagnosis of Hip Pain and Avascular Necrosis

HISTORY: A 31-year-old man with continuous hip pain of 1 year's duration was referred for evaluation of possible avascular necrosis. The patient was a former college football linebacker. (Figs. 5-1 through 5-3: coronal body coil contiguous 7.0-mm T1-weighted images.)

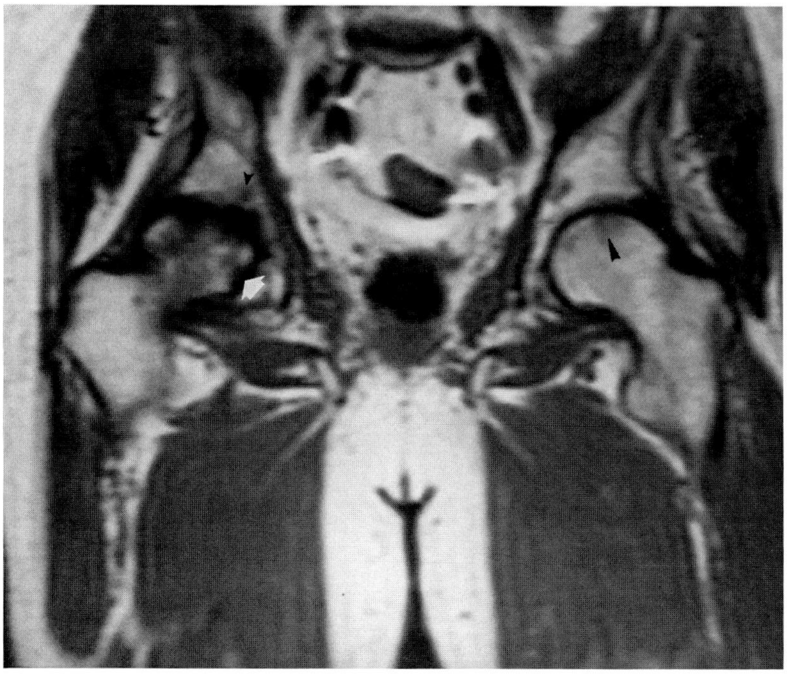

FIGURE 5-1

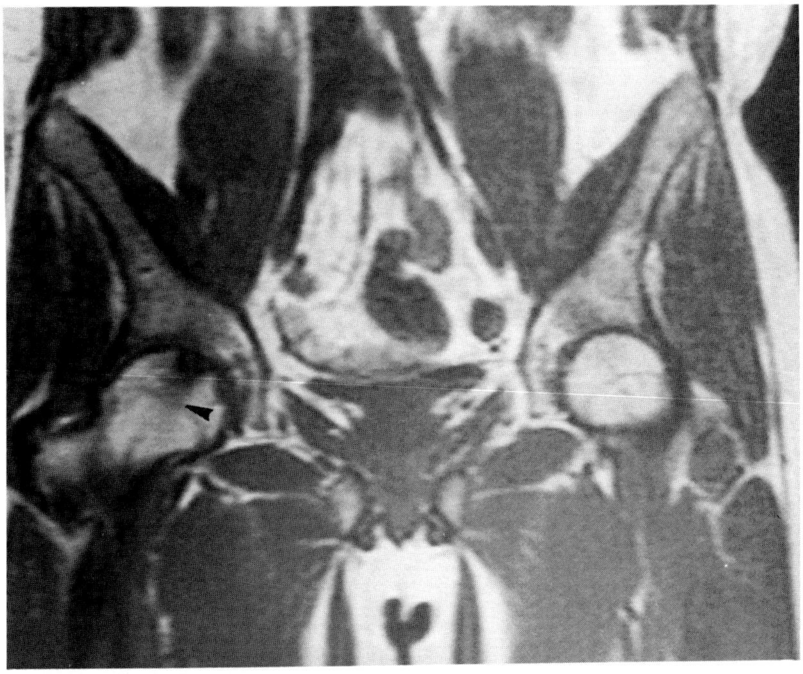

FIGURE 5-2

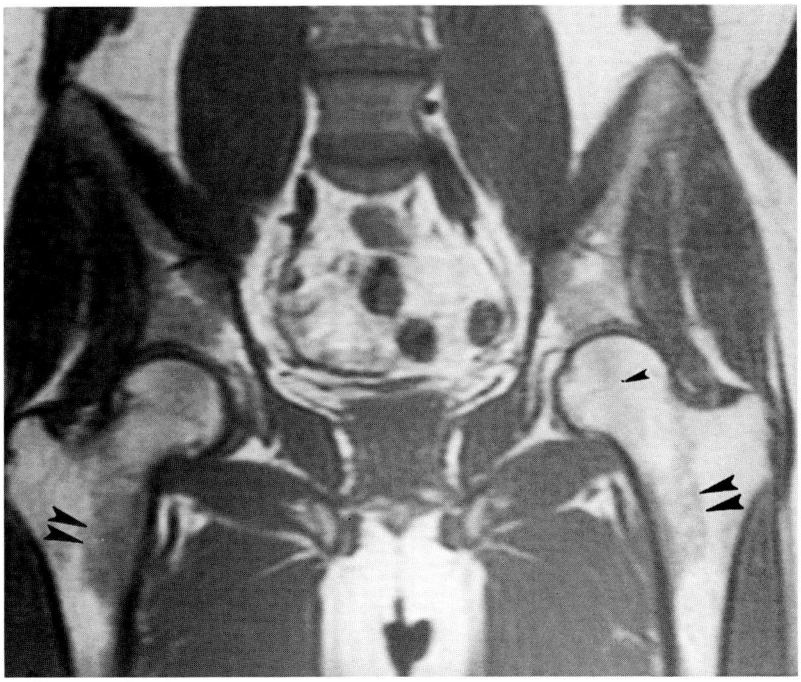

FIGURE 5-3

DISCUSSION: The diagnostic criteria and MRI appearance of avascular necrosis (AVN) were discussed in cases 1 through 4. The images in this case show patchy areas of signal hypointensity that are poorly defined, multifocal, and involve both right and, more subtly, left (medium arrowhead in Fig. 5-1) hips. Both sides of the joint are involved (small arrowhead in Fig. 5-1), a finding present only in late AVN with head collapse. Head collapse is not yet apparent. An important observation is the involvement on non-weight-bearing surfaces (white arrows in Fig. 5-1). This would be unusual in AVN. Also apparent are normal variations in the signal intensity of the hip, including (1) normal weight-bearing trabeculae that course superomedially to inferolaterally (arrowhead in Fig. 5-3), and (2) normal islands of red or hematopoietic marrow (paired arrowheads in Fig. 5-3).

In the right hip in Figure 5-2 is a large, subarticular, hypointense ulcer that does not exhibit the elliptical shape of AVN. It is associated with an exaggerated appearance of the weight-bearing trabeculae (arrowhead in Fig. 5-2), a phenomenon possible with any inflammatory or edema-producing process in the hip.

Involvement of both sides of the hip joint (see Fig. 5-6) that is multifocal, bilateral, chronic, and affects the non-weight-bearing and weight-bearing surfaces is most compatible with osteoarthritis.

MRI evaluation of the hip is incomplete without conventional radiography.

DIAGNOSIS: The patient has osteoarthritis.

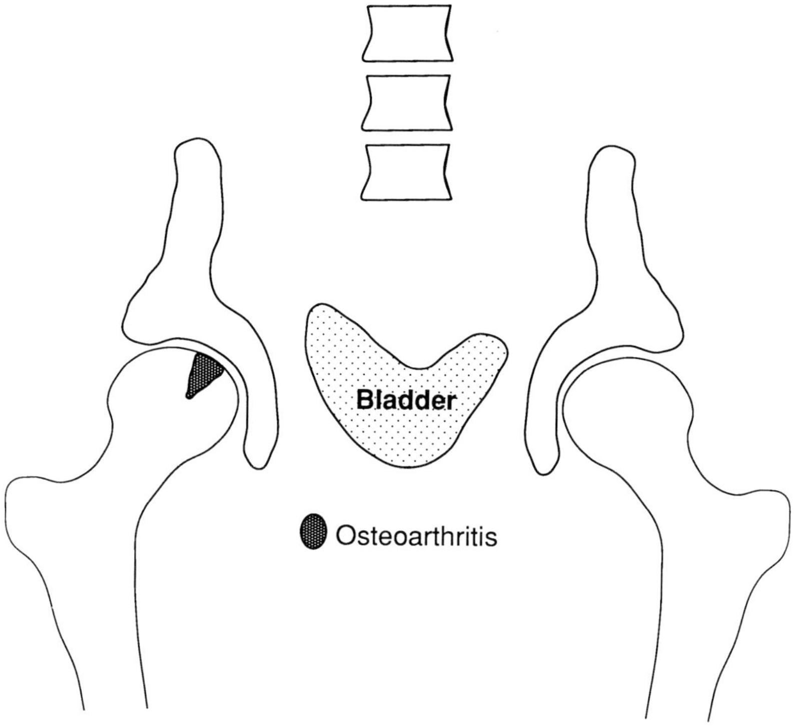

FIGURE 5-4

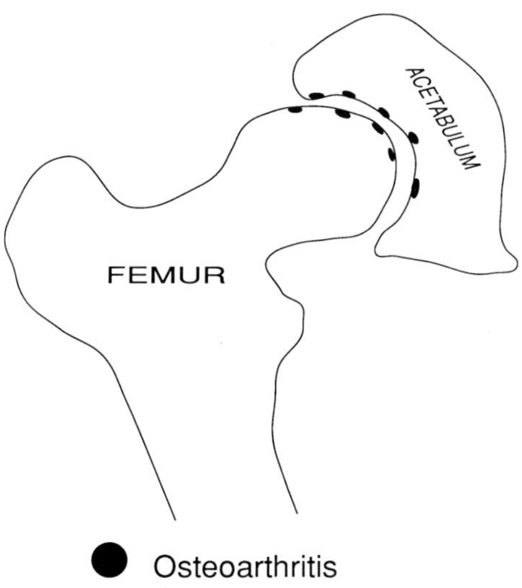

FIGURE 5-5

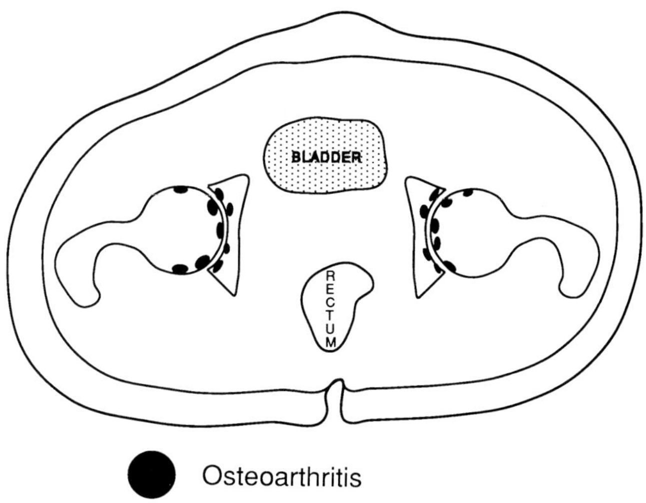

FIGURE 5-6

CASE 6

Differential Diagnosis of Hip Pain and Avascular Necrosis

HISTORY: A 9-year-old gymnast who experienced sudden pain after dismounting from the uneven parallel bars subsequently had continuous hip pain for 6 weeks. The diagnosis was apparent immediately after injury (based on clinical examination and conventional radiographs), and the patient was referred for evaluation of secondary posttraumatic avascular necrosis. What is the MRI diagnosis? (Fig. 6-1: coronal T1-weighted image.)

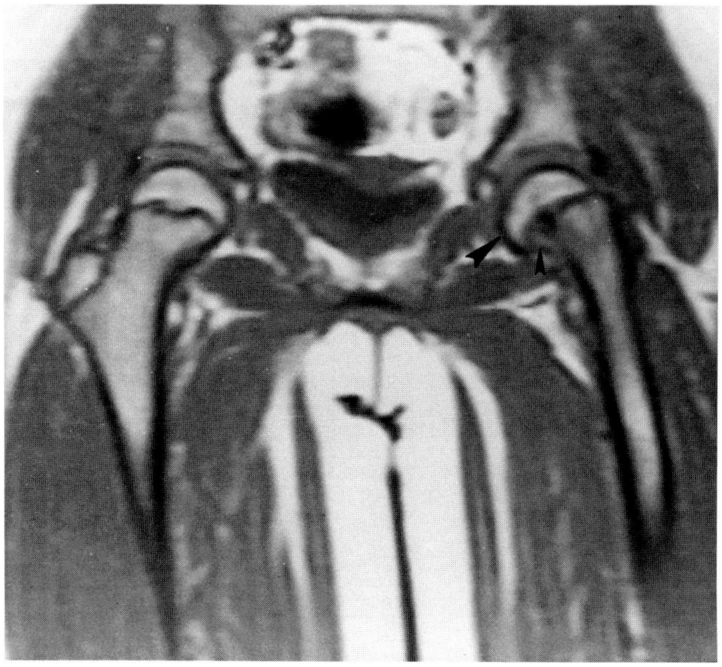

FIGURE 6-1

DISCUSSION: The left femoral head is displaced medially (large arrowhead) and posteriorly (not shown). The findings are typical of slipped capital femoral epiphysis. The patient and her physician were aware of this diagnosis immediately after her injury. The diagnosis at that time was determined from a conventional radiograph. The referral was to exclude avascular necrosis (AVN). The left femoral epiphysis is relatively homogeneous and hyperintense. However, it is slightly hypointense relative to the normal right epiphysis, owing to the presence of mild edema. No evidence of AVN is present.

In patients less than 12 years old the epiphysis normally stands out because of the abundance of red marrow in the subepiphyseal femur (isointense to hypointense), whereas yellow marrow predominates in the epiphyses. Red marrow persists homogeneously in the prepubescent patient and then as patchy islands of hypointensity up to age 50. After age 50, yellow marrow predominates throughout the subepiphyseal femoral region.

Slipped capital femoral epiphysis is a disorder of adolescents, with boys affected more frequently than girls. Affected children are often overweight. In boys, the left hip is affected with twice the frequency of the right. The exact traumatic event may be difficult to ascertain. This injury is a Salter-Harris I fracture. Usually the epiphysis is displaced posteroinferomedially, as in this case. A varus deformity with external rotation and adduction results.

In addition to displacement and edema of the femoral head, the conventional radiographic signs (see Fig. 6-2) are also visible on MRI. These radiographic signs include

1. The triangle sign of Capener (small arrowhead in Fig. 6-1): an intracapsular area of the medial femoral neck overlaps the posterior acetabulum and produces plain film sclerosis or MRI hypointensity;
2. loss of femoral head height;
3. intersection of the epiphysis with a lateral cortical line of the femoral neck no longer visible (see Fig. 6-2), and
4. widening or prominence of the physis, particularly well seen medially in this case.

DIAGNOSIS: The patient has slipped capital femoral epiphysis.

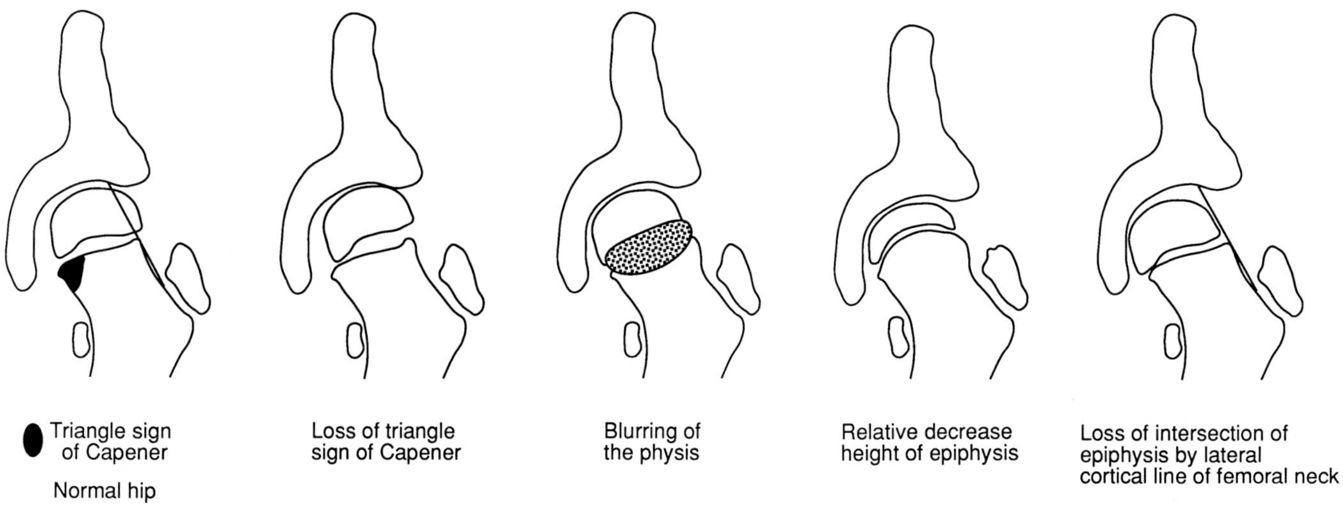

FIGURE 6-2

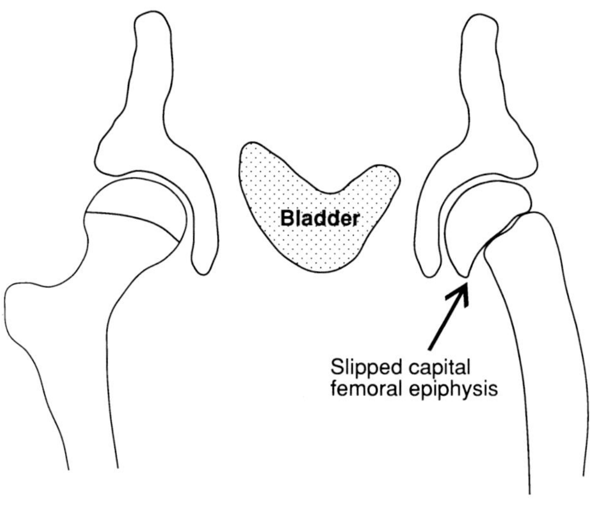

FIGURE 6-3

CASE 7

Differential Diagnosis of Hip Pain and Avascular Necrosis

HISTORY: A 34-year-old man underwent radiologic evaluation for hip pain of 5 weeks' duration. Conventional radiographs were normal. What is the MRI diagnosis? (Fig. 7-1: coronal T1-weighted image.)

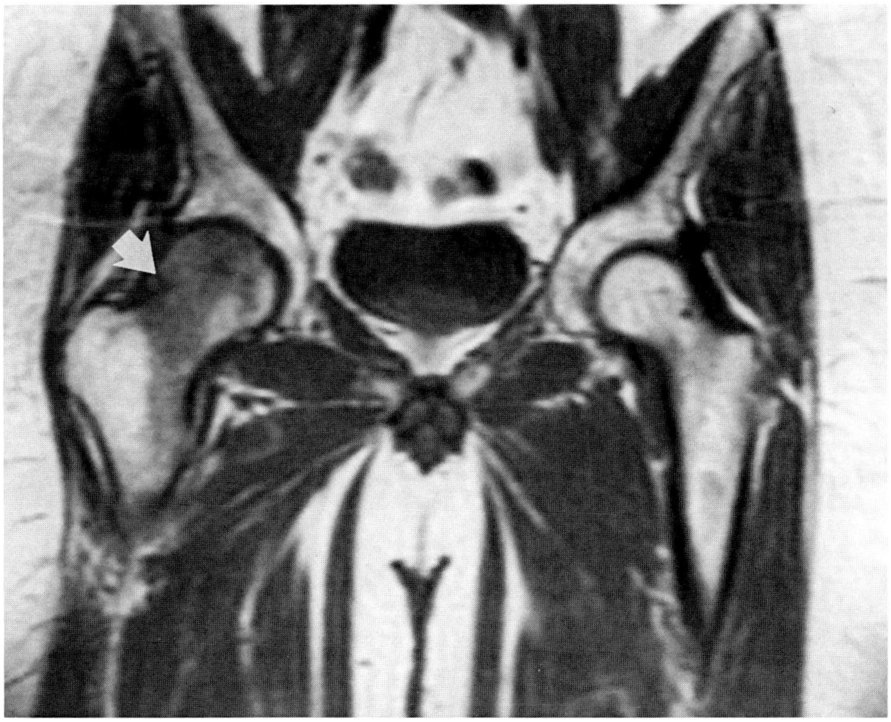

FIGURE 7-1

DISCUSSION: Transient osteoporosis is the most likely diagnosis. Transient osteoporosis was originally described in pregnant women but has since been found to affect middle-aged men. Insidious hip pain occurs over several months to a year. Hyperintense edema may be present on T2-weighted or fast scan imaging, and small joint effusions are almost always found. Demineralization on computed tomography or conventional radiography and increased uptake on bone scintigraphy are characteristic findings. Other conditions that may produce extensive bone edema in the hip and intertrochanteric region include extended pattern avascular necrosis (AVN), osteomyelitis or septic arthritis, stress fractures, and metastatic neoplasm.

The diffuse signal hypointensity in the right hip (arrow in Fig. 7-1), is not typical of AVN. AVN has a subcapital distribution; however, an extended pattern of AVN can produce diffuse low signal on T1-weighted imaging. Metastases appear as focal lesions with or without an associated soft tissue mass. Osteomyelitis is associated with irregular signal hypointensity on T1-weighted imaging.

Stress fractures produce horizontal foci of hypointense signal on T1-weighted imaging, particularly in the intertrochanteric region. In septic arthritis, joint effusions with surrounding hyperintense T2 soft tissue edema predominate. The etiology of this condition is related to hyperemia, marrow edema, and subsequent increased bone mineral turnover; thus the term *transient bone marrow edema syndrome* has been used to describe this condition. The pathophysiology is similar to that of regional migratory osteoporosis or reflex sympathetic dystrophy. In this disorder, transient patchy osteoporosis is found in an extremity or extremities. Migration to contiguous bones or joints is common.

DIAGNOSIS: The patient has transient osteoporosis or bone marrow edema syndrome of the hip.

CASE 8

Differential Diagnosis of Hip Pain and Avascular Necrosis

HISTORY: A 27-year-old man presented with hip pain of 3 months' duration. What is the MRI diagnosis? (Fig. 8-1: coronal T1-weighted image. Fig. 8-2: axial multiformat, multiecho proton-density (*A*) and T2-weighted (*B*) images.)

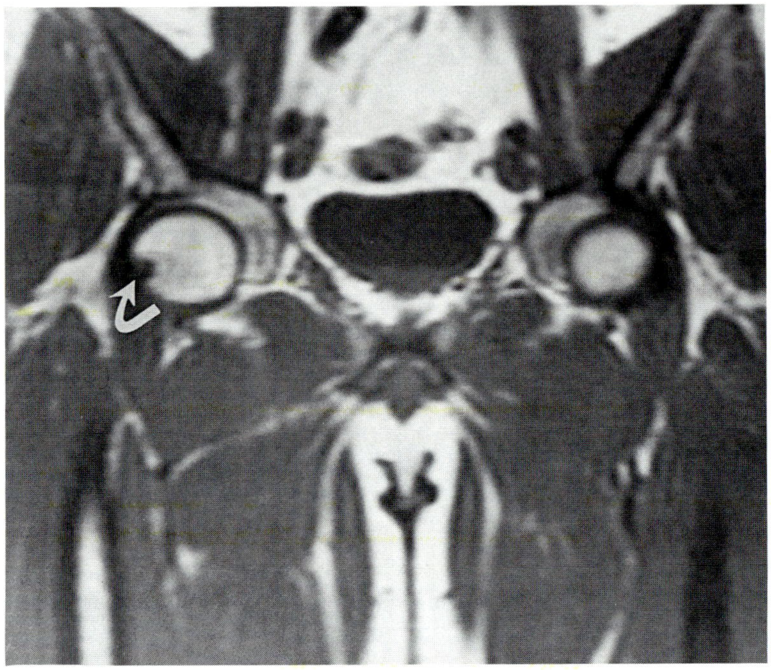

FIGURE 8-1

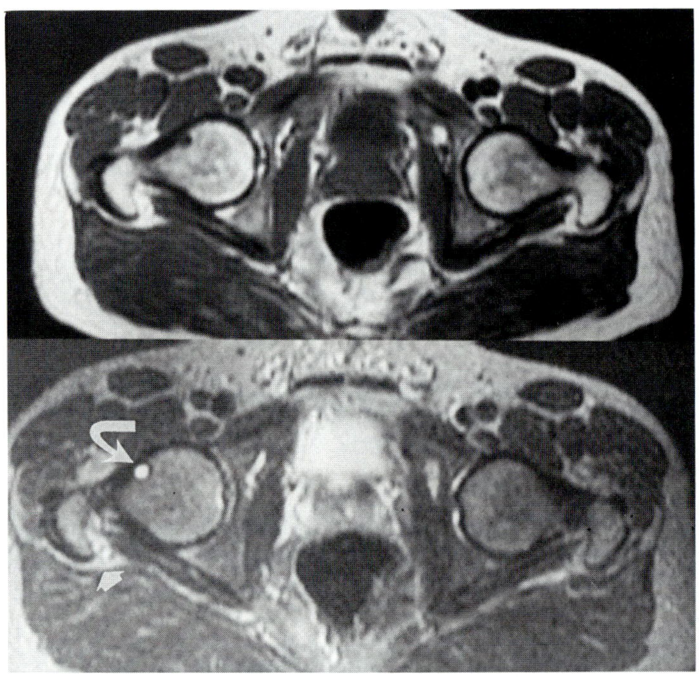

FIGURE 8-2

DISCUSSION: Not to be confused on MRI with avascular necrosis, cyst, or neoplasm, herniation pits are incidental asymptomatic findings that occur in 4% of the population. Mechanical effects of the anterior hip capsule produce this reactive phenomenon on the anterosuperior femoral neck surface. After the soft tissue reaction, the trabecular and medullary bone becomes exposed, allowing adjacent soft tissues to form a subcortical pit.

On MRI, lesions are round (curved white arrows in Fig. 8-1 and 8-2*A*) or oval and bright on T2-weighted images if they contain fluid (80%). Occasionally the lesions may not contain fluid but just fibrous tissue producing low signal (20%) on all pulse sequences. On T1 or fat suppression images, a markedly hypointense ring of sclerotic, reactive new bone may be seen surrounding the pit.

The key to the diagnosis of herniation pit and its differentiation from osteoid osteoma is communication of the hyperintense T2 pit with the cortical surface. Brodie abscess might mimic a herniation pit in signal intensity, but the location of the pit assists in differentiation. Intraosseous ganglia may also mimic the signal intensity of a herniation pit. Ganglia are subarticular and produce pain, but unlike pits, they are lined by synovial-like cells and do not communicate with the articular surface. Location in the anterosuperior quadrant of the femoral neck favors herniation pit over other diagnoses, including intraosseous ganglion. Metastases typically do not exhibit the hypointense pit ring, are not as bright on T2-weighted imaging, and do not communicate with the cortical surface.

DIAGNOSIS: The patient has a herniation pit.

CASE 9

Differential Diagnosis of Hip Pain

HISTORY: A 60-year-old woman with persistent left hip pain and tenderness for 2 weeks presented with fever and a white blood cell count of 20,000/mm^3. What is the MRI diagnosis? (Fig. 9-1: external rotation radiograph of the right hip. Fig. 9-2: coronal T1-weighted image. Fig. 9-3: axial multiformat (two-on-one), multiecho proton-density (*A*) and T2-weighted (*B*) images.)

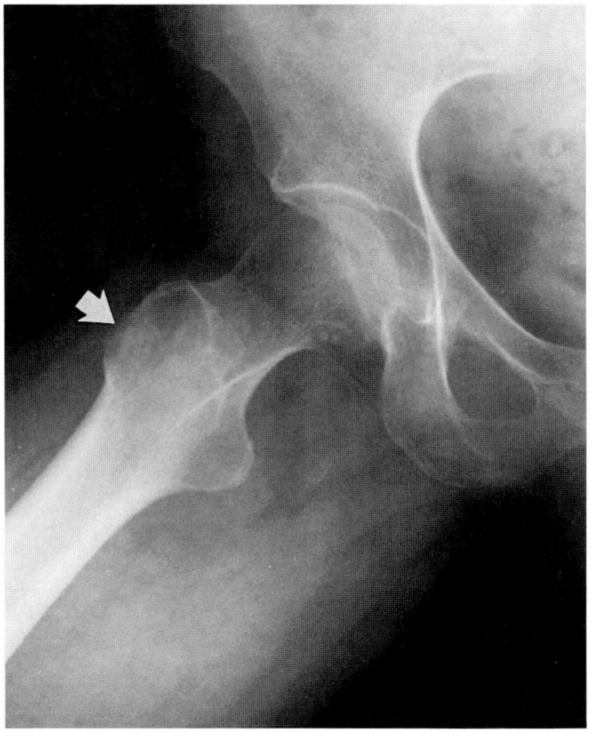

FIGURE 9-1

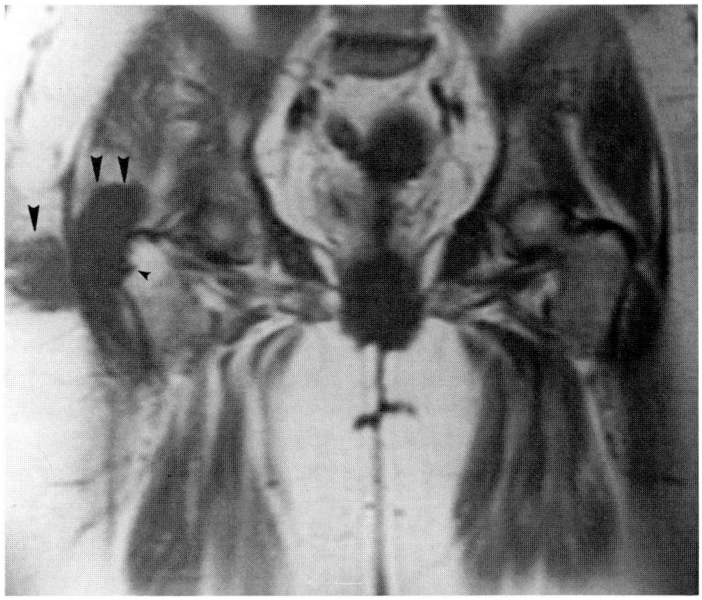

FIGURE 9-2

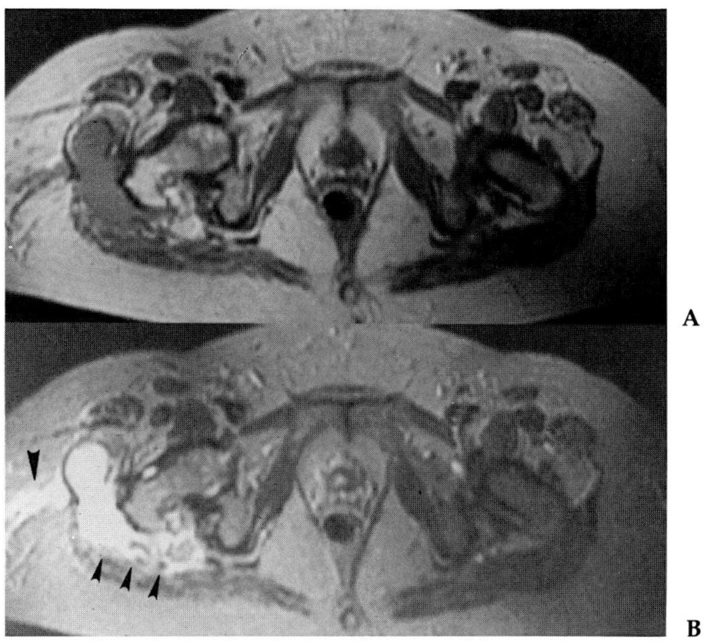

FIGURE 9-3

DISCUSSION: The conventional radiograph shows a subtle area of cortical irregularity without obvious bone destruction (arrow). On the coronal T1-weighted image, a notch or defect in the greater trochanter (small arrowhead in Fig. 9-2) lies deep to a fluid collection that is hypointense on T1-weighted imaging (paired arrowheads in Fig. 9-2) and hyperintense on T2-weighted imaging. The signal of the collection on T1-weighted imaging is not as hypointense as water, as would be the case for cerebrospinal fluid or urine in the bladder. More important, the fluid collection extends around the greater trochanter (triple arrowheads in Fig. 9-3*B*) to involve the posterior myofascial tissues. This process has begun to point to the surface (single arrowheads in Figs. 9-2 and 9-3*B*). The findings are typical of trochanteric bursal abscess with septic arthritis. The changes in the underlying bone suggest concomitant osteomyelitis. Simple bursitis would not be expected to invade or involve adjacent myofascial tissues and extend into the subcutaneous space. Simple bursitis produces a homogeneous signal intensity of water, virtually identical to the MRI appearance of urine in the bladder. Aspiration of this collection revealed frank pus.

DIAGNOSIS: The patient has septic arthritis with a trochanteric bursal abscess and underlying osteomyelitis.

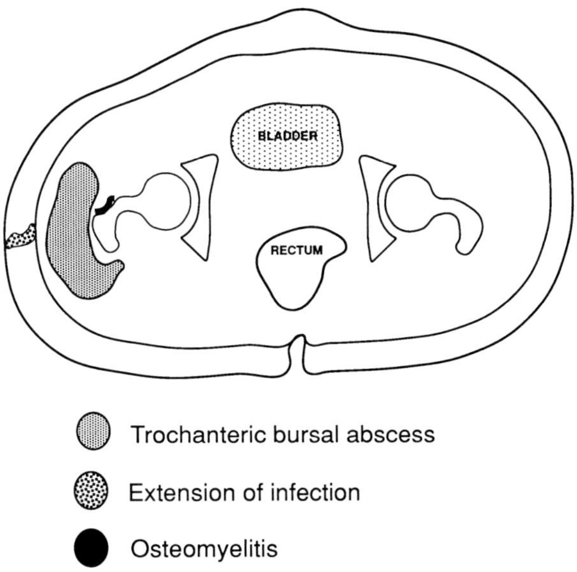

FIGURE 9-4

CASE 10

Differential Diagnosis of Hip Pain

HISTORY: This case study presents four cases of hip pain. The diagnosis was similar in each case but was not known or suspected before MRI was performed. What is the common MRI diagnosis, and what are the MRI signs of this entity? (Patient 1—Fig. 10-1: coronal T1-weighted image. Patient 2—Fig. 10-2: axial multiformat (four-on-one), multiecho proton-density (*A, C*) and T2-weighted (*B, D*) images. Patient 3—Fig. 10-3: axial multiformat (four-on-one) T1-weighted images, and Fig. 10-4: coronal multiformat (two-on-one) T1-weighted images. Patient 4—Fig. 10-5: coronal T1-weighted image; Fig. 10-6: axial multiformat (two-on-one), multiecho proton-density (*A*) and T2-weighted (*B*) images; and Fig. 10-7: conventional anteroposterior radiograph.)

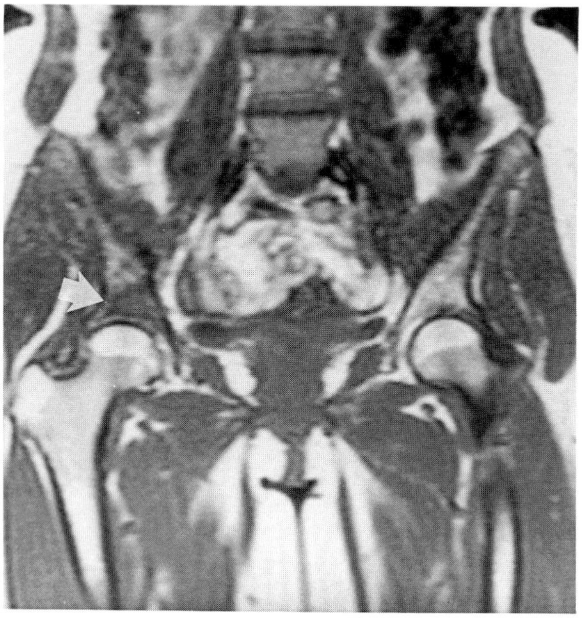

FIGURE 10-1

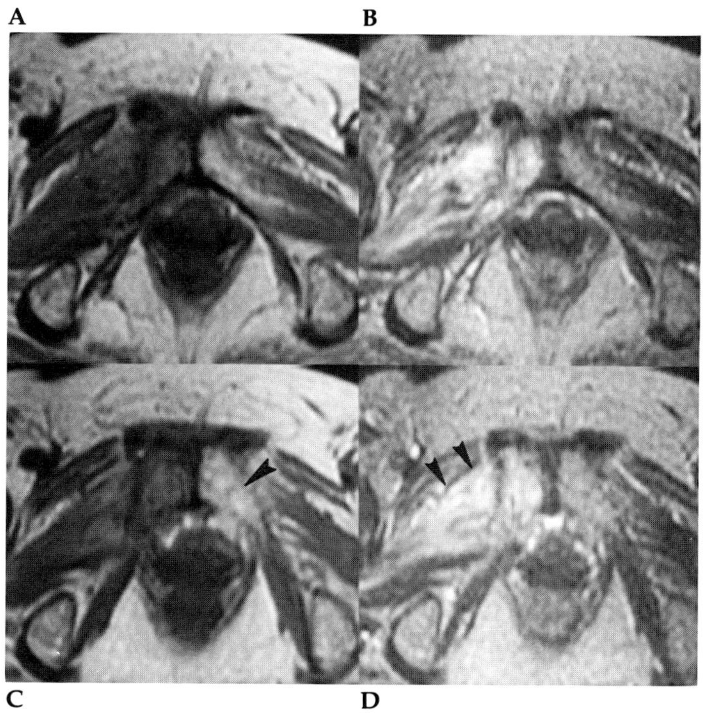

FIGURE 10-2

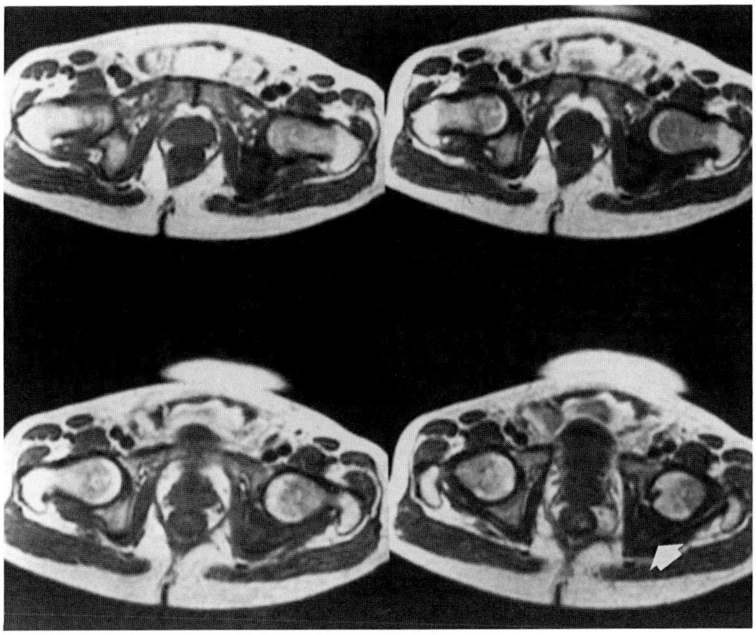

A B C D

FIGURE 10-3

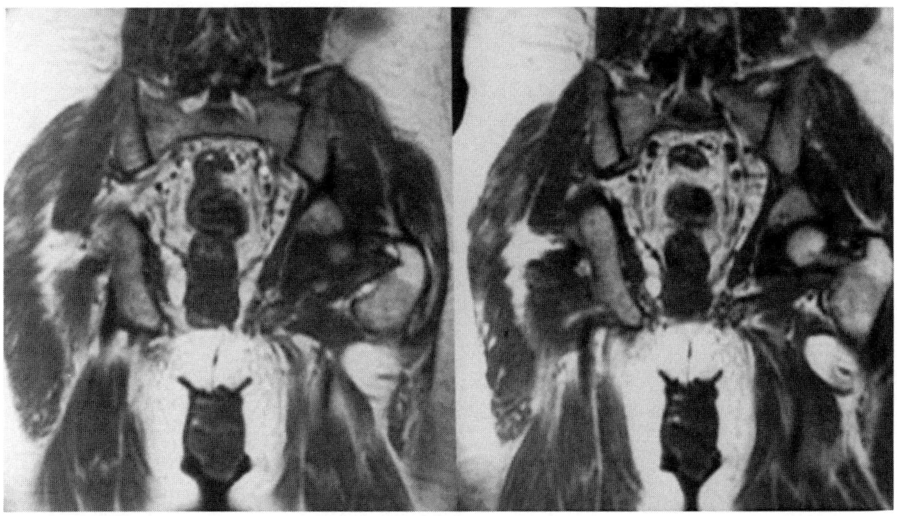

A B

FIGURE 10-4

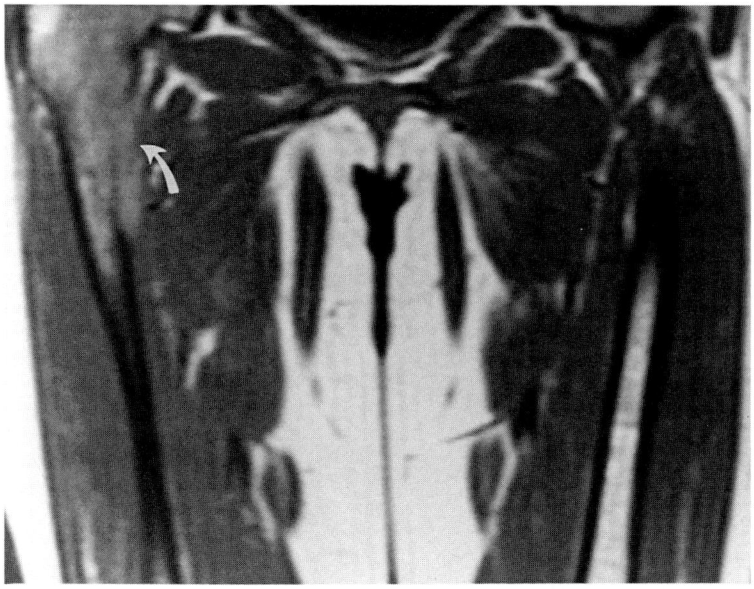

FIGURE 10-5

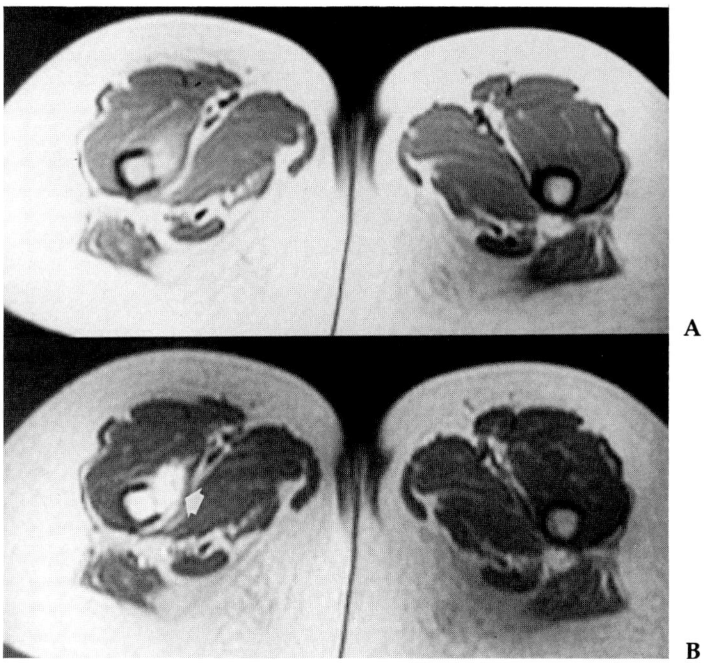

FIGURE 10-6

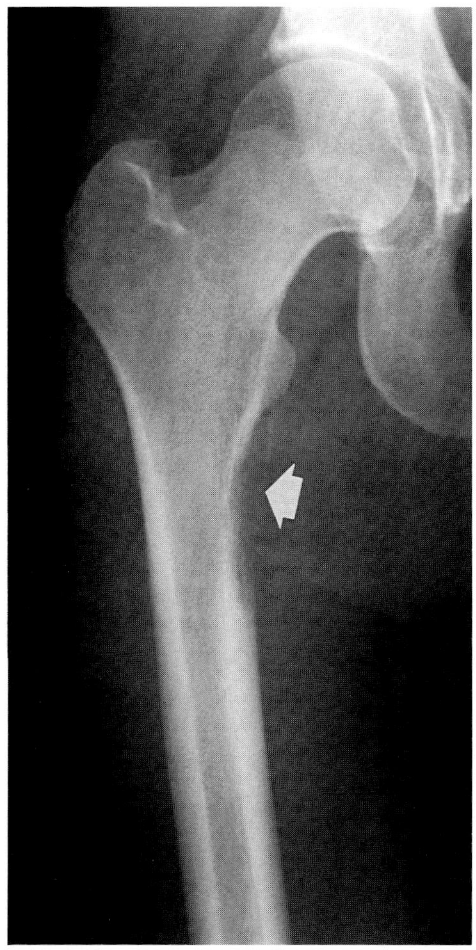

FIGURE 10-7

DISCUSSION: While islands of red marrow are common in the intertrochanteric and subtrochanteric regions, these areas are patchy, not well defined, hypointense on T1-weighted imaging, and do not increase in signal intensity on T2-weighted imaging. The cases presented have numerous features of aggressive neoplastic disease, including:

1. definite marrow asymmetry (white arrows in Figs. 10-1 and 10-3*D*),
2. well-defined lesions with oblique or rounded margins,
3. areas of homogeneous marrow replacement that become hyperintense on T2-weighted imaging (arrowheads in Fig. 10-2*D*, white arrow in Fig. 10-6*B*), and
4. cortical interruption with soft tissue involvement (curved white arrow in Fig. 10-5).

It is common to scrutinize the femoral head during hip evaluations, particularly for avascular necrosis. A subtle skeletal asymmetry is noticeable in the T1-weighted coronal images (Figs. 10-4*A* and *B*, arrows intentionally omitted), with marked signal hypointensity in the left ischium compared with the right. Metastatic disease is always hypointense on T1-weighted imaging and variable in signal intensity on T2-weighted imaging. Various fat suppression techniques have been used to increase the sensitivity of MRI in the detection of skeletal lesions by making areas of edema and marrow replacement hyperintense and normal yellow marrow hypointense. These techniques include two basic pulse sequences: short-time inversion-recovery (STIR), and chemical saturation. STIR works by the selection of an inversion time (T1) that corresponds to the zero or null zone of fat; therefore, fat-containing structures will appear hypointense. Chemical saturation works by selectively saturating the hydrogen protons in fat and sparing the hydrogen protons in water. This is possible because the resonant frequency of the two varies slightly, allowing selective excitation of one without the other.

Critical to the assessment of metastatic disease is knowledge of the pulse sequence used. Note that in Figures 10-2*C* and *D* the left inferior pubic ramus is hyperintense on T1-weighted images (arrowhead in *C*) but the right ramus and adductor muscle group are hyperintense (paired arrowheads in *D*). A useful rule of thumb to follow is: "White is benign on T1-weighted imaging." In other words, the bright signal marrow is almost always the nonpathologic or nonmalignant marrow on T1-weighted images. Although the T2 signal of metastatic disease varies, most lesions are hyperintense. Therefore, the right inferior pubic ramus and muscle group are involved by neoplasm.

The last lesson to be derived from this group of cases relates to the statement "white is right on T1-weighted imaging" and to the lesion in patient 4 (Fig. 10-5). Although I have not seen a truly hyperintense metastasis on T1-weighted imaging, the potential exists for such a phenomenon to occur, particularly with melanoma. Melanin itself can be paramagnetic, but for the most part, the hyperintensity on T1-weighted images and hypointensity on T2-weighted images seen in melanoma are related to hemorrhage. The lesion in patient 4 is exophytic, not as hypointense as most metastatic lesions but not as hyperintense as fat on T1-weighted imaging, and extremely hyperintense on T2-weighted imaging. Pathologically, it contained melanin and foci of hemorrhage. The aggressive nature of this lesion is best appreciated as corticomedullary bone destruction on the conventional radiograph (arrow in Fig. 10-7).

Finally, MR examination of the hip is not complete without conventional radiographs. Hemorrhagic metastases to the skeleton usually have been previously irradiated or are very large, with soft tissue involvement or cortical destruction, so that their identification as aggressive lesions is easy at this point. Smaller lesions do not usually bleed unless irradiated. However, bone irradiation makes detection of metastases easier on MRI and more difficult on conventional radiography. Bone becomes more lucent and subsequently sclerotic on plain films, and either appearance may simulate neoplasm. However, radiation produces pronounced red to yellow marrow reconversion. Whiter marrow aids both the detection of hypointense metastases and the identification of margins of hemorrhagic metastases.

DIAGNOSIS: These cases represent multiple examples of skeletal metastases first evident as hip pain.

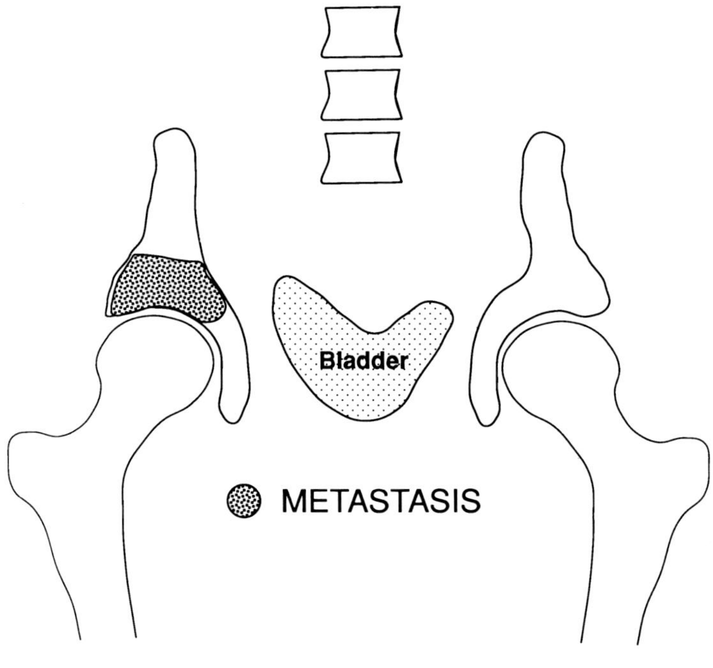

FIGURE 10-8

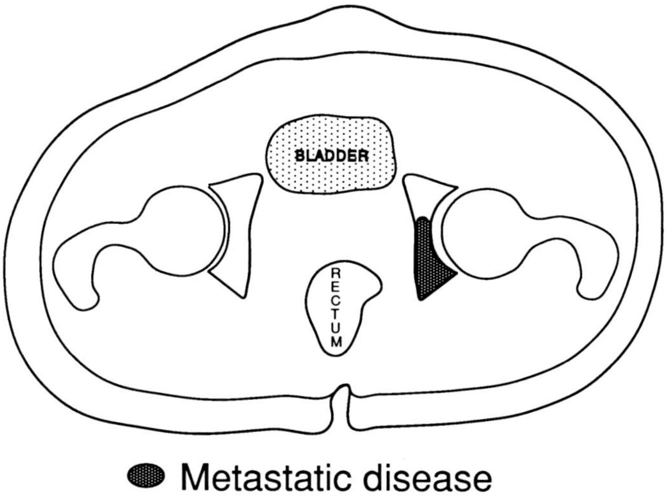

FIGURE 10-9

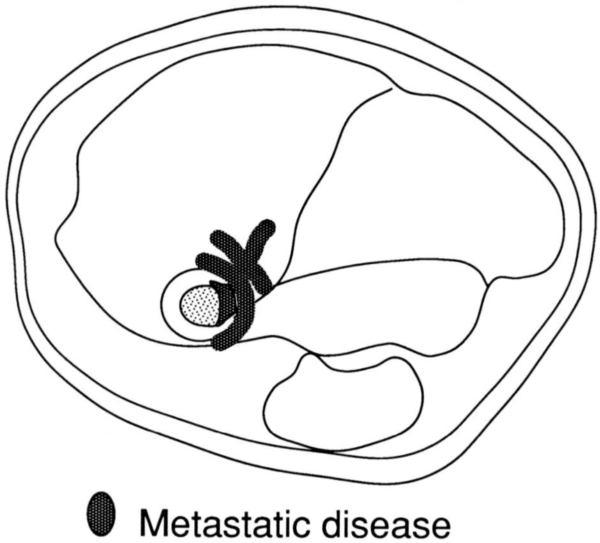

FIGURE 10-10

CASE 11

Differential Diagnosis of Hip Pain

HISTORY: A 31-year-old woman presented with hip pain but was otherwise well. What is the MRI diagnosis? (Fig. 11-1: coronal T1-weighted image. Fig. 11-2: axial multiformat (two-on-one), multiecho proton-density (*A*) and T2-weighted (*B*) images.)

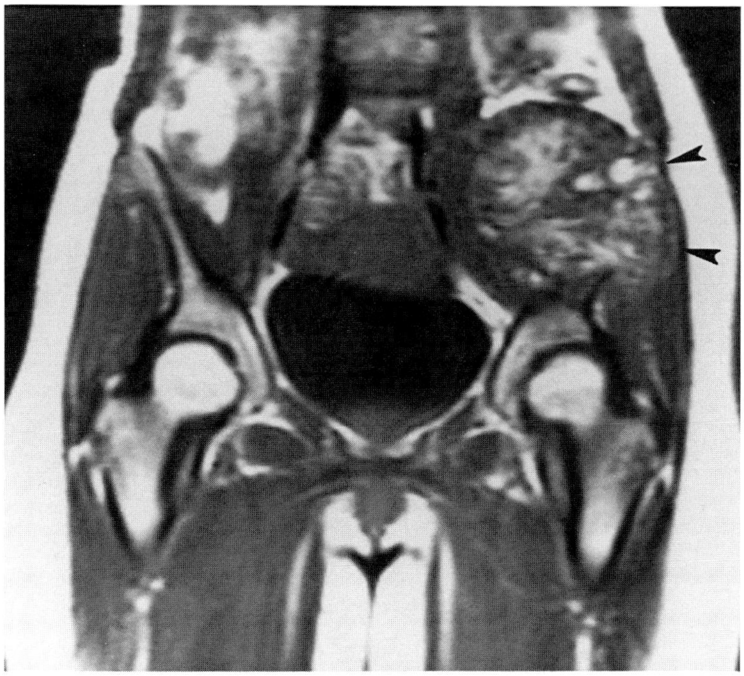

FIGURE 11-1

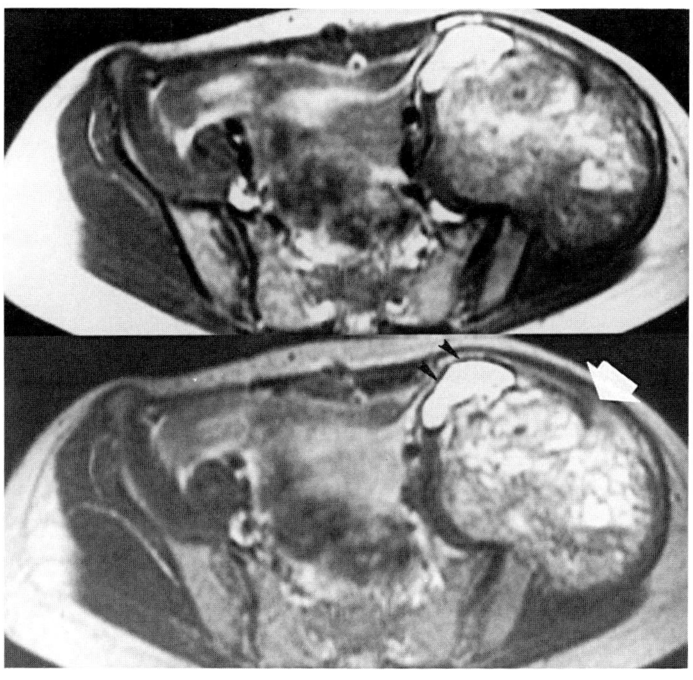

FIGURE 11-2

DISCUSSION: A large mass has replaced and grown through the ilium (arrowheads in Fig. 11-1). It was palpable and produced an apparent bulge or visible protrusion on the patient (white arrow in Fig. 11-2*B*) and contained mixed foci of hyperintensity on T2-weighted imaging, some quite large (paired arrowheads in Fig. 11-2*B*). This mixed "bowl of fruit" or "popcorn" signal inhomogeneity has been classically described in malignant fibrous histiocytoma; however, we have observed the same phenomenon in chondrosarcoma and synovial sarcoma. This particular lesion is destroying a flat bone, and statistically it is far more likely to represent chondrosarcoma than the other two lesions, which are neoplasms of soft tissue. Osteogenic sarcoma tends not to appear so inhomogeneous on MRI, and cystic areas as well as flat bone involvement are far more common with chondroid malignancy.

Chondrosarcomas usually originate in bone (central type), but extracortical lesions do occur (peripheral or juxtacortical chondrosarcoma). They may arise as primary neoplasms or secondary to other processes including Paget's disease, irradiated bone, chondroma or enchondromas, and osteochondromas. Syndromes such as hereditary exostoses and multiple enchondromatosis are prone to chondrosarcoma. In these instances MRI may prove useful in mapping out sites of cyst formation, eccentric growth, or signal asymmetry.

Primary chondrosarcomas may be divided into central, periosteal, mesenchymal, dedifferentiated, or clear cell types, and those secondary to chondroblastoma.

1. *Juxtacortical lesions* are rare, involve the femoral shaft, affect young patients, and may arise from or be the malignant counterpart of juxtacortical chondroma.
2. *Mesenchymal lesions* are rare, often multicentric, arise from the soft tissues, and have a terrible prognosis.
3. *Clear cell chondroblastoma* is an expansile, noncalcified, rare lesion that has a predilection for the epiphyses (especially femoral). This lesion may be expansile and may mimic chondroblastoma or giant cell tumor (see case 91 in Chapter 1, The Knee).
4. *Dedifferentiated chondrosarcomas* have a poor prognosis and arise from preexisting lesions. Specifically, the chondrosarcoma arising from Paget's disease has large exophytic cysts associated with it that look benign and contain gelatinous material that is extremely hyperintense and multilobulated on T2-weighted imaging.
5. *Central chondrosarcoma* is the most likely diagnosis in this case, even though 50% of cases occur after age 50. Generally, this lesion has a better prognosis than osteogenic sarcoma; however, the prognosis worsens the closer the lesion lies to the axial skeleton. The pelvic and shoulder regions are most commonly affected, and lesions may recur long after excision, migrating up or down the body to new sites years later. This lesion spreads hematogenously; therefore, lymphadenopathy is extremely rare for this reason.

DIAGNOSIS: The patient has a central chondrosarcoma.

CASE 12

Differential Diagnosis of Hip Pain

HISTORY: A 64-year-old woman with known Paget's disease reported progressive severe pain in the right hip and thigh of 3 months' duration. A secondary malignant neoplasm was suspected from the conventional radiograph. Do the MRI findings support this diagnosis? (Fig. 12-1: conventional anteroposterior radiograph of the right femur. Figs. 12-2, 12-3, and 12-4: respectively axial T1-weighted image, proton-density image, and T2-weighted image obtained directly through the area of lysis or rarefaction on the plain radiograph.)

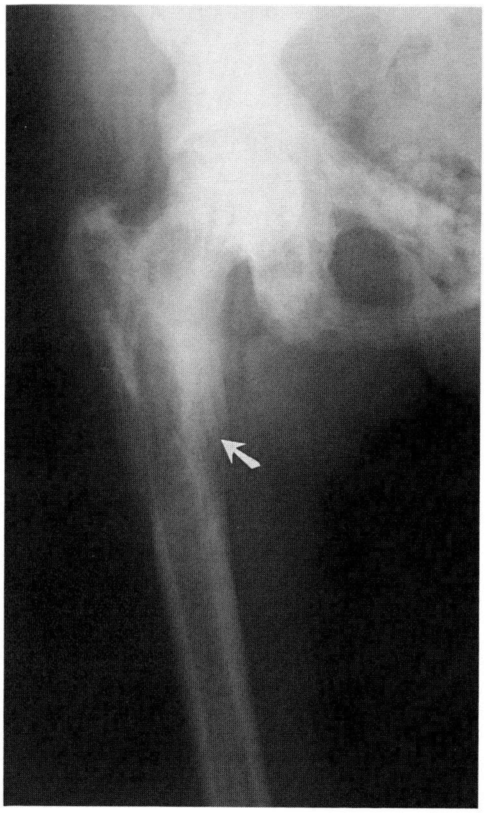

FIGURE 12-1

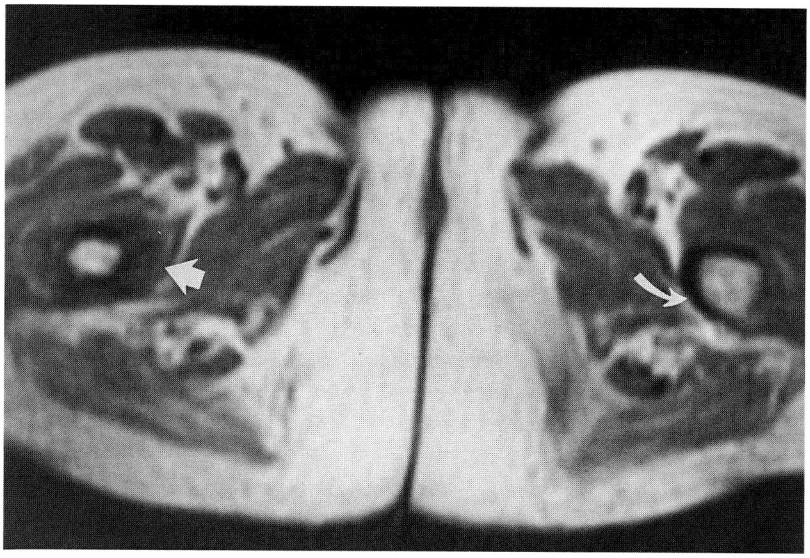

FIGURE 12-2

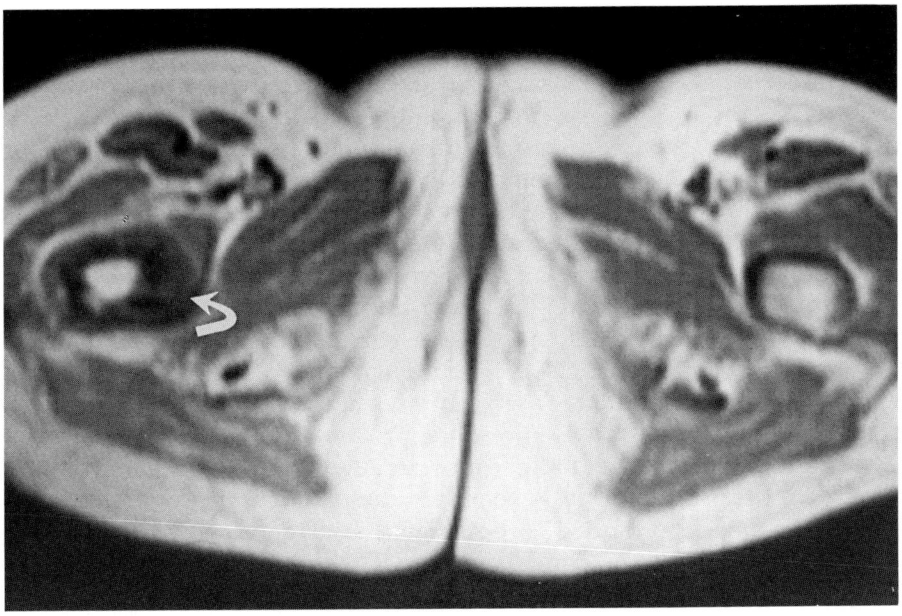

FIGURE 12-3

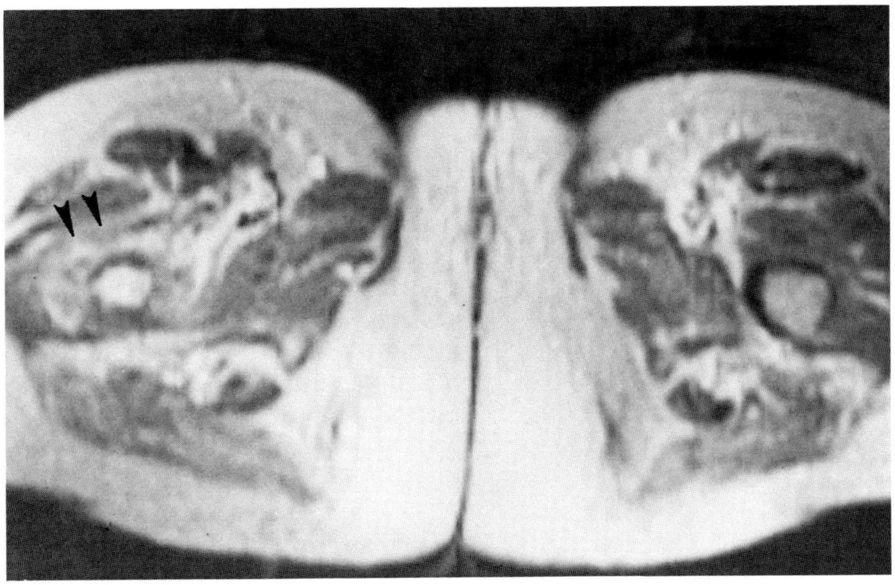

FIGURE 12-4

DISCUSSION: Rarefaction or lucency in the subtrochanteric medial femur (arrow in Fig. 12-1) was cause for concern in this patient, who was experiencing increasing pain from Paget's disease. The cortex of the left femur appears as a circumferential hypointense thin rim around the hyperintense homogeneous medullary bone on the T2-weighted image. The normal left cortex maintains its signal hypointensity on the T2-weighted image, and the medullary bone becomes less intense (curved arrow in Fig. 12-2). The right femoral medullary cavity is shrunken and encroached on by the cortex, a thick circumferential band of intermediate signal intensity on the T1-weighted and proton-density images (arrow in Fig. 12-2, curved arrow in Fig. 12-3). The cortical thickening seen on the proton-density image encircles the femur without focal protrusion or destruction of the medullary cavity center.

Despite the marked rarefaction of the proximal femur on the conventional radiograph, tumors do not grow circumferentially and symmetrically. With preservation of the medullary cavity, circumferential growth, and homogeneous expanded cortical signal, a diagnosis of accelerated Paget's disease without secondary malignant degeneration was made. The patient was treated with metabolic therapy for 6 months and subsequently followed for 3 years, with marked improvement in radiographic and clinical status.

Paget's disease is a metabolic bone disorder that occurs in midlife (45 to 55 years). Radiographically it appears as areas of lysis, sclerosis, or mixed lysis and sclerosis. Men predominate slightly (3 : 2 ratio), and the disease has a geographic predilection peaking in Great Britain, Australia, and New Zealand. This suggests an infectious or viral etiology. The pelvis is the most common site of involvement and is usually affected in the sclerotic phase of the disease. A lucency that becomes focal after the sclerotic phase has occurred may be related to lytic Paget's disease, cystic degeneration, fracture, sarcomatous degeneration, giant cell tumor, and coincidental lesions.

In the early phases (lytic or mixed lytic sclerotic phase) of Paget's disease, the cortex is widened and assumes a less hypointense T1 signal that becomes hyperintense on T2-weighted imaging (paired arrowheads in Fig. 12-4), due to hypervascularity and edema. Enhancement has been consistent with intravenous MRI contrast agents, so the sheetlike hyperintensity occurs at the affected location on contrast-enhanced MRI.

As the disease becomes more sclerotic, the cortex widens further and begins to encroach on the medullary cavity; however, the T2 cortical hyperintensity wanes and may become hypointense. The medullary signal may exhibit slight hyper- or hypointensity on T2-weighted imaging, depending on the degree of encroachment. In the calvarium the intradiploic hyperintense T1 fat signal is diminished in Paget's disease and in osteoporosis circumscripta. The T2 signal is diffusely intermediate, and the inner and outer hypointense tables of the skull widen and remain black. Diffuse enhancement is consistent in CEMR in the affected skull.

DIAGNOSIS: The patient has mixed lytic and sclerotic Paget's disease.

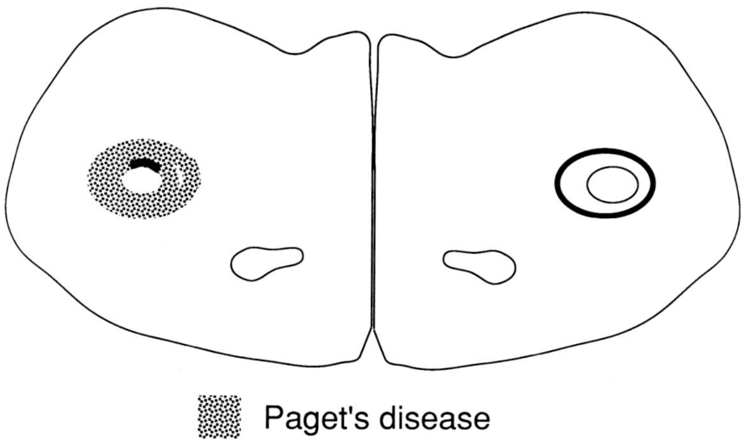

FIGURE 12-5

CASE 13

Differential Diagnosis of Thigh Masses

HISTORY: A 54-year-old man presented with a nontender but annoying soft tissue mass that he had first noticed after playing three sets of tennis. The patient had no systemic symptoms. What is the MRI diagnosis? For comparison, MR images from a 57-year-old man with a similar presentation and diagnosis are shown. Are the masses in these two patients benign or malignant, traumatic or neoplastic? The findings are virtually pathognomonic and give tissue specificity. (Patient 1—Fig. 13-1: axial, and Fig. 13-2: coronal T1-weighted images. Fig. 13-3: coronal T2-weighted image, 1.5 T. Patient 2—Fig. 13-4: axial, and Fig. 13-5: coronal T1-weighted images, 1.5 T.)

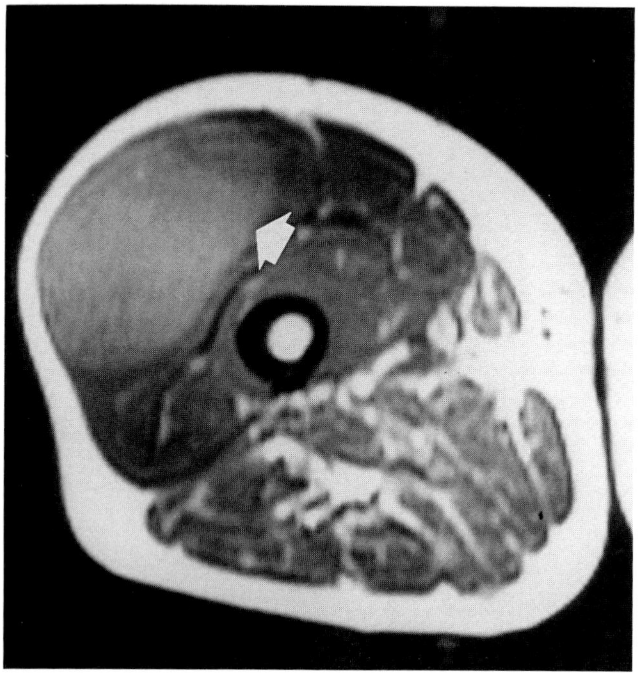

FIGURE 13-1

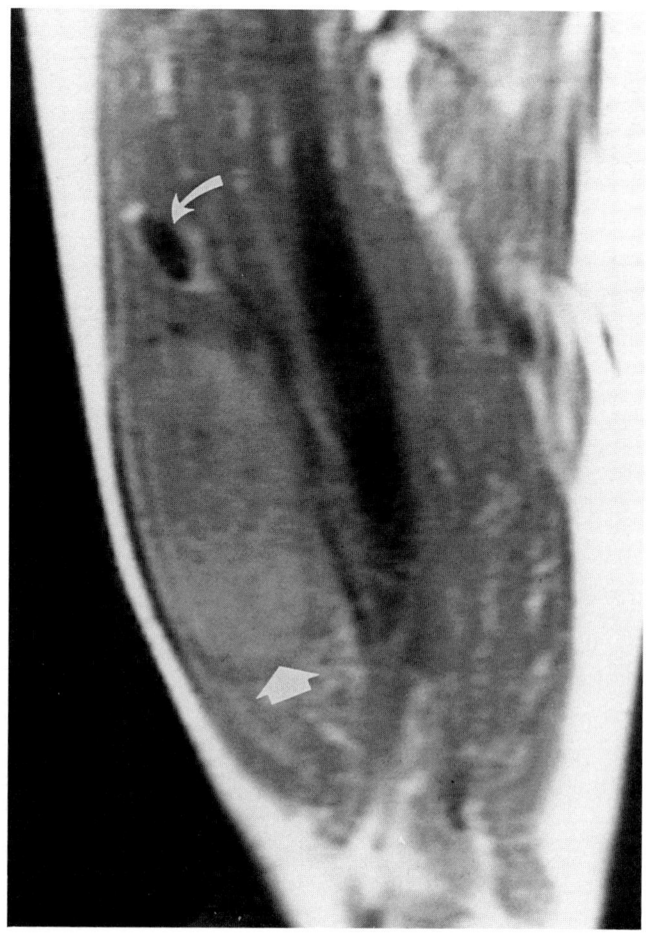

FIGURE 13-2

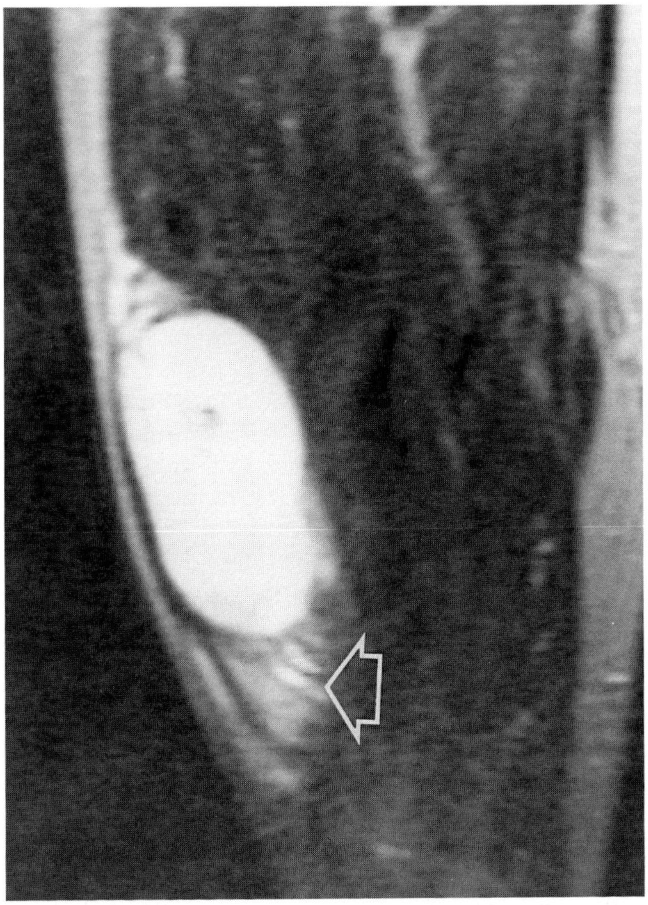

FIGURE 13-3

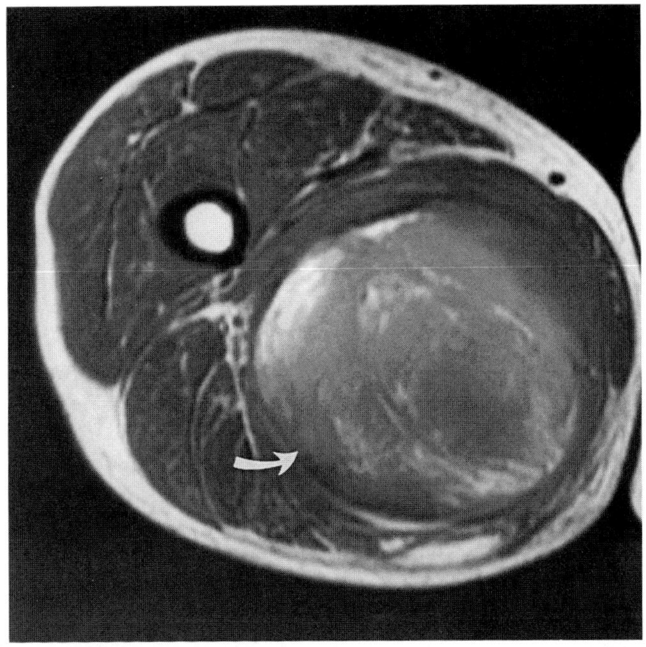

FIGURE 13-4

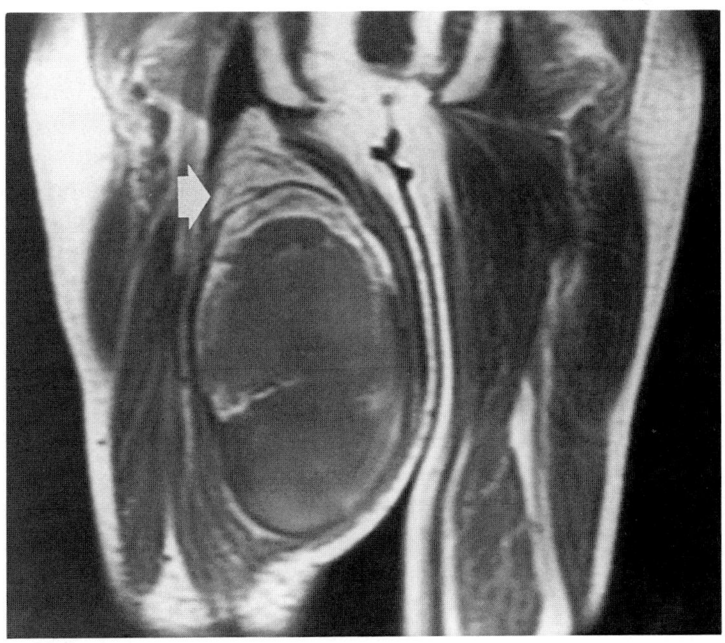

FIGURE 13-5

DISCUSSION: A soft tissue mass involves the vastus lateralis muscle of the thigh of patient 1. The size of the mass alone is ominous, since a hemorrhagic or posttraumatic mass of this size should be quite tender. A diagnosis of hematoma was entertained simply because the mass was hyperintense on T1 and T2. However, the degree of hyperintensity on T1 is not pronounced and not as bright as might be seen in the subacute phase of hemorrhage.

In addition, the peripheral white rim and intermediate signal intensity center of a true subacute hematoma are not present. If this were an early subacute or midsubacute lesion, the T2 signal should be less bright and contain mixed T2 shortening effects along with foci of signal hyperintensity. Bear in mind that the signal changes on T2 due to preferential shortening are less consistent and less pronounced in the body than in the brain and less apparent at low field. These are 1.5 tesla (T) images.

The signal characteristics of this lesion are typical of either proteinaceous or myxoid tissue. A calcification noted on the radiographs is demonstrated on the coronal MR images (curved arrow in Fig. 13-2). The calcification lies outside and above the lesion, an incidental finding unrelated to the lesion. The lesion is surrounded by subtle hyperintense edema below (open arrow in Fig. 13-3) and above. The findings are virtually pathognomonic of a myxoid form of liposarcoma. Pure myxoid tumors (myxosarcomas) do occur, but myxoliposarcomas are more common. These tumors tend to achieve large size and, while appearing well circumscribed radiographically, are quite infiltrative histologically. Myxosarcomas have a worse prognosis than myxoliposarcoma. These are all mesenchymal neoplasms.

Another sarcoma with a propensity for thigh involvement is the alveolar soft part sarcoma; however, these lesions would not produce hyperintense T1 myxoid signal. Malignant fibrous histiocytomas are not bright on T1-weighted imaging and exhibit marked signal inhomogeneity. Likewise, synovial sarcomas exhibit markedly inhomogeneous MR signal intensity on all pulse sequences. Epithelioid sarcomas appear less well circumscribed radiographically, do not exhibit T1 hyperintense signal, and affect the upper extremity, tending to grow around tendons or ligaments. Lymphosarcomas tend not to have bright signal on T1 images. Primary chondroid and osteogenic sarcomas of the soft tissues do not typically appear bright on T1 images but can appear quite hyperintense on T2 images and often contain calcification or matrix. The chondrosarcoma is an inhomogeneous lesion. The calcification in this patient was not related to the neoplasm.

The images from patient 2 show a mass containing mixed areas of intermediate and hyperintense signal, a myxoid liposarcoma (curved white arrow in Fig. 13-4). Benign tumors that contain fat are relatively homogeneous. The more visible are the intermediate signal intensity foci of gray streaks within the lesion, the less likely the lesion is to be benign and the more undifferentiated its histology. Nevertheless, in rare instances homogeneous benign lipomatous lesions have shown malignant behavior on follow-up examinations. Therefore, large lipomatous lesions over 5 to 6 cm in size must be considered for removal.

The triangular area of dedifferentiated fat associated with this neoplasm (white arrow in Fig. 13-5) assists in confirming the fatty origin of this neoplasm. We have referred to this as the "witch's hat sign": the triangle resembles the hat and the neoplasm the witch's face.

DIAGNOSIS: Both patients have a myxoid liposarcoma.

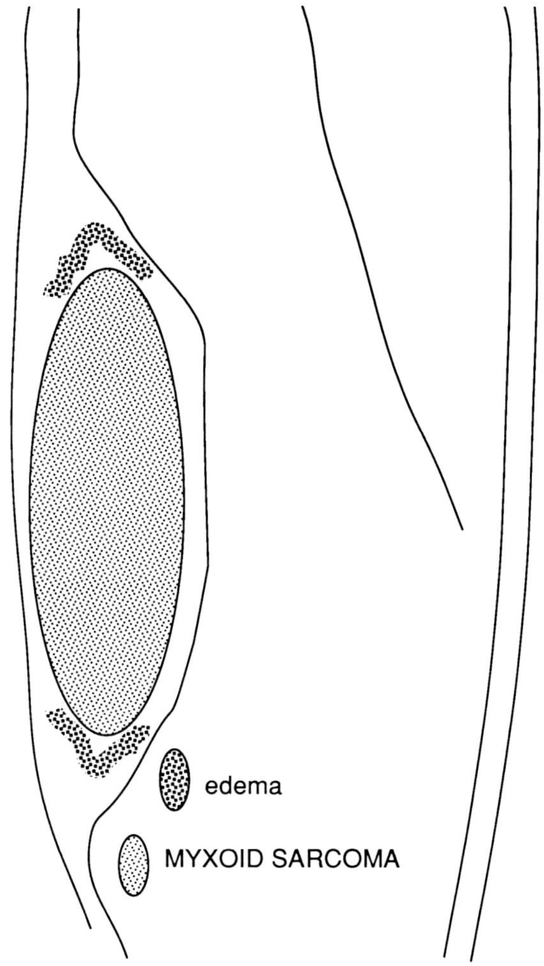

FIGURE 13-6

CASE 14

Differential Diagnosis of Thigh Masses

HISTORY: A 30-year-old man presented with painless swelling in the right medial thigh. He played light contact football weekly and was extremely athletic. Is the lesion benign or malignant, traumatic or neoplastic? (Fig. 14-1: axial multiformat (four-on-one) multiecho proton-density (*A*, *C*) and T2-weighted (*B*, *D*) images.)

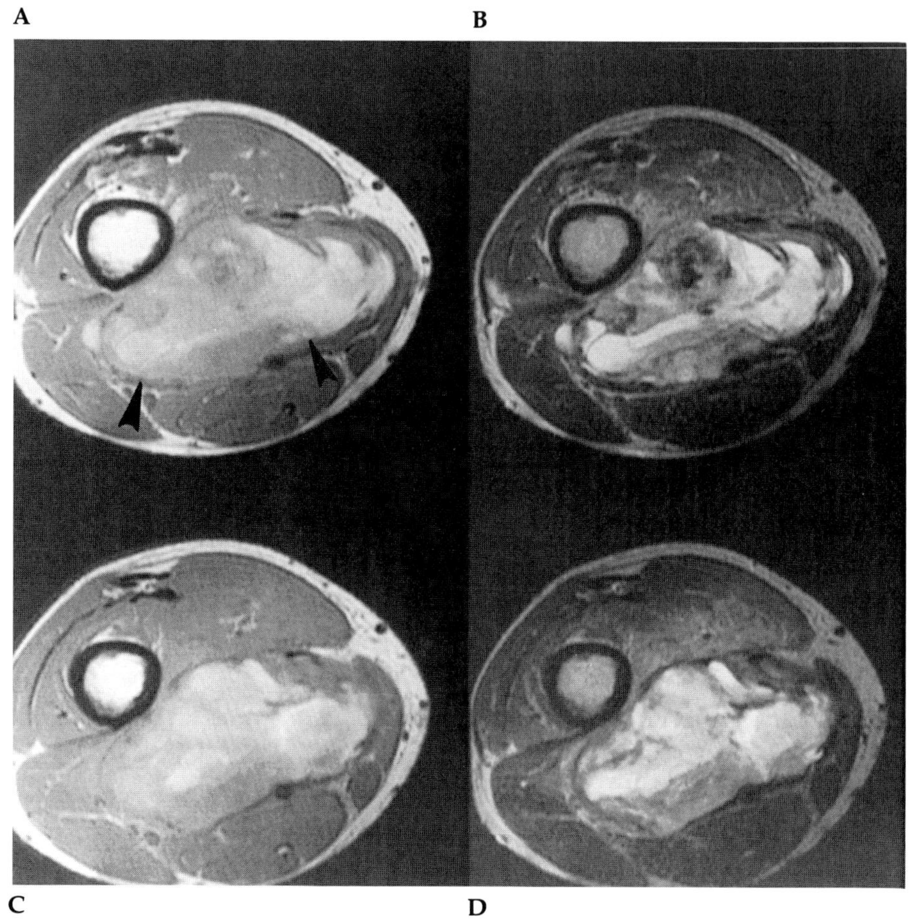

FIGURE 14-1

DISCUSSION: A large soft tissue mass (arrowheads in Fig. 14-1*A*) exhibits marked signal inhomogeneity most apparent on the T2-weighted images. The mixture of hyperintensity and hypointensity on T2-weighted imaging is compatible with a hemorrhagic component. The areas of low signal intensity become increasingly hypointense as T2 weighting is emphasized. However, a simple hematoma of this size should be extremely tender; therefore, the history is critical in deciding that this is a neoplasm even though it does contain areas of hemorrhage. This "bowl of fruit" appearance can be seen in malignant fibrous histiocytoma and synovial sarcoma. When these lesions reach large size, they frequently are found to contain hemorrhagic foci histologically.

Malignant fibrous histiocytomas are the most common soft tissue sarcomas in adults. Their mixed signal is related to the presence of hemorrhage, myxoid tissue, and fibrous tissue. Although appearing well marginated, the lesions tend to grow along fascial planes; therefore, local recurrence is common. Invasion or secondary involvement of adjacent bone is not rare, and lung metastases are seen in 50% to 60% of cases. An inflammatory variant exists that may mimic retroperitoneal fibrosis but is more masslike and presents with systemic symptoms, including fever, malaise, weight loss, and leukocytosis. The lesions are rare in childhood. The peak age range of occurrence is 50 to 70 years.

Synovial sarcoma is a disorder seen in younger patients, 30 to 40 years old, and usually men. There is a predilection for the lower extremity, particularly the knee. However, its name is a misnomer, since the lesion is extraarticular in 90% of cases. In fact, synovial sarcoma does not arise from synovium; rather, the name is derived from the wheellike appearance histologically that resembles synovial cells. This tumor, like epithelioid sarcoma, tracks along tendon sheaths; however, epithelioid sarcoma has a predilection for the upper extremity. A cystic appearance with homogeneous T2 signal has been described with this lesion, in addition to the mixed or "bowl of fruit" appearance.

DIAGNOSIS: The patient has a sarcoma, a malignant fibrous histiocytoma.

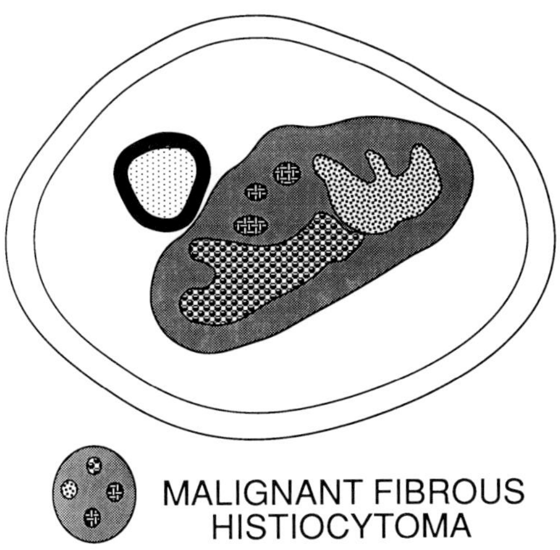

FIGURE 14-2

CASE 15

Differential Diagnosis of Thigh Masses

HISTORY: A 54-year-old woman presented with a full sensation in the medial thigh. No mass could be palpated. Is the lesion benign or malignant? (Fig. 15-1: coronal multiformat (four-on-one) contiguous T1-weighted images, 5-mm sections.)

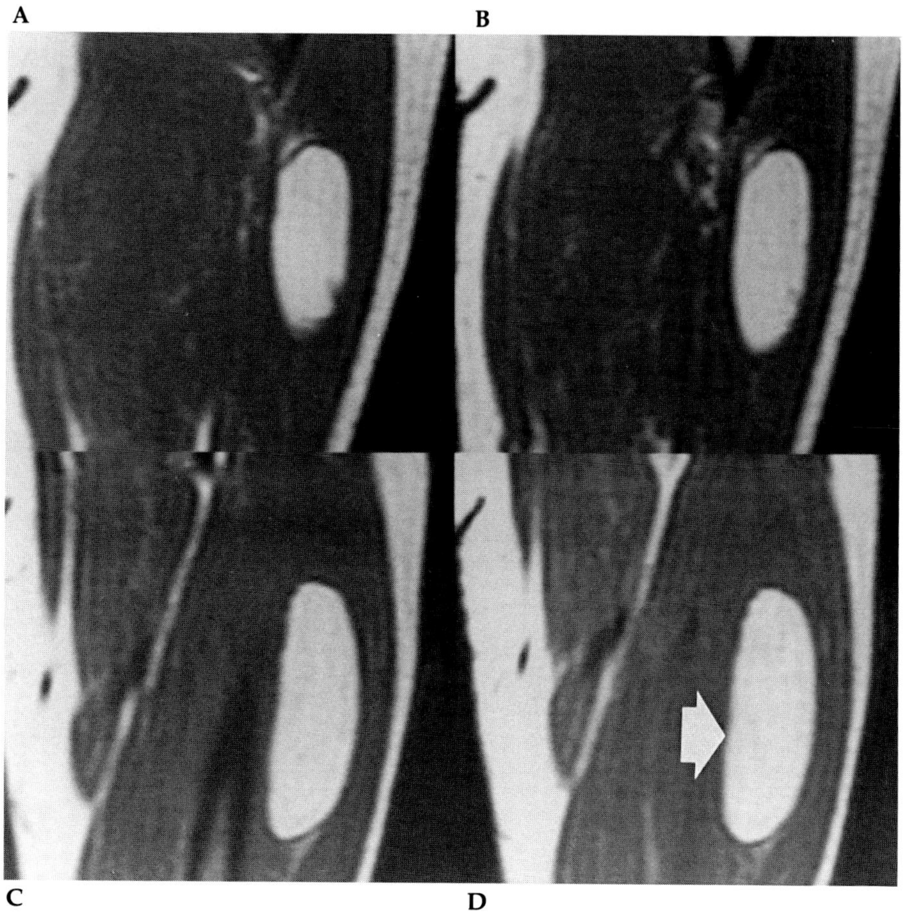

FIGURE 15-1

DISCUSSION: A homogeneously hyperintense mass (arrow in Fig. 15-1*D*) is present on T1-weighted imaging. The lesion is well circumscribed and located in the medial muscular compartment. The diagnosis is easily confirmed in such cases by comparing the lesion with a known tissue standard, in this case the subcutaneous fat. If the lesion signal matches fat on T1- and T2-weighted images, a diagnosis of lipoma is certain. Lesion benignity is difficult to confirm absolutely on MRI, however, lesion homogeneity and the absence of solid tissue or intermediate signal streaks on T1-weighted images support a well-differentiated lesion. Although size alone does not allow differentiation of benign from malignant lesions, lesions over 5 to 6 cm in size are removed. More than 95% of all liposarcomas arise de novo, not from preexisting lipomas.

Lipoma is the most common tumor of the body. Most occur in the subcutaneous space but intramuscular, intraosseous, parosteal, and intermuscular locations may also be seen.

Brown fat lipomas or hibernomas have the same signal intensity on T1-weighted imaging as conventional lipomas but tend to occur in the axillary and interscapular areas. Congenital lipomatosis is a diffuse, fatty, infiltrative, hamartomatous disease that manifests in infancy. It usually begins in a hand or foot and progresses proximally. Overgrowth of the affected limb is referred to as *macrodystrophia lipomatose.* Lipoblastoma is a rare benign tumor of embryonal fat that affects patients in the first year of life. Both a circumscribed type (benign lipoblastomatosis) and a diffuse type (benign lipoblastoma) may occur. Intermediate signal intensity septations are common in these lesions. Histologically, both mature and immature fat cells are involved.

DIAGNOSIS: The patient has an intramuscular lipoma.

CASE 16

Differential Diagnosis of Thigh Masses

HISTORY: A 27-year-old man presented with medial thigh and hip pain of 2 years' duration. A conventional radiograph eventually taken in the clinician's office prompted an extended radiologic examination. Is this lesion benign or malignant? (Fig. 16-1: axial bone window setting CT scan made through the upper thigh. Fig. 16-2: axial T1-weighted image. Fig. 16-3: coronal T1-weighted image.)

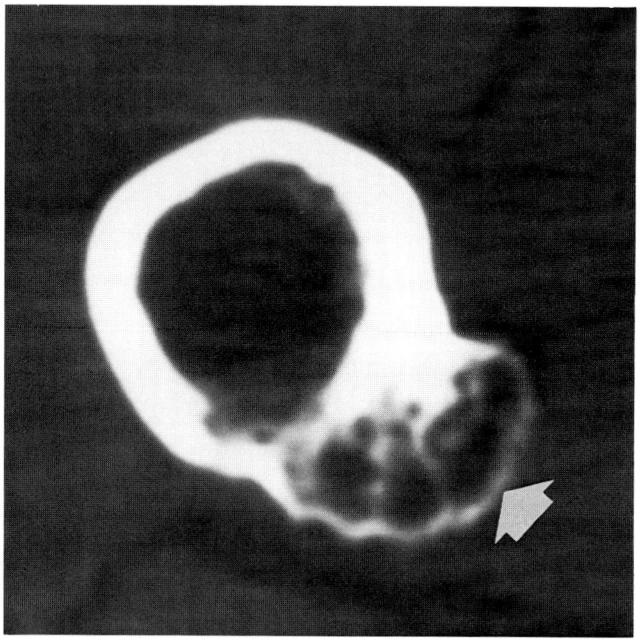

FIGURE 16-1

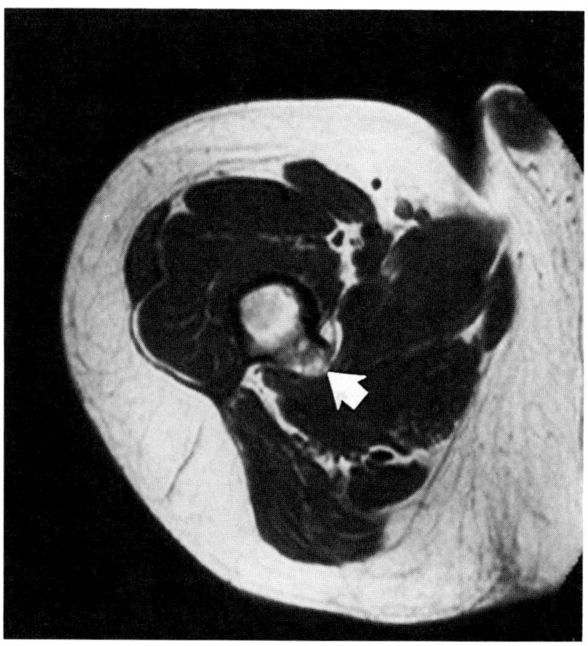

FIGURE 16-2

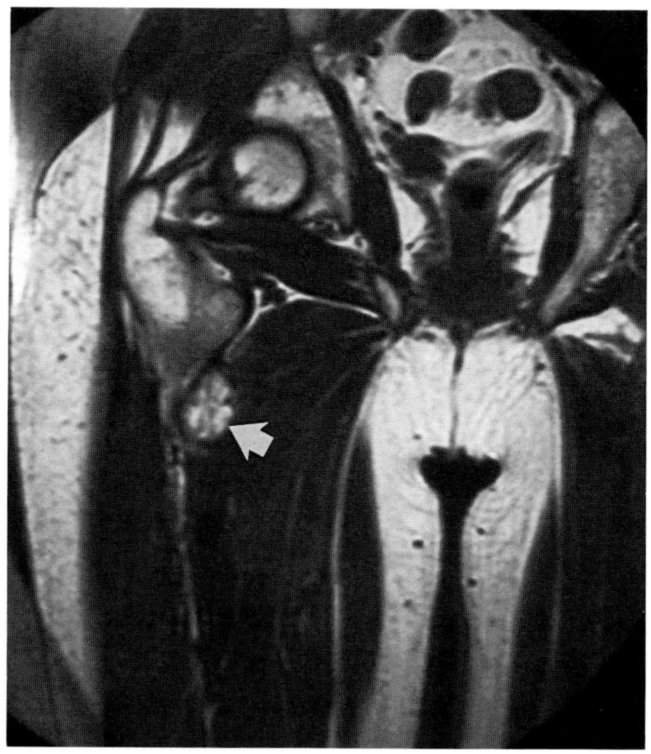

FIGURE 16-3

DISCUSSION: A protuberance or excrescence extends from the medial surface of the subtrochanteric femur (arrows in Figs. 16-1, 16-2, and 16-3). A lucency on the CT scan and hyperintensity on the T1-weighted MR image are reminiscent of fat signal. The lesion is well circumscribed, does not appear to invade adjacent structures, and appears to have a flat attachment to the underlying femur. The differential diagnosis of a protuberant fat-containing lesion attached to bone lies between osteochondroma and parosteal lipoma. Heterotopic calcification secondary to remote hemorrhage could have the same signal intensity; however, pronounced fusion to the underlying bone (even in the "en plaque" type of posttraumatic calcification) without associated clefting would be unusual.

Most osteochondromas have an overlying cartilaginous cap of intermediate signal intensity. This is not a reliable differential feature, since the cap frequently involutes and becomes hypointense or barely visible.

Parosteal lipoma is a deep soft tissue tumor that arises directly adjacent to the underlying bone, occasionally appearing to uplift the underlying periosteum. A hypointense cleft is usually present between the lesion and the underlying bone; however, such lesions may be impossible to differentiate from the en plaque type of posttraumatic calcification.

DIAGNOSIS: The patient has an osteochondroma simulating a parosteal lipoma.

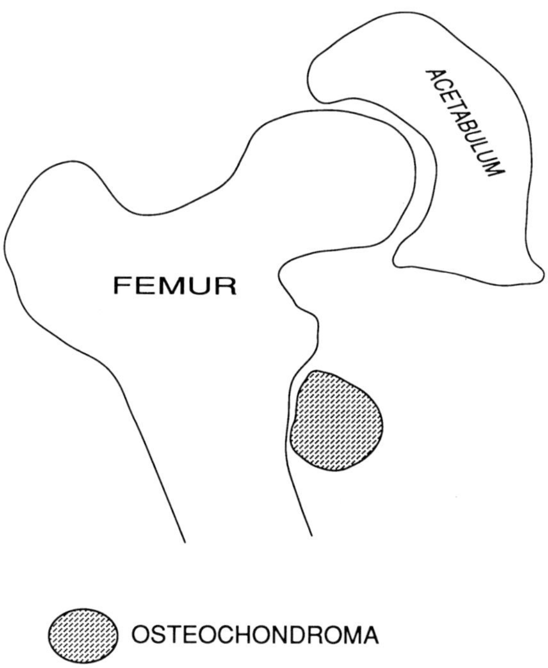

FIGURE 16-4

CASE 17

Differential Diagnosis of Thigh Masses

HISTORY: A 26-year-old man with sickle cell trait had anterior thigh pain after painting a house for 7 hours. What is the MRI diagnosis? (Fig. 17-1: axial multiformat (two-on-one), multiecho proton-density (*A*) and T2-weighted (*B*) images.)

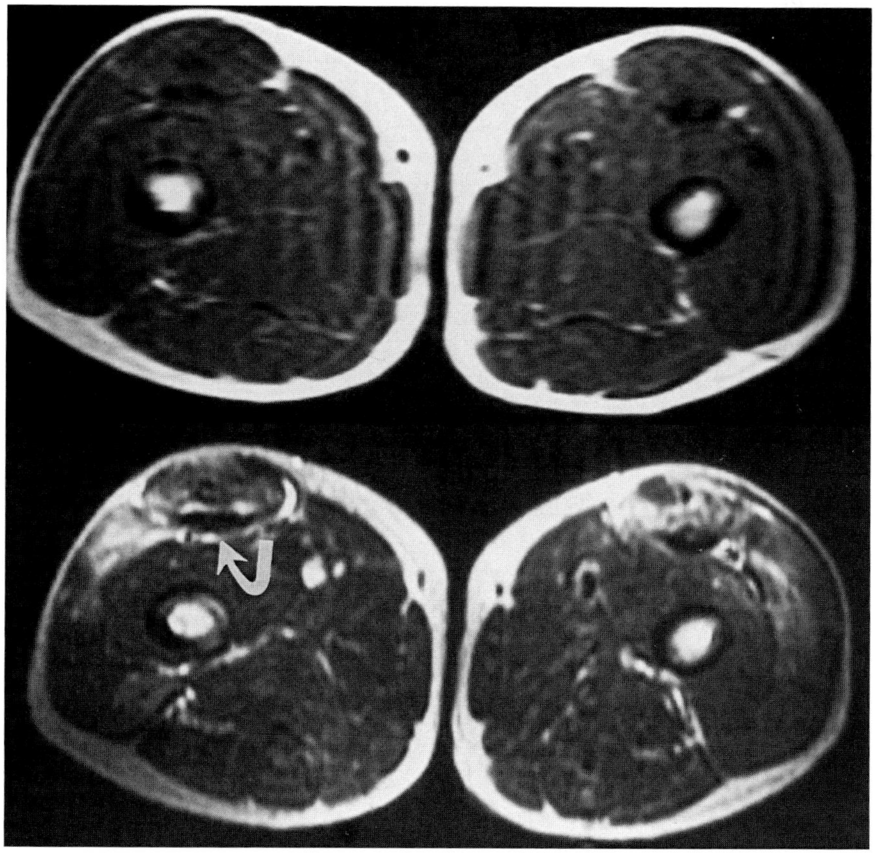

A

B

FIGURE 17-1

DISCUSSION: The rectus femoris muscles appear normal on the first echo image; however, mixed areas of high and low signal intensity are present bilaterally on the T2-weighted images (curved arrow in Fig. 17-1*B*). Slight extension into the lateral compartment (hyperintense on T2) on the right side is noted, but the process is relatively symmetric. Sickle cell trait is not associated with ischemic phenomena, infarction, or other symptomatic events except in the most extreme circumstances of hypoxia. The symmetry of this process is pathognomonic of a stress-related injury to both rectus muscles.

Similar types of lesions are seen in the soleus and gastrocnemius muscles of runners and in the vastus lateralis muscles in competitive bicycle riders. This patient squatted for hours at a time before he took a break from painting. The findings are analogous to stress fractures that occur in the bones of athletes and represent sites of micro- and macrohemorrhage and edema. The contribution of the patient's underlying hemoglobinopathy to this process is difficult to determine.

DIAGNOSIS: The patient has a stress-related injury of the rectus femoris muscles.

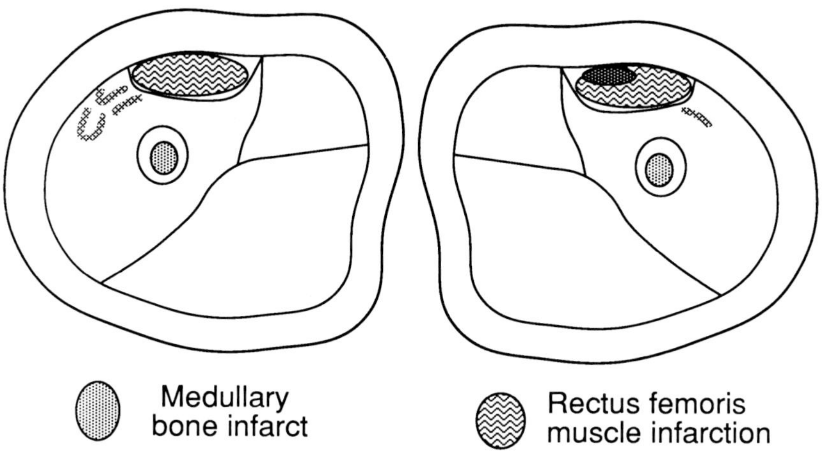

FIGURE 17-2

CASE 18

Differential Diagnosis of Thigh Masses

HISTORY: Three professional athletes were disabled by posterior thigh pain and tenderness. What is the differential diagnosis and the prognosis for each player, based on the MRI findings? (Patient 1, a 25-year-old tight end—Fig. 18-1: sagittal multiformat, multiecho proton-density (*A*) and T2-weighted (*B*) MR images. Patient 2, a 32-year-old second baseman—Figs. 18-2 and 18-3: sagittal and axial MR images. Patient 3, a 27-year-old center fielder—Fig. 18-4: sagittal multiformat, multiecho proton-density (*A*) and T2-weighted (*B*) MR images.)

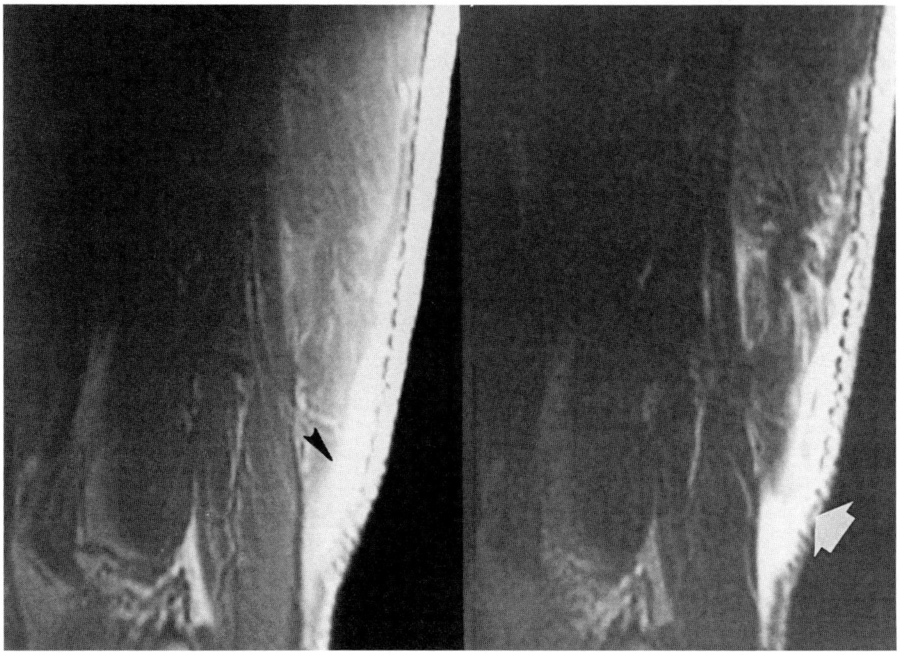

A **B**

FIGURE 18-1

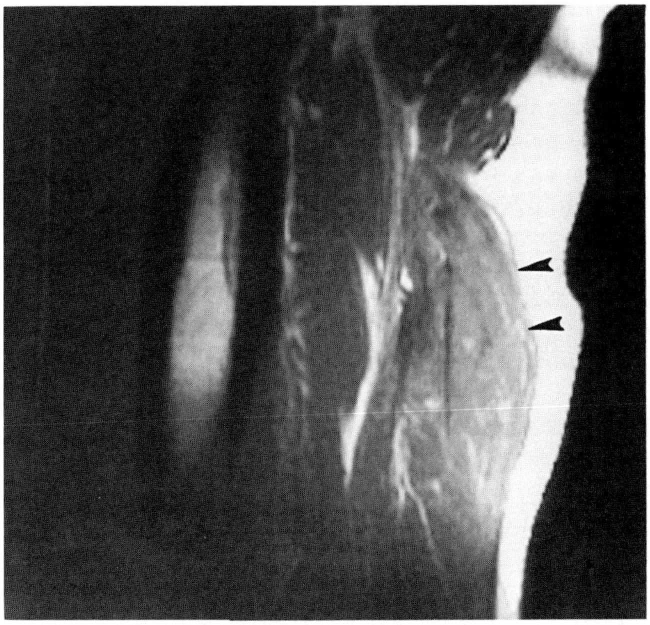

FIGURE 18-2

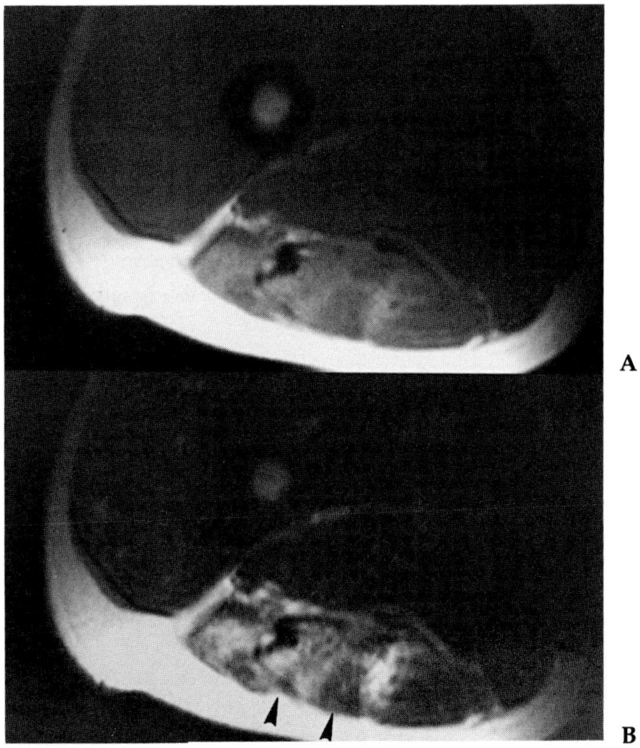

FIGURE 18-3

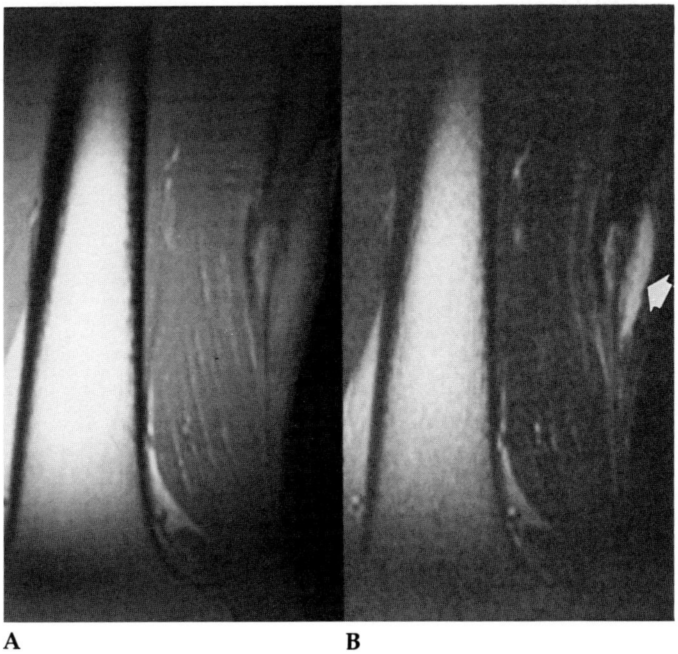

FIGURE 18-4

DISCUSSION

PATIENT 1: The hamstring muscle and complex primarily consist of the biceps femoris muscle. When the biceps muscle undergoes a sudden flexion, particularly when it is cold, muscle fibers can tear, leading to hematoma, ganglion formation, or myofascial edema. In addition, the tendon may rupture near its apex, producing triangular areas of increased signal intensity, as occurred in this case. These areas are particularly apparent on the T2-weighted images at the muscle apex. The distal muscle itself exhibits inhomogeneous density proximal to its insertion.

The sagittal multiecho sequences (Fig. 18-1) show hyperintense signal (arrowhead and arrow) superficially replacing the intermediate signal intensity of the hamstring muscle complex. Mixed hemorrhage and edema contribute to the superficial signal hyperintensity. Superficial fiber muscle loss and replacement by hemorrhagic effusion (partial rupture) has an intermediate prognosis for functional recovery (2 to 5 weeks).

PATIENT 2: The muscle size is not attenuated, but a large, swollen, edematous biceps femoris muscle (paired arrowheads in Fig. 18-2) exhibits its mixed intramuscular signal hyperintensity (paired arrowheads in Fig. 18-3*B*). This phase of hamstring injury (edema phase) has a faster recovery period (2 weeks).

PATIENT 3: The distal hypointense linear biceps femoris tendon is circumscribed by a well-marginated area of signal hyperintensity on the T2-weighted image (arrow in Fig. 18-4*B*). The connective tissue that surrounds tendons and joint spaces may soften or undergo myxoid change over time. This is the presumed mechanism of ganglion formation.

Less well-circumscribed collections may form around chronically injured tendons, resembling ganglion formation but less well circumscribed. This "ganglionic phase" of hamstring injury has an intermediate prognosis for recovery, but recurrent or chronic hamstring tears frequently occur. Complete tendon tear with tendon fiber retraction (not shown) has the poorest prognosis for recovery.

DIAGNOSIS: All three athletes have hamstring injuries: partial rupture in the first, edema phase injury in the second, and ganglionic phase injury in the third.

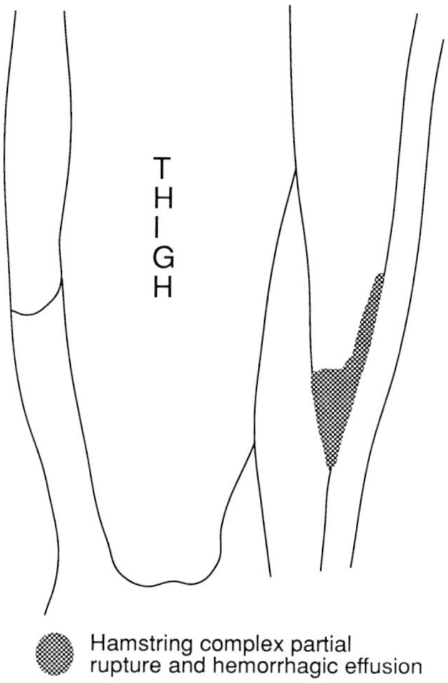

FIGURE 18-5

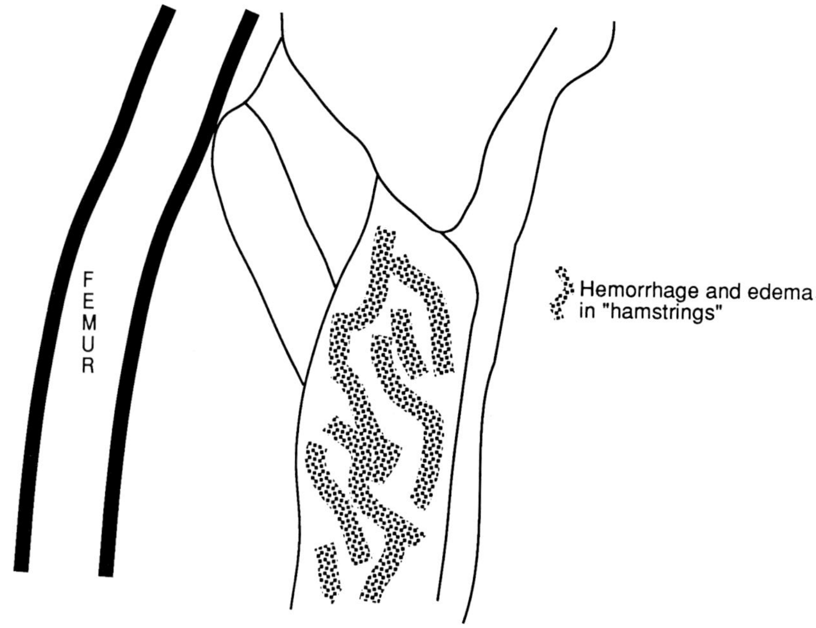

FIGURE 18-6

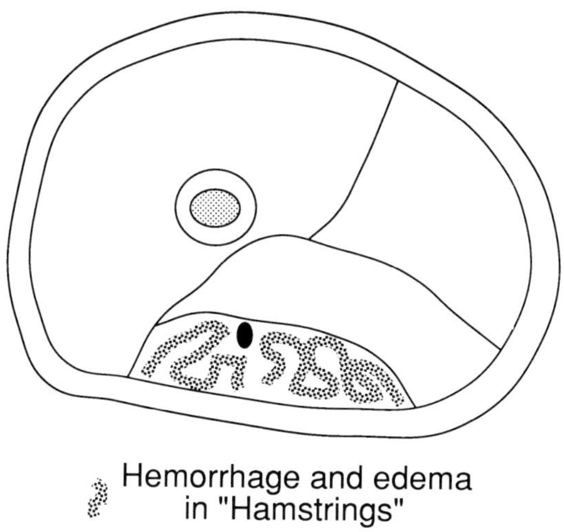

FIGURE 18-7

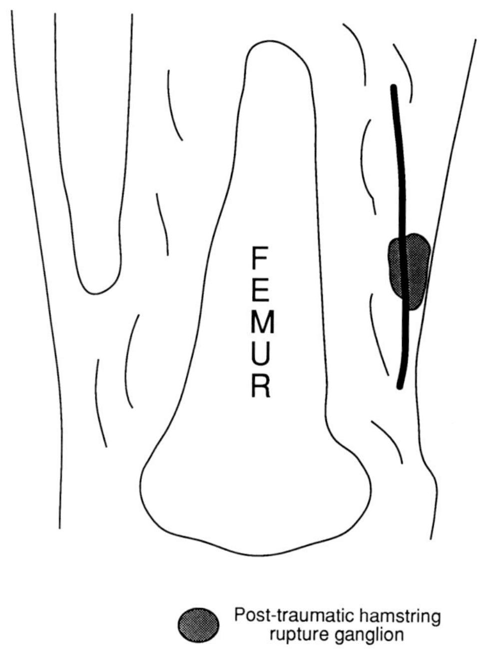

FIGURE 18-8

PART IV

Ankle, Foot, and Lower Extremity

CASE 1

Differential Diagnosis of Chronic Heel Pain

HISTORY: A 48-year-old, physically active woman presented with chronic heel pain and tenderness over the plantar complex and anteroinferior calcaneus. No conventional radiographs were available. The patient declined reexamination. What is the MRI diagnosis? (Fig. 1-1: axial computed tomograph through the calcaneus, bone window setting. Fig. 1-2: sagittal T1-weighted MR image through the midline of the ankle.)

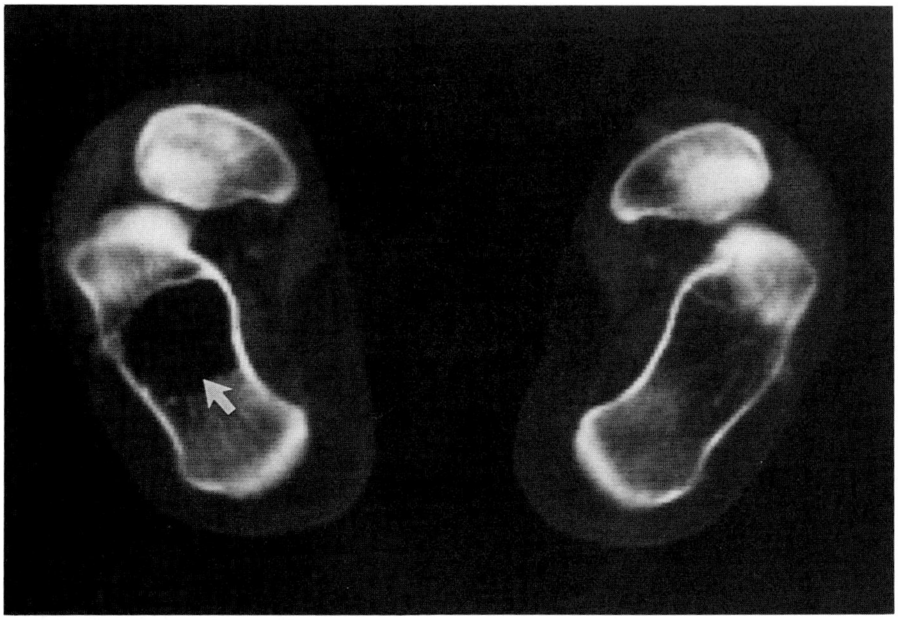

FIGURE 1-1

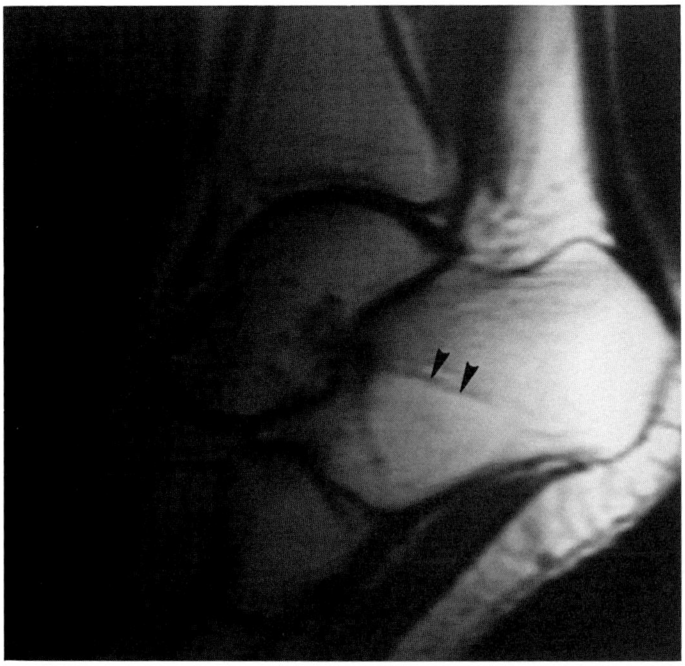

FIGURE 1-2

DISCUSSION: A wedge-shaped area of increased signal intensity, virtually isointense with the surrounding calcaneal medullary bone signal, is demarcated from the remaining medullary bone. Lesion isointensity with fat and its location are typical of intramedullary lipoma. Because this is a T1-weighted image, bone cyst (hypointense) is excluded, even though it is a major diagnostic consideration on conventional radiographs. Intramedullary lipoma is rare and usually asymptomatic. On MRI, the lesion is encapsulated by a distinct hypointense margin (arrowheads in Fig. 1-2). No cortical interruption or evidence of hypointense edema around the lesion should be seen. Nagging pain is less common with intramedullary lipoma than with simple bone cyst. Like giant cell tumor, chondroblastoma, tuberculosis, coccidioidomycosis, pigmented villonodular synovitis, and arthropathic cysts, this tumor often occurs at the ends of bones. The presence of calcification on conventional radiographs or MR images (not present in this case) virtually clinches the diagnosis. The axial CT scan through the calcaneus confirms fat density (arrow in Fig. 1-1) and negative Hounsfield unit measurements (−80).

Parosteal lipoma is a soft tissue tumor that occurs next to bone and may appear subperiosteal. It most commonly occurs in patients 40 to 70 years old, is usually large and nontender, and occasionally will present with local nerve compression.

DIAGNOSIS: The patient has a calcaneal lipoma.

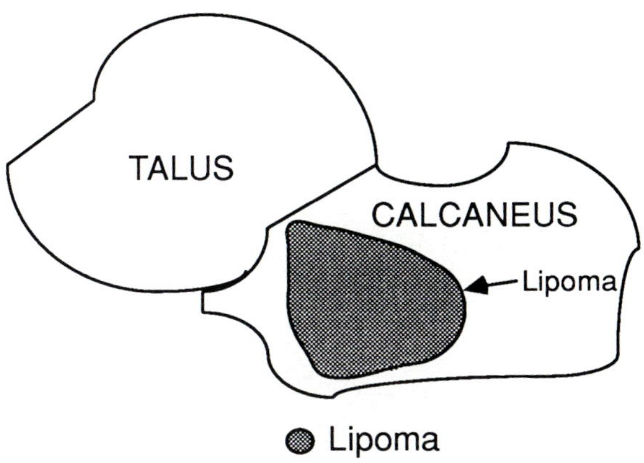

FIGURE 1-3

CASE 2

Differential Diagnosis of Chronic Heel Pain

HISTORY: A 14-year-old presented with chronic heel pain of 4 months' duration. What is the MRI diagnosis? (Fig. 2-1: lateral conventional radiograph. Figs. 2-2 and 2-3: sagittal T1- and T2-weighted MR images, respectively.)

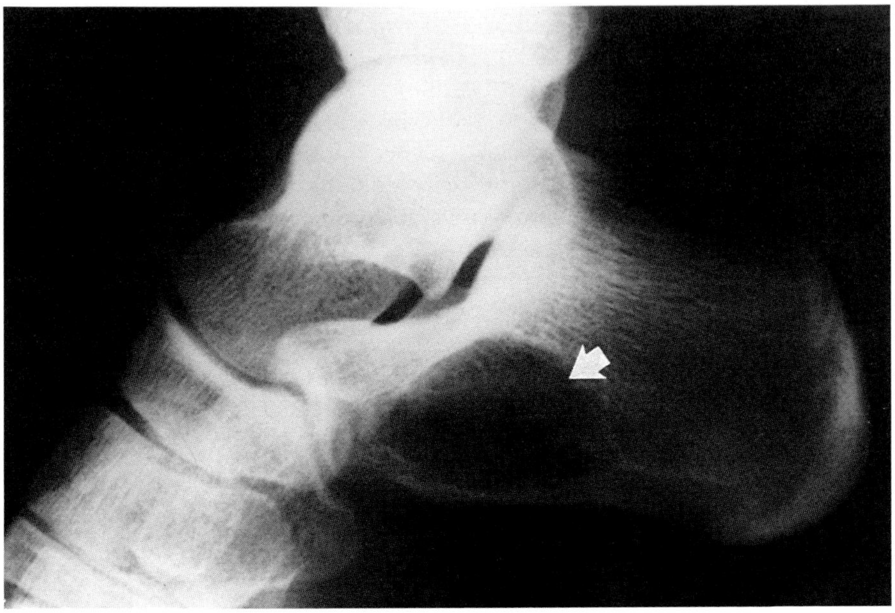

FIGURE 2-1

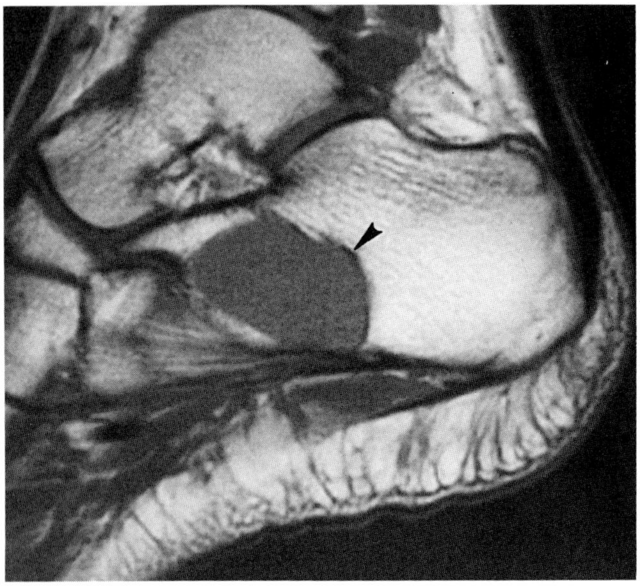

FIGURE 2-2

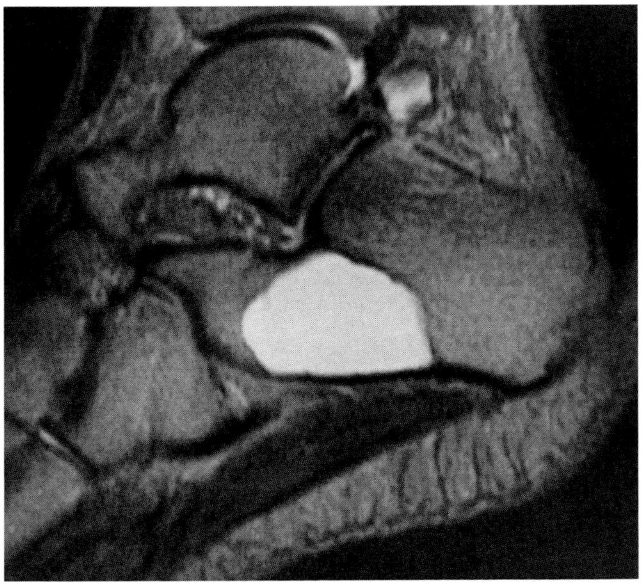

FIGURE 2-3

DISCUSSION: A well-marginated lytic lesion (white arrow in Fig. 2-1) in the calcaneus without calcification, particularly in a young patient, is a simple cyst until proved otherwise. Simple cysts have a propensity to occur in the proximal humerus and proximal femur. On MRI, foci of T1 hypointensity (arrowhead in Fig. 2-2) and T2 hyperintensity with or without septations are typical. These areas of hypointensity in the cyst are not true septations but, rather, ridging on the inner surface of the cyst wall. Sharp lesion margination without surrounding hypointense T1 edema is essential to the diagnosis. Simple bone cysts do not calcify, do not produce cortical destruction (only thinning), and are not associated with soft tissue mass or periostitis. The cysts may abut the epiphyseal plate but rarely interrupt or cross it.

Simple bone cysts occur between the ages of 3 and 14 years (mean age at reporting, 9 years). A male–female ratio of 3:1 exists. Actively growing bone cysts require surgical treatment due to their propensity for fracture. A feature useful for differentiating active from latent cysts is lesion location relative to the epiphyseal plate. Direct flat apposition to this plate is usually seen in lesions with active growth potential, while more latent lesions are separated for a distance from the plate. Curettage and bone grafting may be necessary with large lesions.

DIAGNOSIS: The patient has a simple bone cyst.

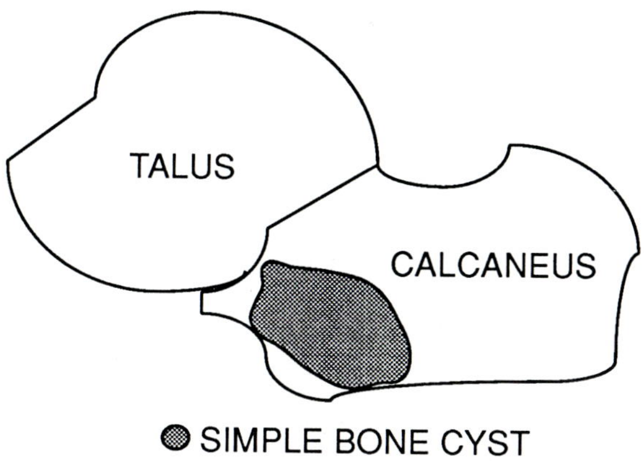

FIGURE 2-4

CASE 3

Differential Diagnosis of Heel Pain

HISTORY: A 21-year-old woman, a competitive runner, presented with heel pain of 1 month's duration. What is the MRI diagnosis? (Fig. 3-1: sagittal multiformat (two-on-one) single-echo T1-weighted images.)

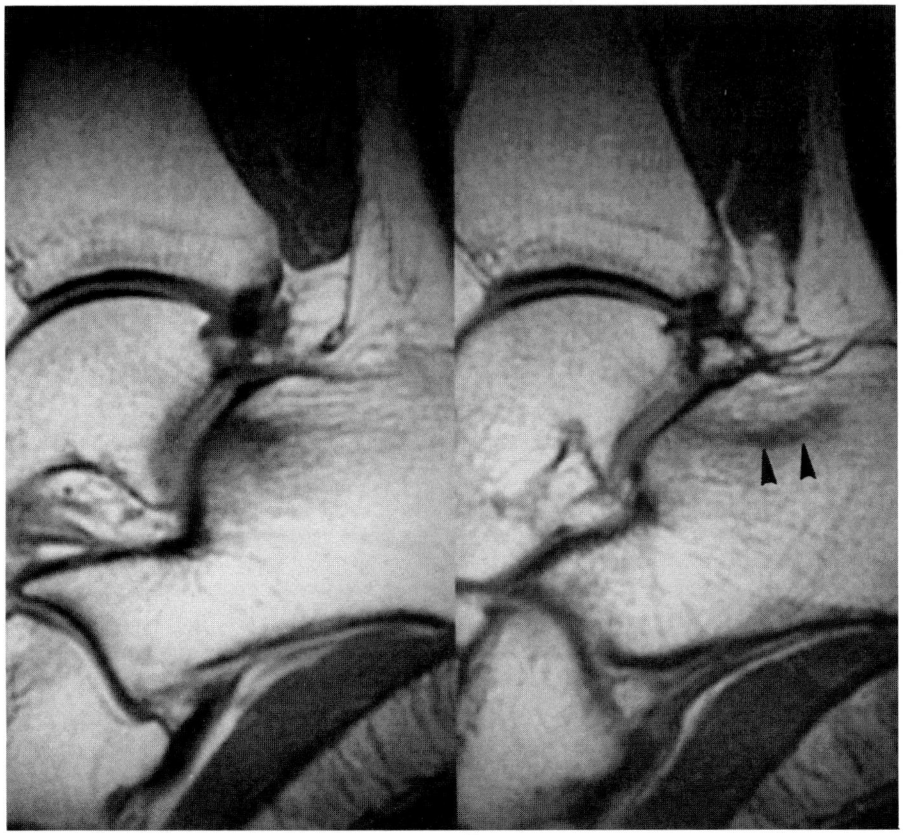

A **B**

FIGURE 3-1

DISCUSSION: A linear area of low signal intensity (arrowheads in *B*) traverses the calcaneus anteriorly to posteriorly. It is surrounded by hypointense edema, vague and poorly defined areas of hypointensity, although not as hypointense as the area defined by the paired arrowheads. The findings are typical of microfracture or stress fracture. Corresponding conventional radiographs and MR images should show no bone separation in stress fracture; otherwise the diagnosis of macrofracture should be made. Stress fractures may appear as linear hypointense foci or as spiderlike areas of low signal intensity, particularly about the knee. Associated bone bruising, contusion, or edema coexists and may be seen as poorly defined areas of low T1 signal and bright T2 signal on T2 spin-echo, gradient-echo fast scan, short-time inversion-recovery (STIR), or chemical saturation (CS) sequences. Increased sensitivity in the detection of small microfractures or stress fractures may be achieved by using fat suppression or "white water" techniques (CS or STIR).

DIAGNOSIS: The patient has a stress fracture of the calcaneus.

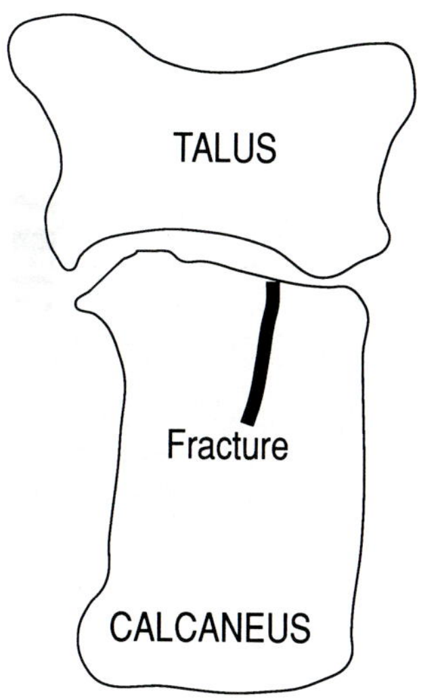

FIGURE 3-2

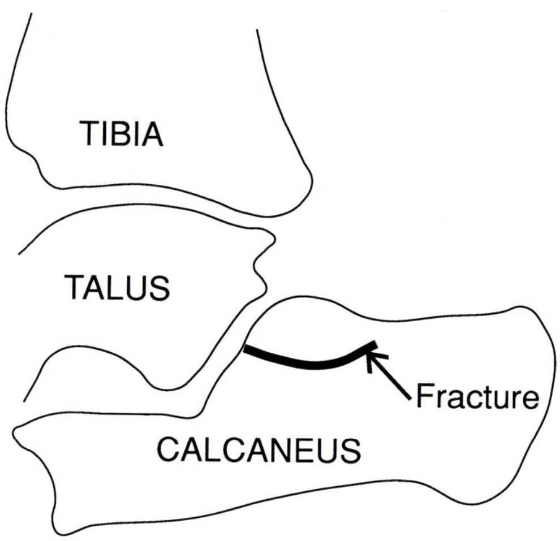

FIGURE 3-3

CASE 4

Differential Diagnosis of Heel Pain

HISTORY: A 26-year-old woman with a history of synovial sarcoma of the knee presented with heel pain and bilateral knee and ankle pain of 4 months' duration. Did she have recurrent synovial sarcoma? Is the lesion benign or malignant? What entities are in the differential diagnosis? (Fig. 4-1: sagittal multiformat (two-on-one) single-echo T1-weighted (*A*) and T2-weighted (*B*) MR images.)

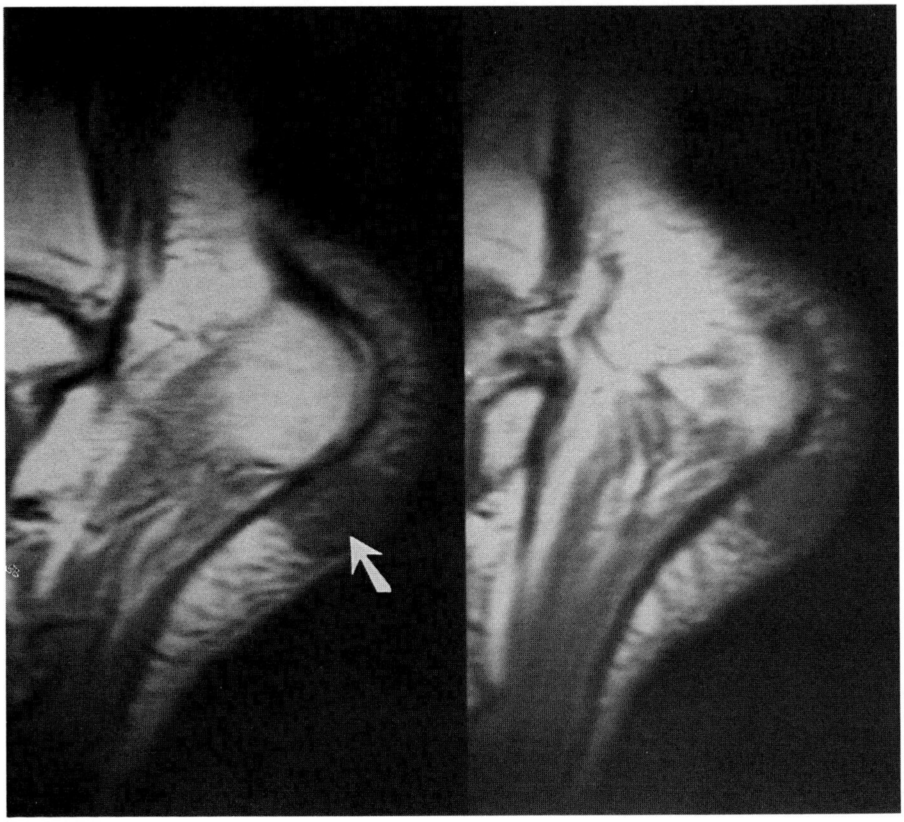

A **B**

FIGURE 4-1

DISCUSSION: On both images, a rounded area of intermediate signal intensity is present in the subcutaneous heel pad (white arrow in Fig. 4-1*A*). Synovial sarcoma is an aggressive neoplasm frequently found in the knee but not actually arising from synovial cells. It is usually inhomogeneously hyperintense. The signal intensity of the nodule or mass seen in this patient's heel pad is intermediate on both T1- and T2-weighted images. This suggests a fibrous, dense, or "water-poor" lesion. Although not initially recognized before this lesion was biopsied, a second, similar lesion was present in the contralateral heel. Rheumatoid granulomas were found, and subsequently a diagnosis of systemic rheumatoid arthritis was made.

Granulomas of any kind, particularly the rheumatoid granulomas, are isointense on multiple pulse sequences. Calcified granulomas are isointense on T1-weighted images and iso- to hypointense on T2-weighted images. Fibromas may have the same appearance and shape as the lesion depicted in this case. Desmoids may also be of intermediate signal intensity on all pulse sequences. Rarely, patients with Gardner's syndrome may present with bone pain (osteomas) and desmoid tumors or fibromas. Simple scar formation may produce intermediate signal on all pulse sequences but is infrequently as round as the lesion in this case.

DIAGNOSIS: The patient has rheumatoid granulomas and systemic rheumatoid arthritis.

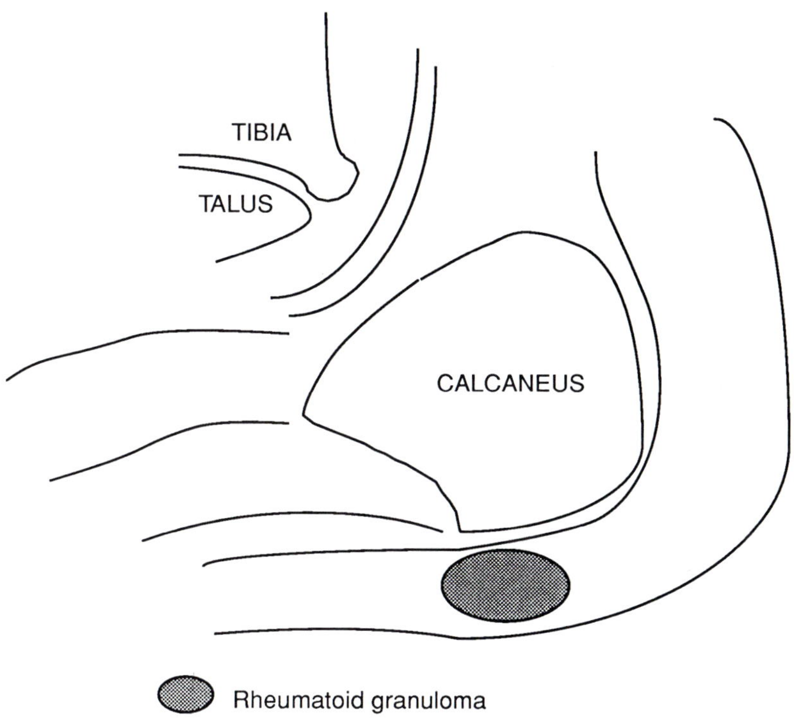

FIGURE 4-2

CASE 5

Differential Diagnosis of Heel Pain

HISTORY: A 9-year-old girl presented with visible irregularity in the heel pad region and the lower extremities bilaterally. What is the MRI diagnosis? (Fig. 5-1: sagittal T1-weighted MR image.)

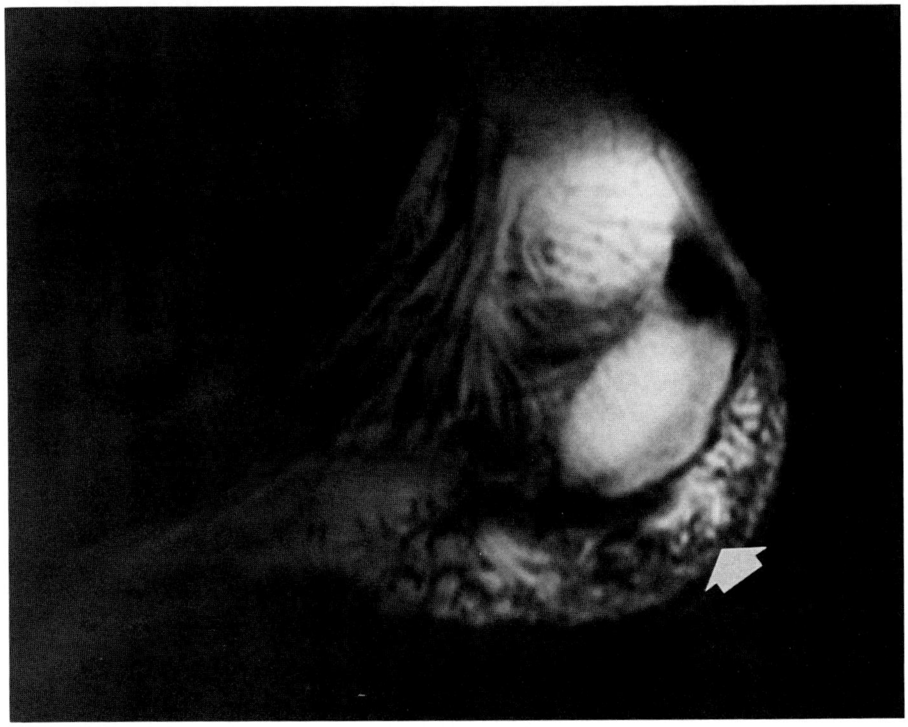

FIGURE 5-1

DISCUSSION: Foci of irregular intermediate signal intensity are present in the subcutaneous space of the heel pad (white arrow). The underlying calcaneal medullary and cortical bone is spared. The low signal intensity, infiltrative appearance, and patient age are compatible with the diagnosis of congenital juvenile fibromatosis. Local infiltration by these lesions is common; however, distant metastases do not occur. Variable differentiation may occur, so that poorly differentiated lesions may histologically resemble fibrosarcoma.

Other fibrous lesions occurring in the soft tissues include fibroma, desmoid, juvenile aponeurotic calcifying fibroma, fibromatous coli, congenital (juvenile) generalized fibromatosis, palmar and plantar fibromatosis, pseudosarcomatous fasciitis, progressive fibrosing myositis, and radiation fibromatosis.

Fibromas frequently occur in the extremities, are well encapsulated, and are hypointense on T1- and T2-weighted imaging.

Desmoid is a locally invasive fibrous growth. It is found in the anterior abdominal walls of women 20 to 40 years old, particularly in the rectus musculature. In 10% of patients, the lesions occur in the second trimester of pregnancy. Extraabdominal desmoids occur in the extremities, more so in the upper (28%) than in the lower (22%) extremities.

Juvenile aponeurotic calcifying fibroma is a rare benign fibrous tumor that originates from the aponeurotic tisses in the hand or foot. The tumors are painless.

Fibromatous coli occurs exclusively in the sternocleidomastoid muscle of newborns and children and may be associated with torticollis.

Congenital juvenile generalized fibromatosis is characterized by dysplastic or hyperplastic connective tissue and may occur in two forms:

a. fatal disease with visceral and bone involvement or
b. multiple fibromatosis without visceral involvement.

Palmar and plantar fibromatosis, or Dupuytren's contracture, is characterized by shortening and thickening of the palmar aponeurosis. The condition is most often seen in middle-aged men. Plantar fibromatosis may be confused with fibrosarcoma, often producing medial contraction of the first and second toes. A familial tendency exists.

Pseudosarcomatous fasciitis occurs in the subcutaneous space near the deep fascia and occasionally invades striated muscle. It is most common in the forearm.

Progressive fibrosing myositis is an intramuscular fibrosis with onset in the first 5 years of life.

Fibrosis and *fibrosarcoma* may occur as complications of radiation. The patient history is critical to making the correct diagnosis.

DIAGNOSIS: The patient has congenital juvenile fibromatosis of the nonvisceral type.

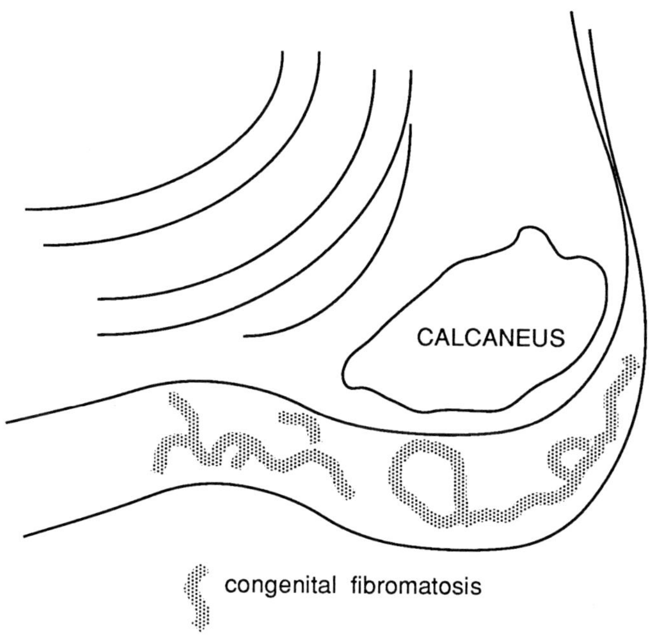

FIGURE 5-2

CASE 6

Differential Diagnosis of Acute Foot Pain

HISTORY: Three different cases are presented, all involving moderate metatarsal pain and tenderness. What is the diagnosis in each case? (Patient 1—Fig. 6-1: coronal T1-weighted MR images; Fig. 6-2: axial multiecho multiformat (four-on-one) proton-density (*A, C*) and T2-weighted (*B, D*) MR images. Patient 2—Fig. 6-3: axial multiecho, multiformat (two-on-one) proton-density (*A*) and T2-weighted (*B*) images. Patients 3—Fig. 6-4: coronal multiecho, multiformat (two-on-one) proton-density (*A*) and T2-weighted (*B*) images.)

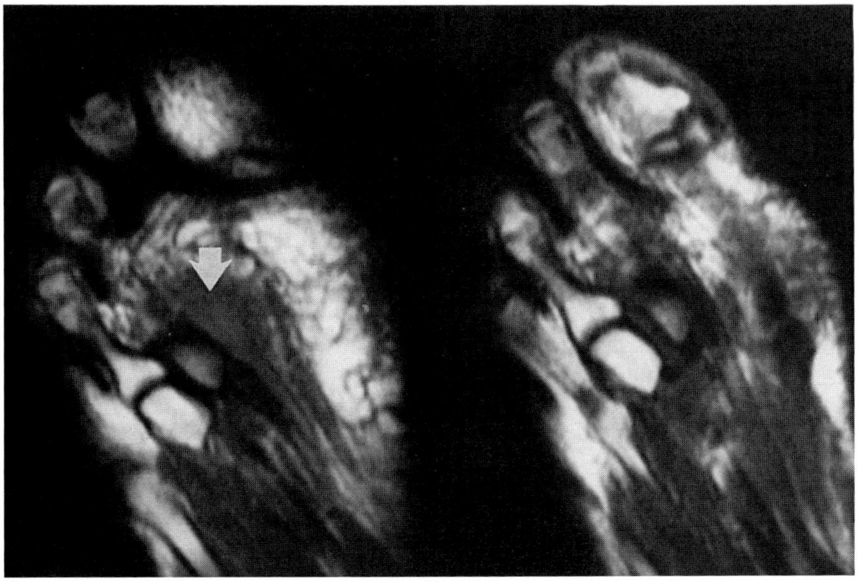

A B

FIGURE 6-1

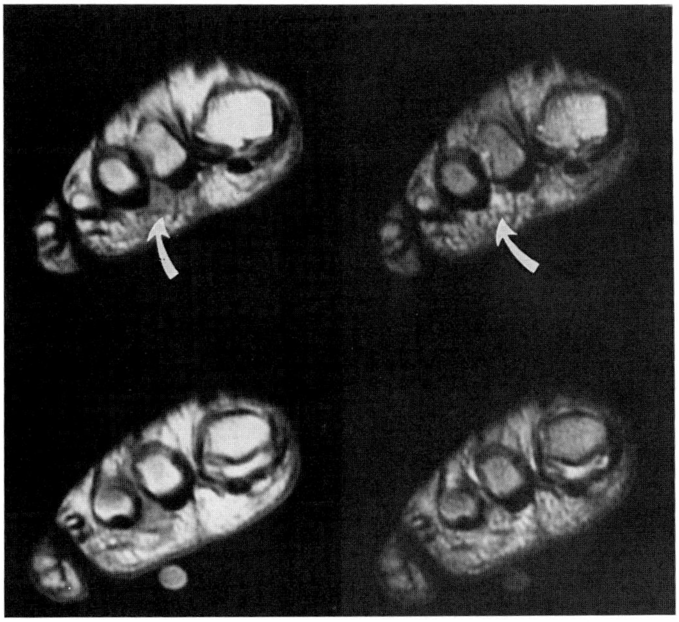

A B C D

FIGURE 6-2

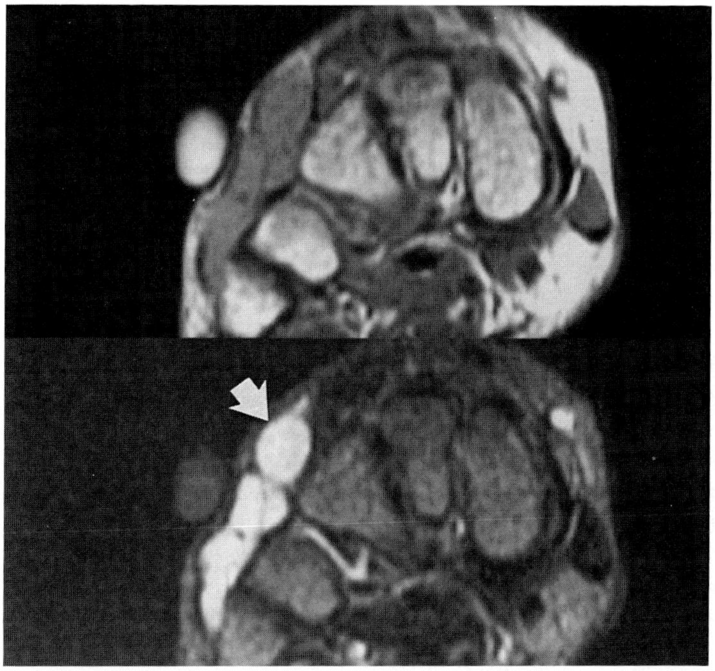

A

B

FIGURE 6-3

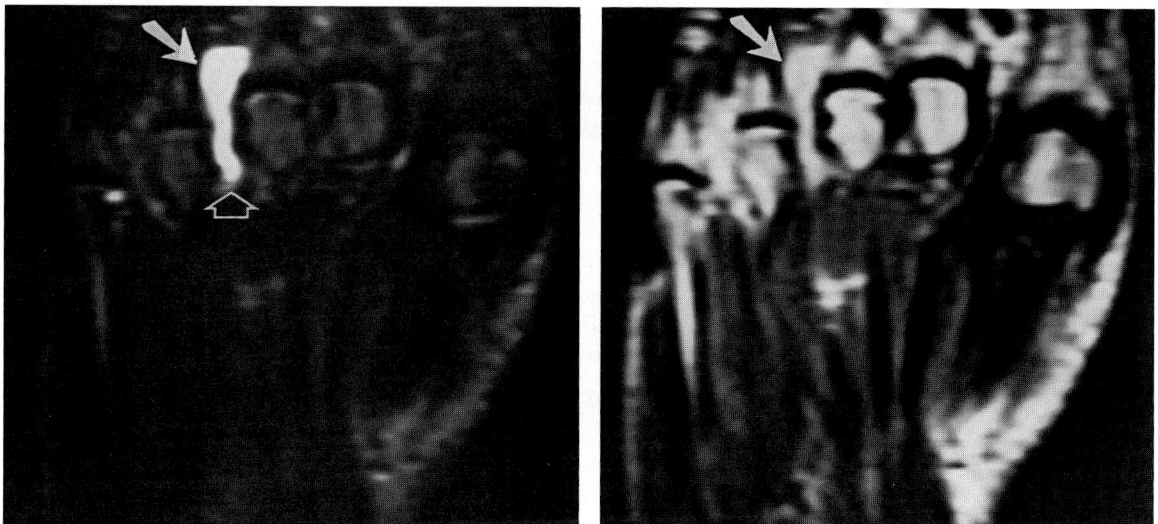

A

B

FIGURE 6-4

DISCUSSION

PATIENT 1: Between the third and fourth metatarsals is a mass of intermediate signal intensity (white arrow in Fig. 6-1*A*) on T1 weighting and slightly hyperintense signal (curved white arrow in Fig. 6-2*B*) on T2 weighting. The T2 signal intensity is not as hyperintense as in Figures 6-3*B* and 6-4*B* and contains subtle ringlike foci of low T2 signal. The intermetatarsal location, history of pain, and signal intensity are typical of perineural fibroma or Morton's neuroma. Typically, affected patients experience more severe pain on weight-bearing, and the condition is more common in women. The other name given to this condition is "perineural fibroma." Reactive fibrosis in the epi- and perineurium circumscribes an area of neural degeneration and is mixed with areas of neuroaxonal myelinoclasis. The fibrous component of this lesion likely accounts for its lack of T2 signal hyperintensity. This lesion must be contrasted with true neurinomas (neurolemmoma) and neurofibromas. Neurofibromas consist of an overgrowth of nerve cells, Schwann cells, and fibroblasts, not fibrous tissue. Therefore, signal hyperintensity on T2-weighted imaging with or without central areas of low signal intensity are most commonly seen. Neurolemmomas do not contain fibroblasts, tend toward a more homogeneous T2 hyperintense signal, and are not associated with neurofibromatosis. Posttraumatic or postamputation neuromas resemble Morton's neuroma histologically, an overgrowth of fibrous and neural tissue with one or the other predominating. Usually these lesions are iso- or only slightly hyperintense on T2-weighted imaging.

PATIENTS 2 and 3: The signal intensity of the lesions in these two cases is homogeneous and much brighter on T2-weighted images than in the prior case or perineural fibroma. The signal (arrows in Figs. 6-3 and 6-4) is typical of ganglion formation. Ganglion was once considered a tumor of tendon sheaths. In actuality, it represents cystic softening and myxoid degeneration of a joint capsule or tendon sheath. Thus, its relationship to joint spaces or tendons is explained. Its communication with these structures may produce the appearance of a tapering tail (open arrow in Fig. 6-4*A*), the so-called tail sign.

DIAGNOSIS: The first patient has a Morton's neuroma. Patients 2 and 3 have a common ganglion.

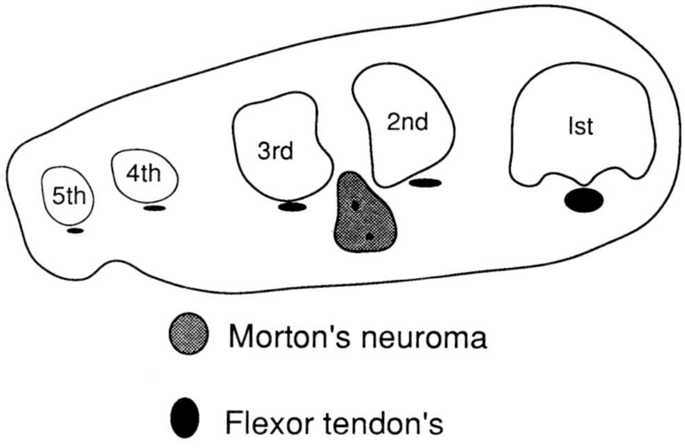

FIGURE 6-5

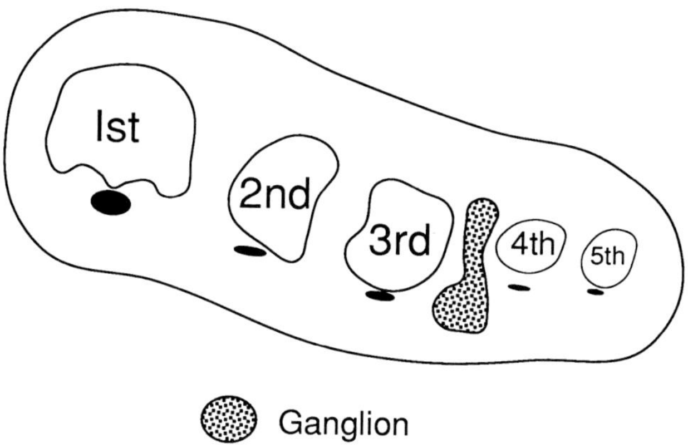

FIGURE 6-6

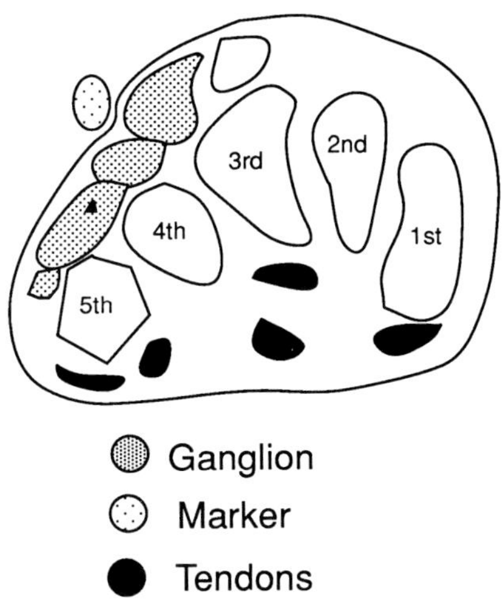

FIGURE 6-7

CASE 7

Differential Diagnosis of Acute Foot Pain

HISTORY: A 44-year-old man, an avid tennis player, fell during a match but felt fine. The following morning he could not walk, owing to extreme pain on the plantar foot surface. What is the MRI diagnosis? (Fig. 7-1: axial multiformat (two-on-one) multiecho proton-density (*A*) and T2-weighted (*B*) MR images.)

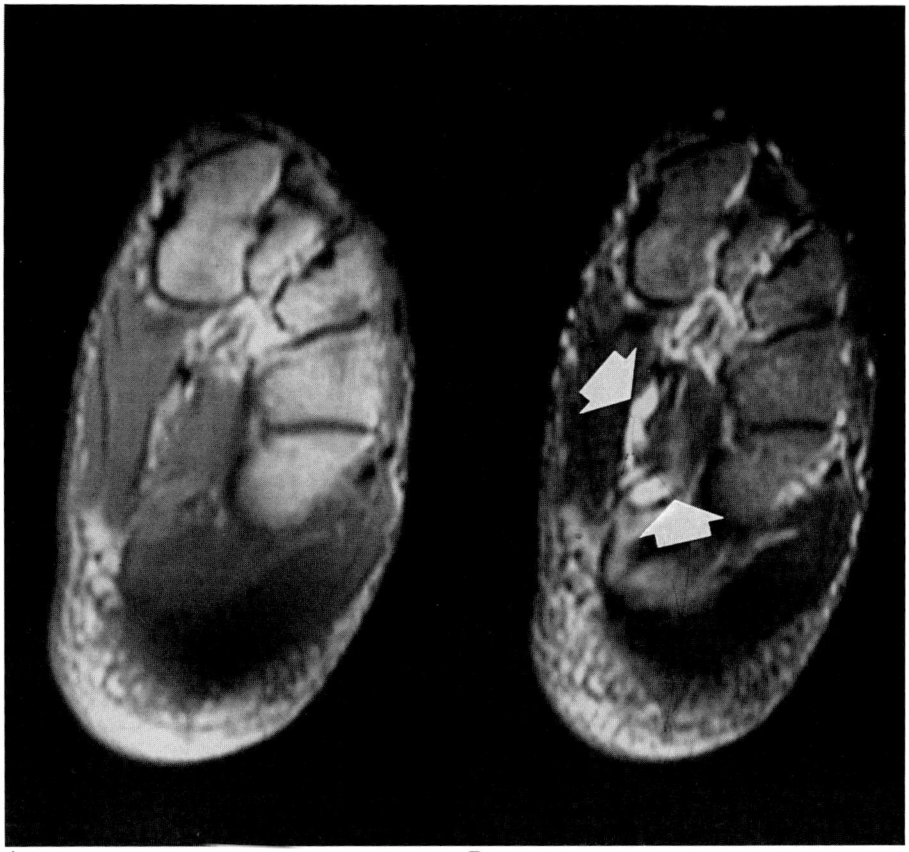

A **B**

FIGURE 7-1

DISCUSSION: Axial sections show increased signal intensity on T2-weighted imaging (white arrows in *B*), compatible with edema or acute hemorrhage. The edema lies directly within the anatomic confines of the calcaneonavicular or spring ligament complex. The plantar fascial complex may be injured in hyperflexion or hyperextension injuries, with the former the more common mechanism. Areas of linear intramuscular or interfascial signal hyperintensity predominate and are best viewed either sagittally or axially. The utility of MRI is in determining the presence of complete muscle rupture and retraction, a condition potentially requiring surgical repair. Rounded areas of hyperintense signal on T1 weighting and hypointense signal on T2 weighting connote a poor prognosis with a prolonged convalescence.

DIAGNOSIS: The patient has an incomplete plantar musculotendinous injury with fasciitis.

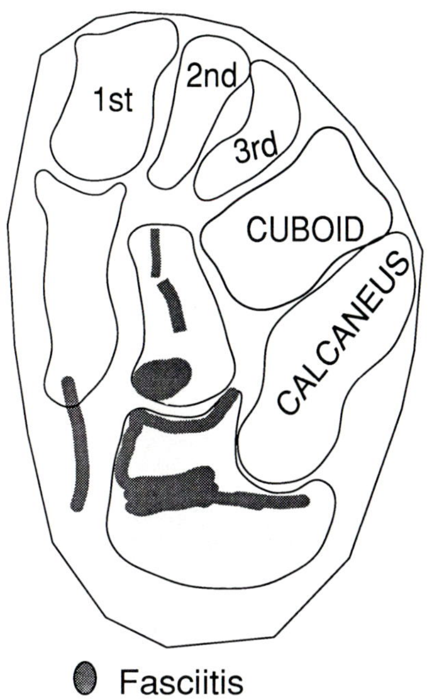

FIGURE 7-2

CASE 8

Differential Diagnosis of Acute Foot Pain

HISTORY: Two women, one 31 years old, the other 52, with diabetes presented with fever and ankle and foot pain. What is the MRI diagnosis in each case? (Patient 1—Fig. 8-1: sagittal T1-weighted MR image. Patient 2—Fig. 8-2: sagittal multiformat (four-on-one) T1-weighted images, and Fig. 8-3: multiecho proton-density (*A, C*) and T2-weighted (*B, D*) MR images.)

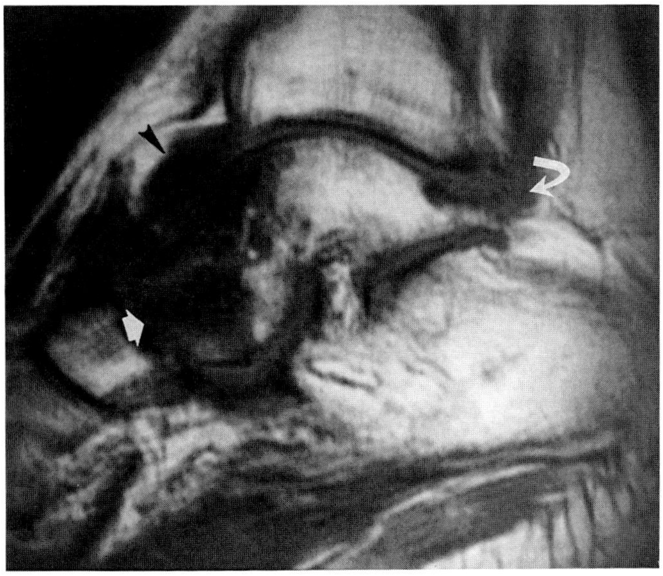

FIGURE 8-1

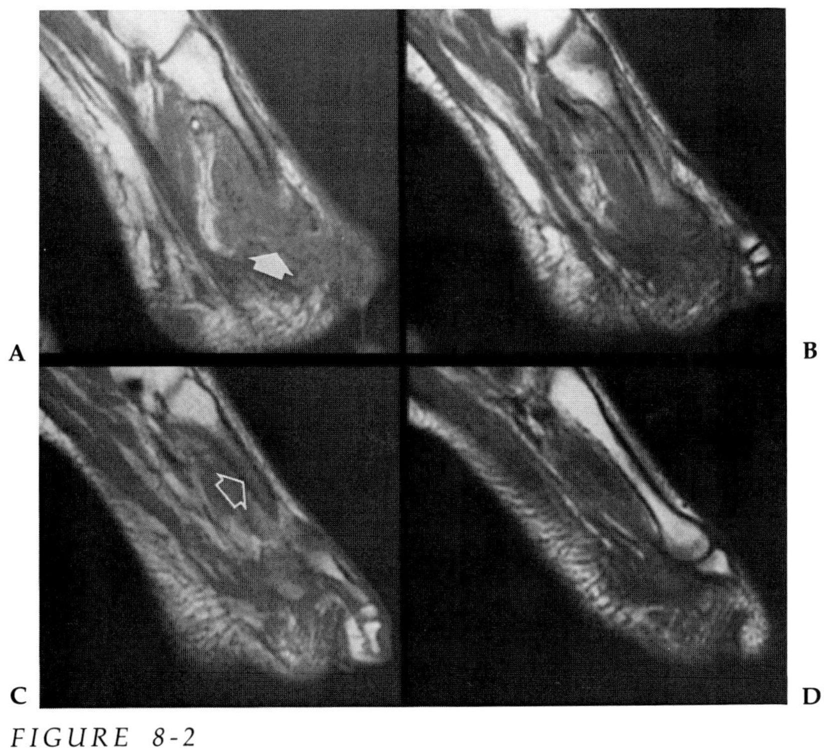

FIGURE 8-2

DIAGNOSIS: Both patients have talar and metatarsal osteomyelitis.

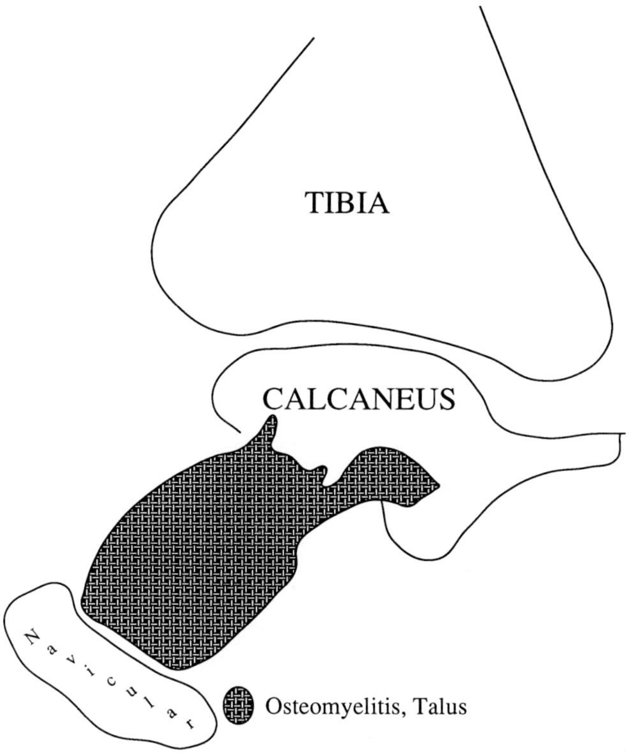

FIGURE 8-4

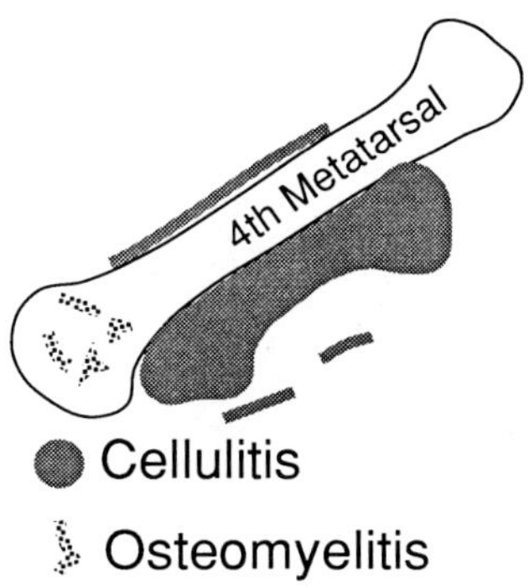

FIGURE 8-5

CASE 9

Differential Diagnosis of Acute Foot Pain

HISTORY: A 26-year-old woman presented with acute foot pain on dorsiflexion the day after a soccer match. What is the MRI diagnosis? (Fig. 9-1: sagittal T1-weighted MR image. Fig. 9-2: sagittal multiecho, multiformat (two-on-one) proton-density (*A*) and T2-weighted (*B*) images.)

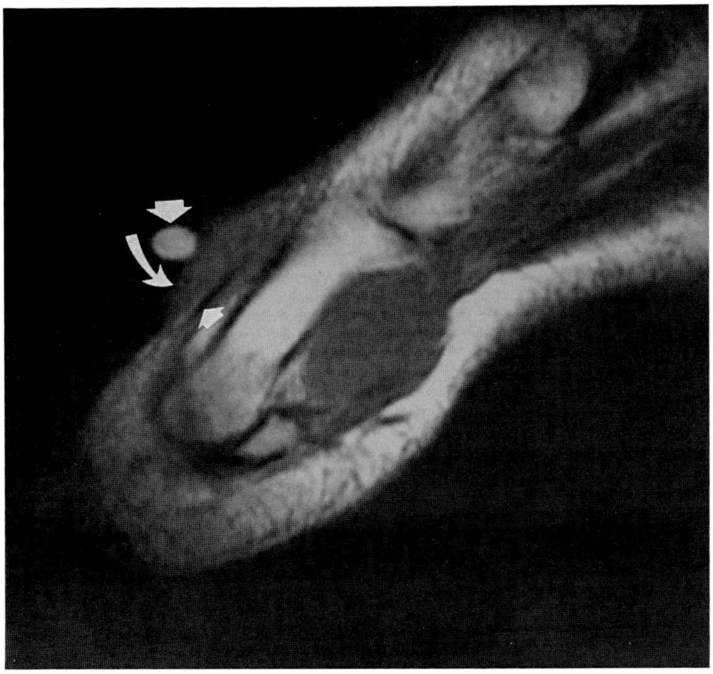

FIGURE 9-1

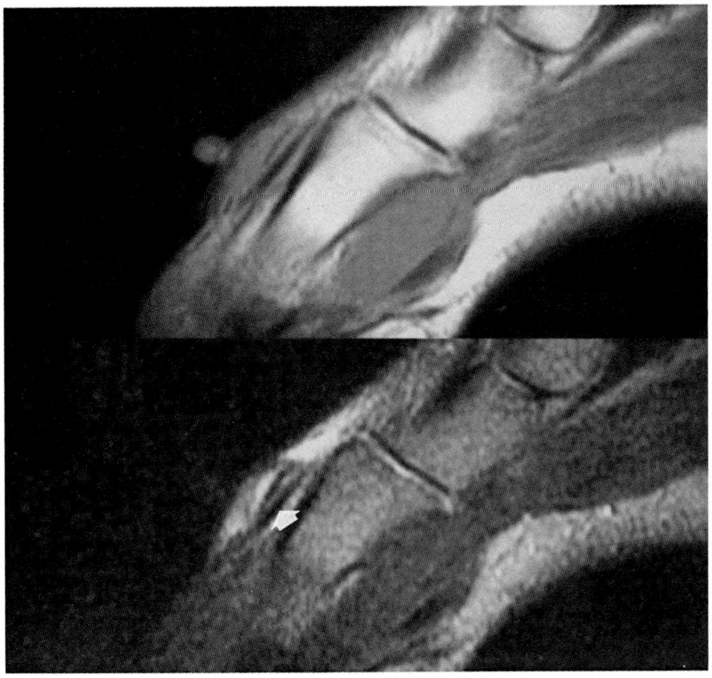

A

B

FIGURE 9-2

DISCUSSION: A gelatin capsule placed over the area of tenderness and swelling appears as a hyperintense round ball on the skin surface (white arrow in Fig. 9-1). Below this capsule is an area of intermediate signal intensity (curved white arrow) that is not well-circumscribed, as is a soft tissue ganglion, but does appear to circumscribe a linear hypointense structure (small white arrow in Fig. 9-1), the injured extensor tendon of the first digit. In addition, on T2-weighted imaging this masslike area appears as a poorly defined hyperintense region that surrounds the tendon but is not as homogeneous or bright as a ganglion formation.

When a tendon ruptures, fluid in the tendinous sheath and adjacent myotendinous anatomy may undergo myxoid change without forming an actual well-circumscribed ganglion. This may be the precursor lesion to ganglion formation. With complete tendon rupture, retraction and an accordianlike appearance may result. Peritendinous hemorrhage is another potential sequela producing foci of T1 signal hyperintensity. This is not uncommon in hamstring injuries (see case 18 in Chapter 3, The Hip).

DIAGNOSIS: The patient has an incomplete rupture of the extensor hallicus longus tendon.

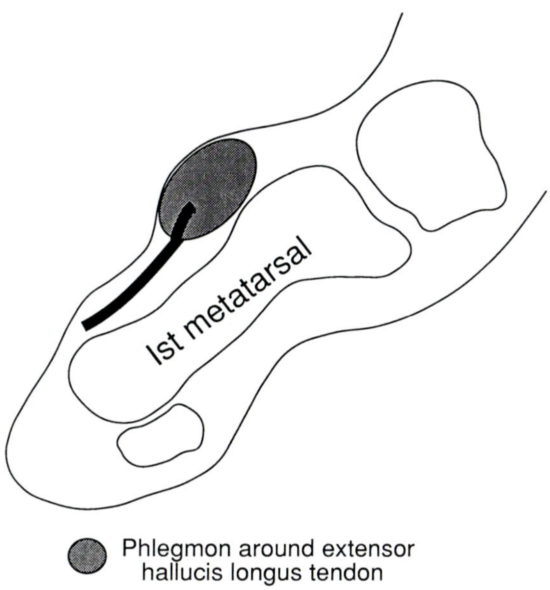

FIGURE 9-3

CASE 10

Differential Diagnosis of Foot Pain

HISTORY: A 13-year-old girl presented with foot and plantar arch pain and discomfort of unknown duration. What is the MRI diagnosis? (Figs. 10-1 and 10-2: respectively, sagittal and axial fast scan gradient-echo free induction decay images, flip angle 15°, TR/TE 400/13 msec.)

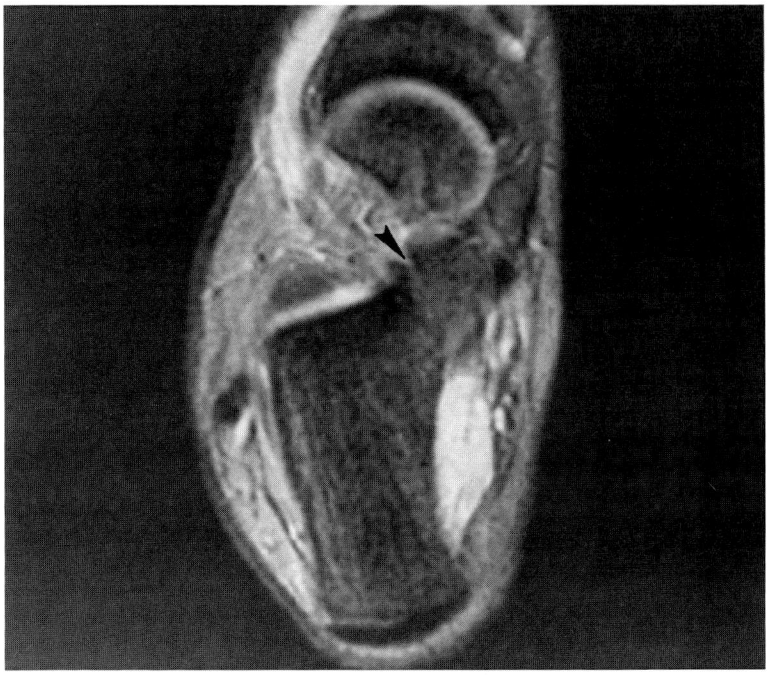

FIGURE 10-1

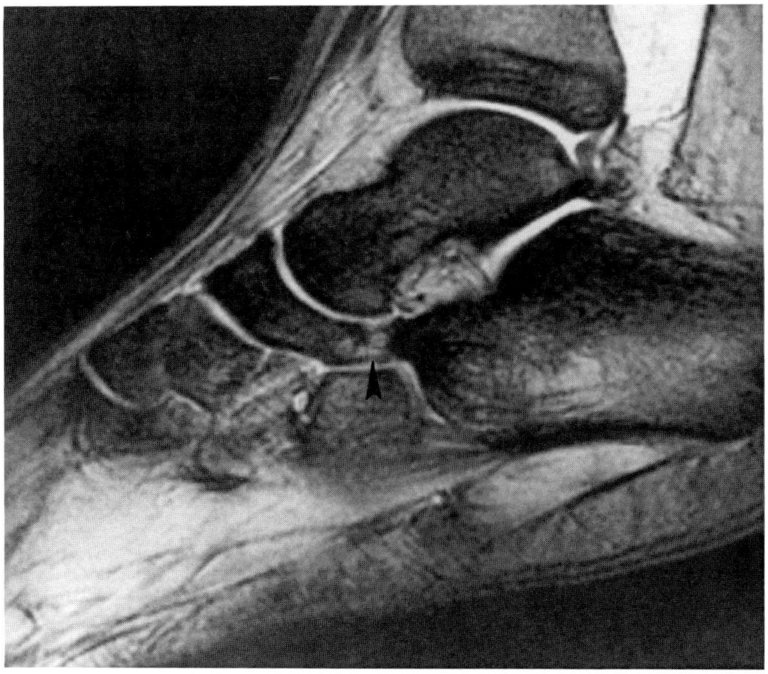

FIGURE 10-2

DISCUSSION: The interface between the calcaneus and the navicular is almost continuous, with a residual area of slight chondral hyperintensity (arrowhead in Fig. 10-1). In the axial projection, the medullary hypointense bone signal is continuous between the two bones. The findings are typical of a combined chondral and bony calcaneonavicular bar. Fast scan imaging is a useful way to assess these bars since this sequence is extremely sensitive to water protons. Hyaline cartilage bar (synchondrosis) will exhibit slight signal hyperintensity, a purely fibrous bar (syndesmosis), hypointensity, and a bone bar (synostosis), hypo- or isointensity with surrounding or adjacent medullary bone.

Our technique for evaluating coalitions includes an axial and parasagittal oblique set of sections utilizing T1 and fast scan imaging. For calcaneonavicular coalition, a 45° parasagittal section through the calcaneonavicular (anteromedially to posterolaterally) interface is best. Talocalcaneal coalitions are best seen with axial and parasagittal sections (superomedially to inferolaterally). These sections are analogous to the 45° medial oblique and Harris–Beath views used in conventional radiography.

The most common coalition occurs between the calcaneus and the navicular, followed by the talus and calcaneus, and least commonly between the calcaneus and the cuboid.

DIAGNOSIS: The patient has a synostotic and synchondrotic calcaneonavicular coalition.

CASE 11

Differential Diagnosis of Foot Pain

HISTORY: A 27-year-old athletic woman presented with nagging medial ankle pain of 4 to 6 months' duration. A preliminary radiographic diagnosis of posttraumatic or arthropathic cyst had been made. What is the MRI diagnosis? (Fig. 11-1: oblique longitudinal radiograph of the left ankle. Fig. 11-2: sagittal T1-weighted MR image. Fig. 11-3: coronal multi-echo, multiformat proton-density (*A*) and T2-weighted (*B*) MR images.)

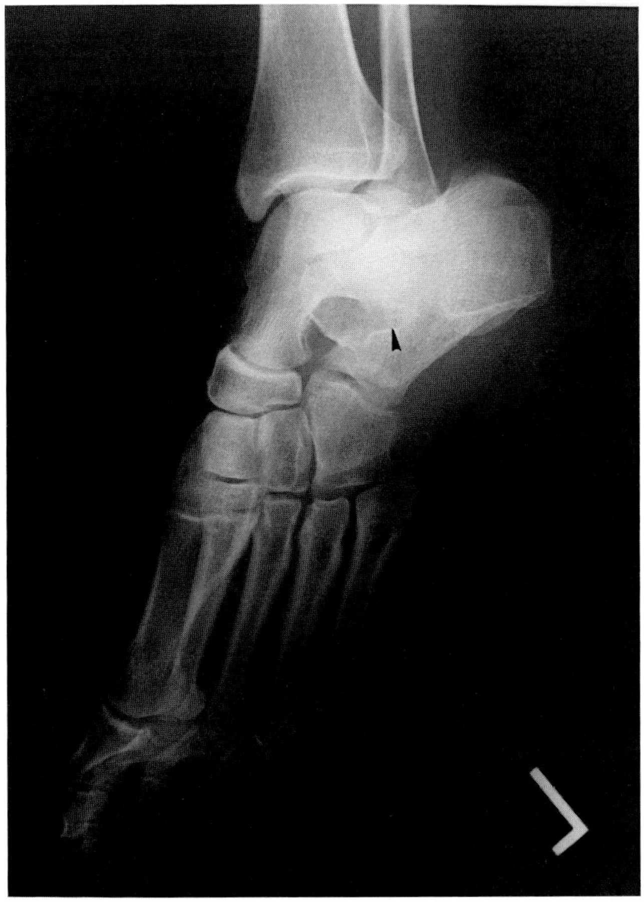

FIGURE 11-1

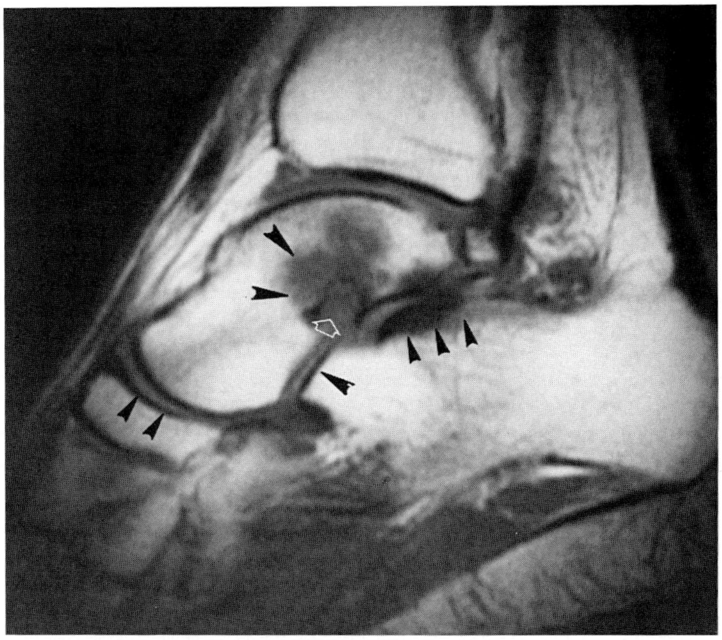

FIGURE 11-2

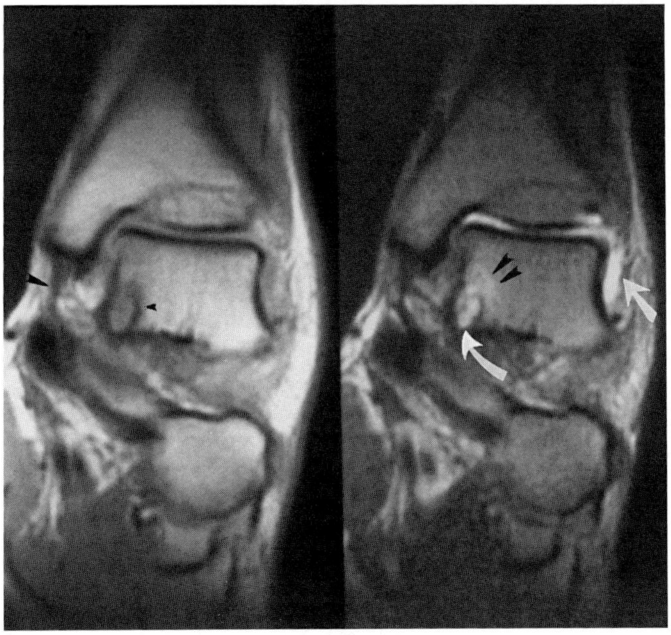

A B

FIGURE 11-3

DISCUSSION: The conventional radiograph reveals a prominent sinus tarsi and a lucency projecting posterior to it (arrowhead in Fig. 11-1). On the sagittal T1-weighted image the normal sinus tarsi fat has been replaced by intermediate signal intensity (open arrow in Fig. 11-2) that extends into adjacent medullary bone (two nonparallel arrowheads in Fig. 11-2). For anatomic purposes, the posterior (triple arrowheads), middle (single arrowhead), and anterior (paired arrowheads) subtalar and talar facets have been identified. Hyperintense signal alteration is apparent on the inferior and medial talar surface (curved white arrow), surrounded by edema.

Because this patient was athletic, posttraumatic cyst with surrounding edema was the favored diagnosis. A history of trauma was not elicited, even though edema (paired arrowheads in Fig.11-3*B*) surrounds the lesion. Both arthropathic cysts and posttraumatic cysts communicate with the articular surface. Arthropathic cysts should be accompanied by other signs of arthropathy, including irregularity and attenuation of cartilaginous interfaces, multifocal disease with geodes and pannus formation, and involvement of weight-bearing surfaces. None of these criteria is present here. The patient did have medial ankle pain, and a diagnosis of deltoid (tibiotalar) ligament injury was considered but excluded on coronal T1-weighted imaging (larger arrowhead in Fig. 11-3*A*).

Unlike intraosseous ganglion, another lesion related to acute or chronic trauma, this lesion communicates with the joint space. Curettage of the lesion revealed an area of cyst formation, secondary to localized nodular synovitis, with scant synovial pigmentation. Pigmented villonodular synovitis (the diffuse articular form), localized nodular synovitis (focal articular form), and giant cell tumor of tendon sheath (local extraarticular form) likely arise as an inflammatory response to recurrent or chronic trauma. Although a neoplastic etiology has been suggested, it is a less likely explanation for this disease.

The three most common joints involved by articular disease are the knee (75%), hip, and ankle. However, tendon involvement is most common about the flexor and extensor tendons of the hand. Such lesions involve the adjacent bone in 25% of the patients. Histologically, the lesions contain variable amounts of lipid, fibrous tissue, and hemosiderin or synovial-laden macrophages.

This explains the heterogeneous MR appearance, which includes mixed areas of bright and intermediate T1 signal due to an admixture of lipid, hemorrhage, and fibrous tissue, and bright and dark T2 signal due to edema, cyst formation, hemorrhage, and hemosiderin.

Cystic lesions are often surrounded by a peripheral hypointense fibrous rim (small arrowhead in Fig. 11-3*A*). Small to moderate joint effusions frequently coexist (white arrow in Fig. 11-3*B*). The intermediate signal intensity hyaline cartilage appears well preserved on sagittal T1-weighted imaging. The appearance of erosive or cystic bone disease is observed in the hip (>90%), shoulder (75%), elbow (60%), ankle (50%), and knee (25%).

MRI serves as a staging tool in this disease for localized resection. Since the incidence of local recurrence after radical resection such as synovectomy is at least 85%, conservative local resections are most commonly performed, with MRI serving as the surgical road map.

DIAGNOSIS: The patient has pigmented nodular synovitis with cyst formation.

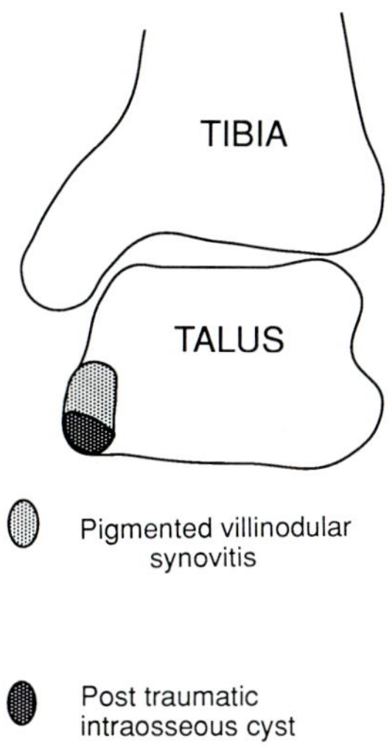

FIGURE 11-4

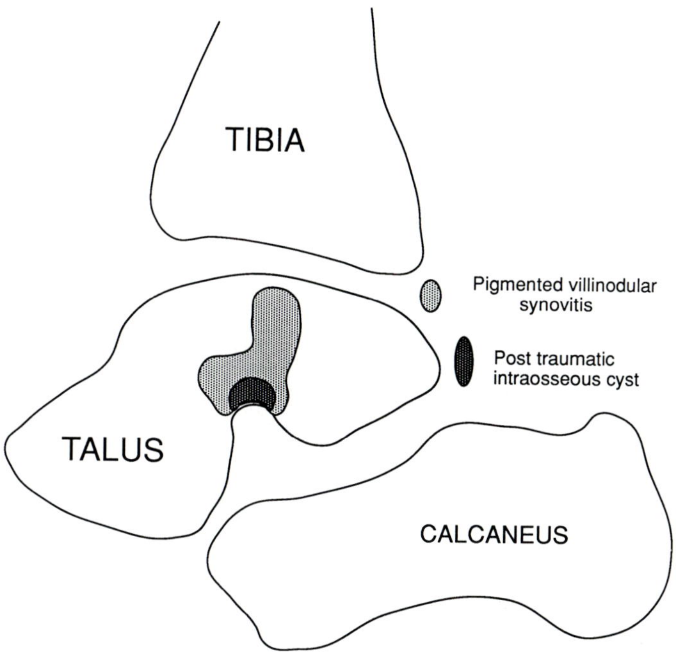

FIGURE 11-5

CASE 12

Differential Diagnosis of Chronic Ankle Pain

HISTORY: A 34-year-old jogger and avid tennis player presented with chronic ankle pain, medial side tenderness, and no evidence of swelling. What is the MRI diagnosis? (Fig. 12-1: anteroposterior radiograph. Fig. 12-2: coronal T1-weighted image. Fig. 12-3: sagittal T2-weighted image.)

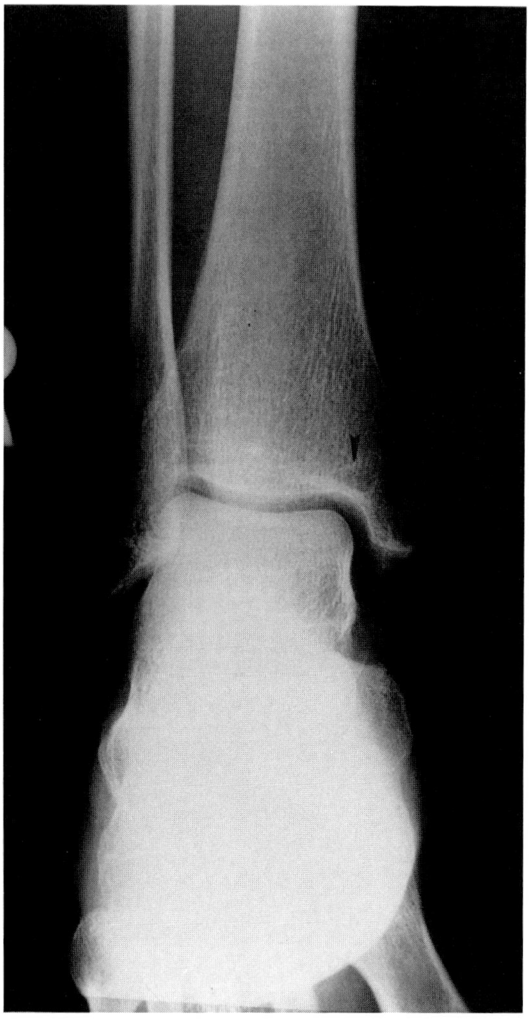

FIGURE 12-1

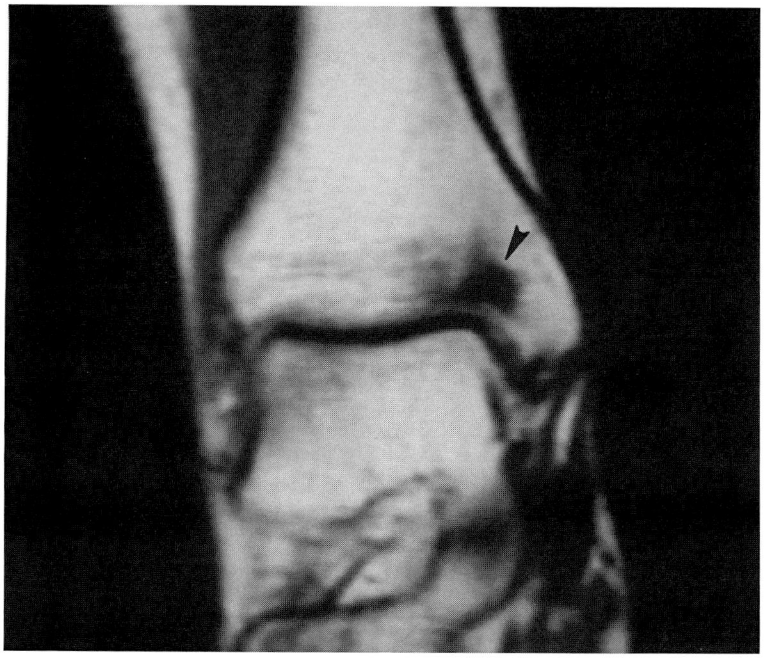

FIGURE 12-2

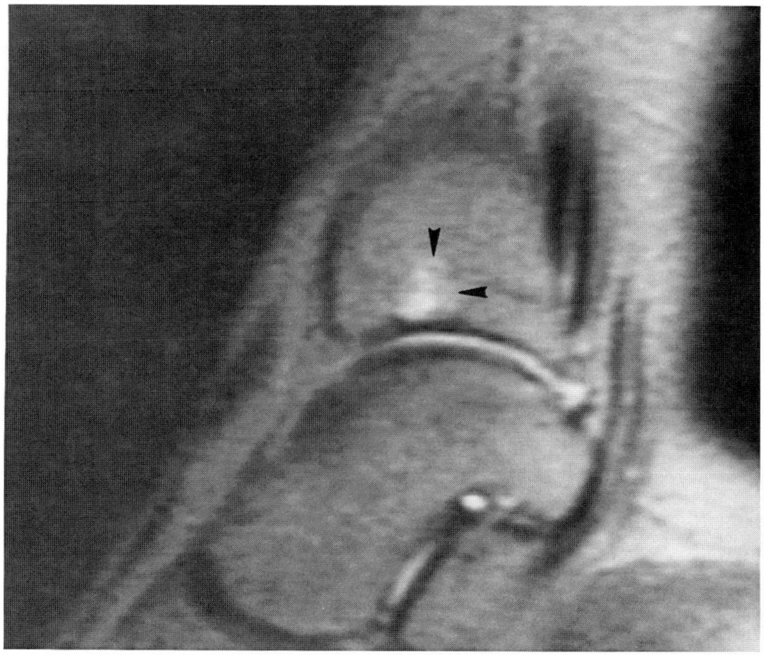

FIGURE 12-3

DISCUSSION: Barely visible on the radiograph is a well-defined lucency in the medial, tibial subchondral bone adjacent to the medial malleolus, with faint sclerotic margins (arrowhead in Fig. 12-1). The lesion is hypointense on T1-weighted imaging arrowhead in Fig. 12-2), easily visible, quite hyperintense on the T2-weighted image (arrowheads in Fig. 8-3), and does not appear to communicate with the articular surface. There is no evidence of joint effusion, and no other direct or indirect signs of arthopathy are present. The findings are typical of intraosseous ganglion. Because these are gelatinous lesions, they are hypointense on T1 and hyperintense on T2, just as is a peritendinous ganglion. They behave as proteinaceous cysts. Supporting the diagnosis in this case is that the most common site of involvement (34% of cases) is the medial aspect of the distal tibia near the medial malleolus.

The lesion is typically eccentric and involves a non-weight-bearing joint surface. It likely has a posttraumatic etiology and is quite rare in persons less than 15 to 20 years old. Unlike posttraumatic or arthropathic cysts, the lesions do not communicate with the joint space, are not accompanied by signs of degenerative arthropathy, and are associated with chronic nagging pain. Degenerative or arthropathic cysts are well marginated, communicate with the joint space, and often are accompanied by other signs of arthropathy, involving hyaline cartilage or bone. Other lesions occurring at bone ends include Brodie's abscess or coccidioidomycosis, lipoma, chondroblastoma, giant cell tumor, arthropathic or posttraumatic cysts, and pigmented villonodular synovitis.

DIAGNOSIS: The patient has an intraosseus ganglion.

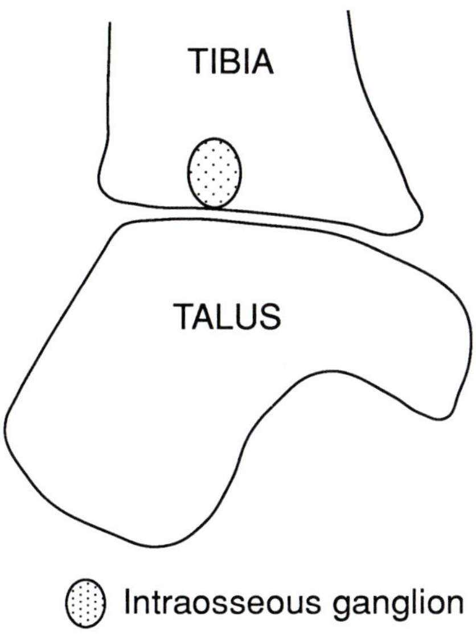

FIGURE 12-4

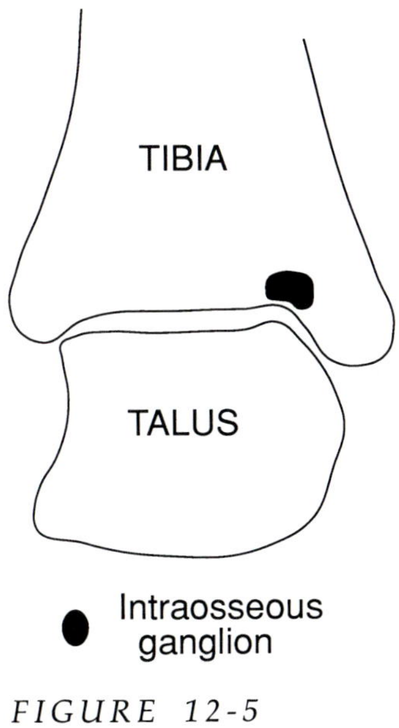

FIGURE 12-5

CASE 13

Differential Diagnosis of Chronic Ankle Pain

HISTORY: A 35-year-old woman on hemodialysis for 4 years and on steroid therapy for 1 year presented with a swollen and tender left ankle joint. What is the MRI diagnosis? (Fig. 13-1: lateral radiograph of the left ankle. Figs. 13-2 and 13-3: sagittal T1-weighted MR images made a year apart.)

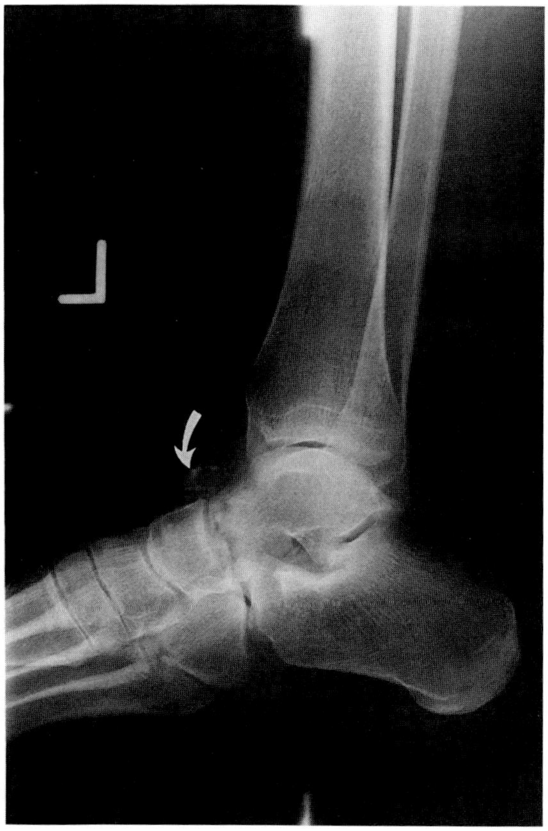

FIGURE 13-1

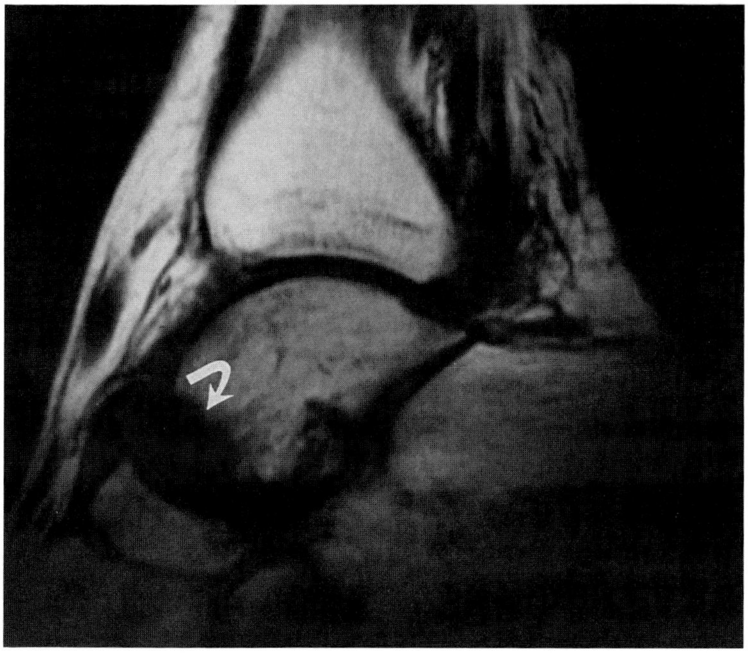

FIGURE 13-2

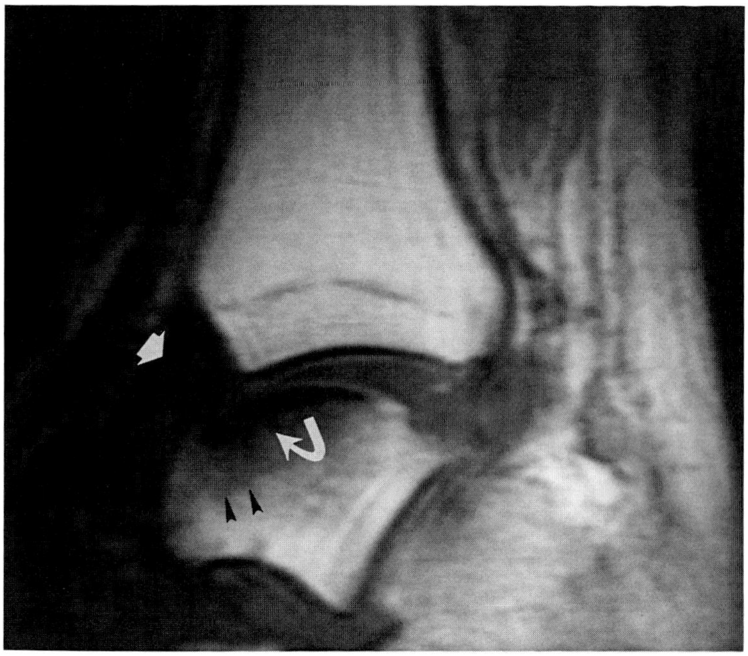

FIGURE 13-3

DISCUSSION: The radiograph shows a calcification projecting dorsad to the talonavicular joint (curved white arrow in Fig. 13-1) and subtle sclerosis in the talar neck. The first T1-weighted image shows confluent hypointense signal in the talar neck that increased little in signal intensity on T2 weighting (image not shown). A confluent T1 signal hypointensity that corresponds to an area of sclerosis on plain radiography and does not increase in intensity on T2-weighted images supports lesion chronicity and a "burned-out" phase of talar avascular necrosis (AVN). One year later, a sagittal T1-weighted image showed confluent, poorly defined, homogeneous hypointense signal in the talar dome (curved white arrow in Fig. 13-3). This signal was hyperintense on T2 (not shown), implying a more recent event. Surrounding areas of poorly defined edema (paired arrowheads in Fig. 13-3) circumscribe the more hypointense subarticular area of necrosis. A large hypointense joint effusion is also present (white arrow in Fig. 13-3). The talar dome is the most common site of steroid-induced AVN, followed by the talar neck.

On conventional radiography, foci of sclerosis occur late; however, with an intact talar vascular supply, acute osteolysis or bone rarefaction may be seen (Hawkin's sign). Because the talus is surrounded by articular cartilage on 60% to 70% of its surface, the talar blood supply is marginal. The artery of the tarsal canal, a branch of the posterior tibial artery, is the major blood supply. Branches of the anterior tibial artery, peroneal, and perforating small branches from synovium of adjacent bones contribute smaller branches.

Fractures are the most common cause of talar AVN. Complete talar dislocations with tibiotalar, subtalar, and talonavicular interruption are associated with AVN in all cases. The other fracture commonly associated with talar AVN (50% of cases) is the vertical fracture that extends into the subtalar joint between the posterior and middle facet.

MRI can demonstrate associated cartilage abnormalities, AVN multiplicity, and approximate disease stage. Lesions that are consistently hypointense on all pulse sequences are not likely to respond to aggressive surgical therapy.

DIAGNOSIS: The patient has steroid-induced acute talar dome osteonecrosis and remote talar neck osteonecrosis.

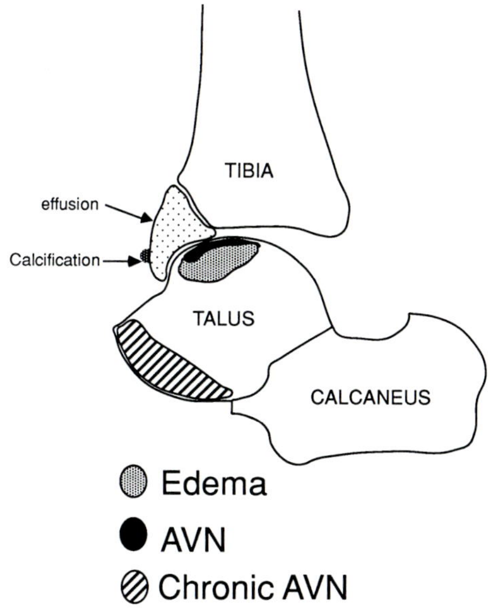

FIGURE 13-4

CASE 14

Differential Diagnosis of Chronic Ankle Pain

HISTORY: Two cases are presented for study. Patient 1, a 17-year-old athletic woman, presented with an acute inversion and dorsiflexion injury after catching her foot on a fence 9 months earlier. Patient 2, a 39-year-old man, sought medical attention for chronic ankle pain and an aching sensation along the medial joint line 4 months' duration. No focal traumatic event was elicited. What is the MRI diagnosis in each case? (Patient 1—Fig. 14-1: sagittal T1-weighted MR image. Fig. 14-2: sagittal multiecho, multiformat proton-density (*A*) and T2-weighted (*B*) MR images. Fig. 14-3: coronal T1-weighted image. Patient 2—Fig. 14-4: coronal multiformat, multiecho proton-density (*A*) and T2-weighted (*B*) images.)

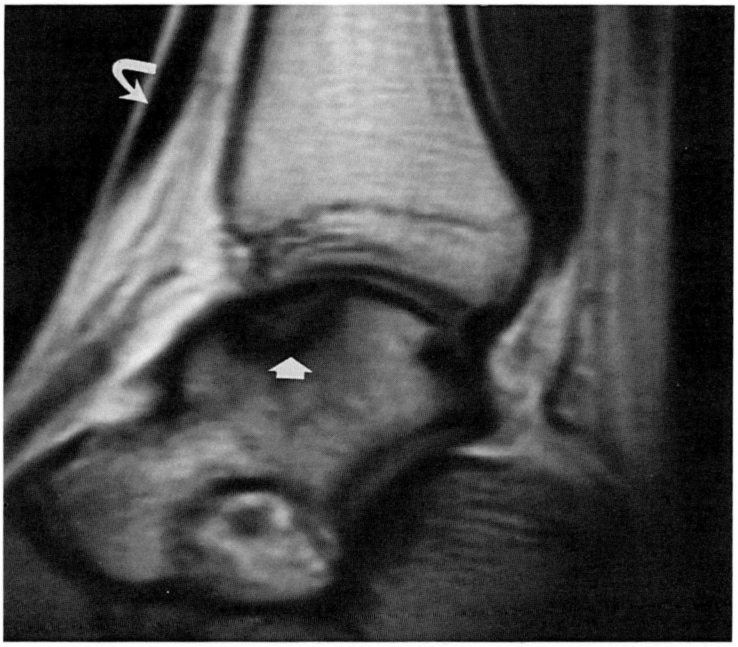

FIGURE 14-1

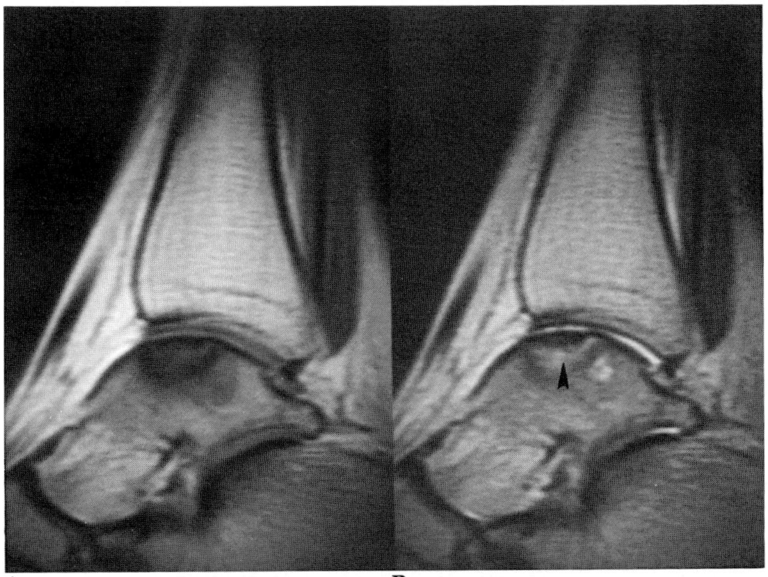

A B

FIGURE 14-2

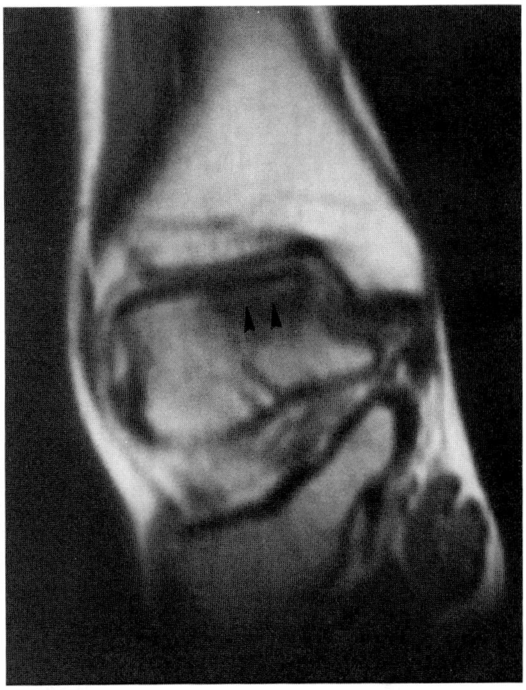

FIGURE 14-3

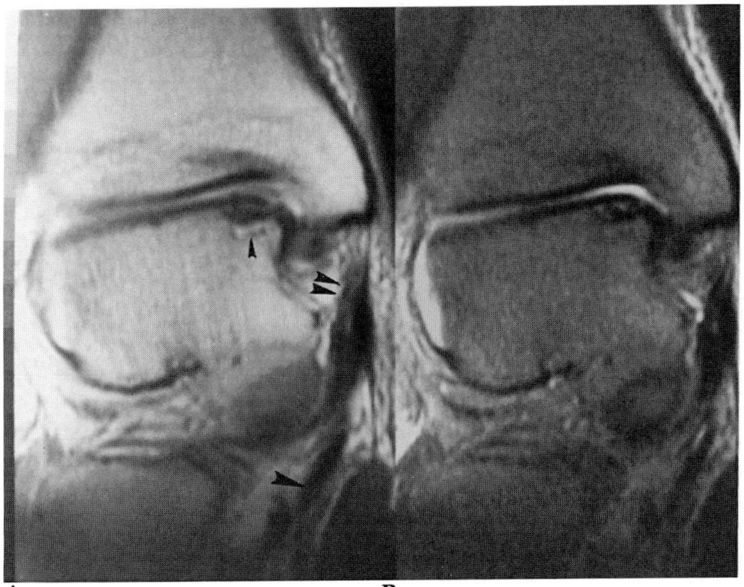

A B

FIGURE 14-4

DISCUSSION

PATIENT 1: A plain radiograph in this case was normal. A posttraumatic etiology is clear for two reasons: the patient's history and the cortical depression visualized on the sagittal T2-weighted image (arrowhead in Fig. 14-2*B*). While one is tempted to make a diagnosis of avascular necrosis (AVN), osteochondral injury or osteochondritis dissecans is more likely. The area of signal alteration is extensive, heterogeneous, and surrounded by a hypointense fibrous rim (white arrow in Fig. 14-1) and a hyperintense reactive interface (arrowhead in Fig. 14-2*B*) similar to that seen in AVN of the hip.

Areas of low signal intensity on the T2-weighted image corresponded pathologically to areas of fibrosis and avascular granulation tissue. The reactive area of hyperintense signal on the T2-weighted image corresponded to hemorrhagic and edematous bone. This patient was virtually asymptomatic 2 years following surgical correction of bone depression. An osteochondral fracture with 6 mm of depression was found surgically. The normal tibialis anterior tendon (curved white arrow in Fig. 14-1) is identified. The transverse extent of the lesion is best assessed on the coronal image (arrowheads in Fig. 14-3).

PATIENT 2: In contrast to the first case a focal, well-circumscribed smaller area of hypointense signal is surrounded by a hyperintense rim. With medial ankle pain, the status of the deltoid ligament is relevant; it is intact (paired arrowheads in Fig. 14-4*A*). Osteochondritis dissecans is most commonly seen in adolescents and may involve bone, bone and cartilage, or cartilage alone. Therefore, terms such as osteochondral injury, osteochondral fracture, or transchondral fracture are used synonymously.

These lesions may remain in their normal position (in situ), or undergo cartilage migration or bone and cartilage migration. Because there is both bone and cartilaginous signal change but without clear detachment of bone and cartilage, this would be categorized as a grade 2 lesion. Clearly detached osteochondral fragments are considered grade 3, and dislodged, migrated osteochondral fragments are grade 4. Grade 1 simply represents bone injury or signal alteration without cartilaginous signal change. The fact that the lesion is hyperintense on T2 weighting with minimal surrounding edema and small joint effusion supports an acute or subacute injury. Remote osteochondral injury tends to remain hypointense on T1 spin-density imaging.

Osteochondral lesions may resorb, may increase in size (owing to heterotopic bone formation), may become embedded in synovium, or may act as a loose body. The medial posterior talar dome is by far the most common site involved. The mechanism is commonly eversion and hyperextension so that the talar dome is compressed against the tibia. Medial lesions tend to be larger and deeper than lateral lesions. The function of MRI is to detect in situ and migrated bone and cartilage fragments. Normal conventional radiographs and grossly abnormal MRI findings are common in osteochondral injury to the talus.

DIAGNOSIS: Both patients have osteochondral injury or osteochondritis dissecans.

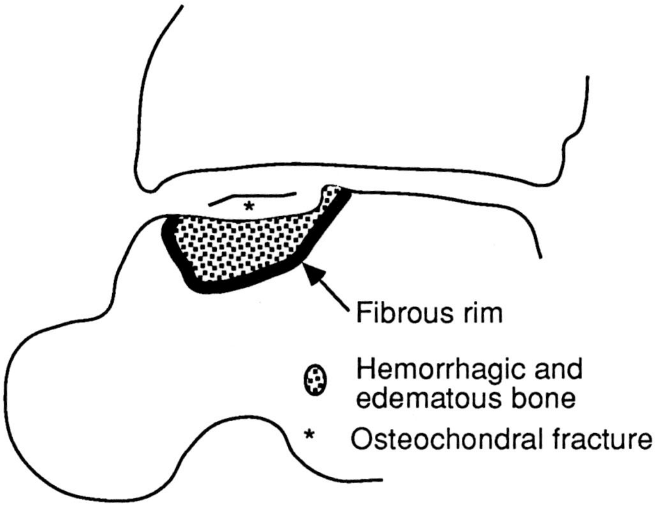

FIGURE 14-5

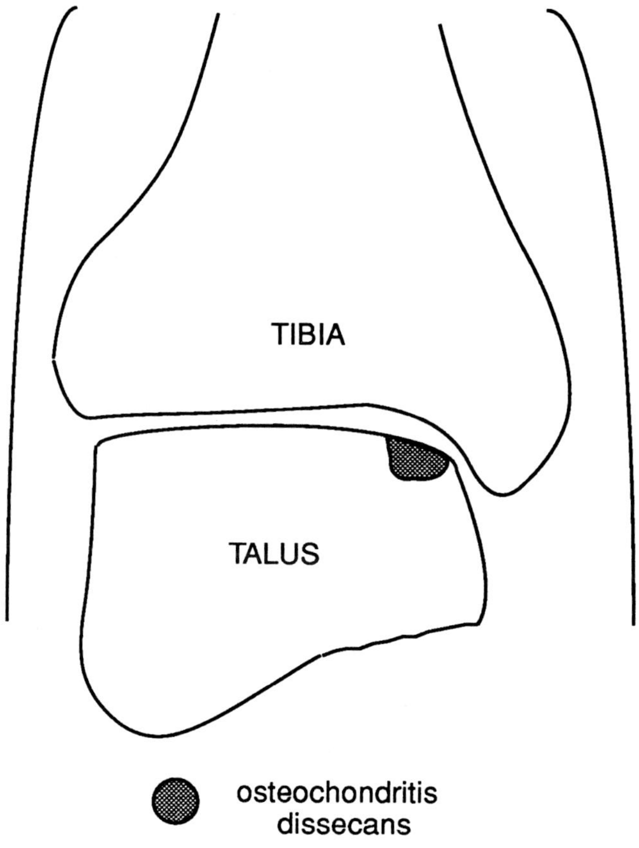

FIGURE 14-6

CASE 15

Differential Diagnosis of Chronic Ankle Pain

HISTORY: A 21-year-old football player presented with chronic ankle pain and swelling of 1 year's duration and was referred for evaluation of possible avascular necrosis. What is the MRI diagnosis? (Fig. 15-1: axial multiformat (two-on-one), multiecho proton-density (*A*) and T2-weighted MR images. Fig. 15-2: similar imaging sequence, sagittal views.)

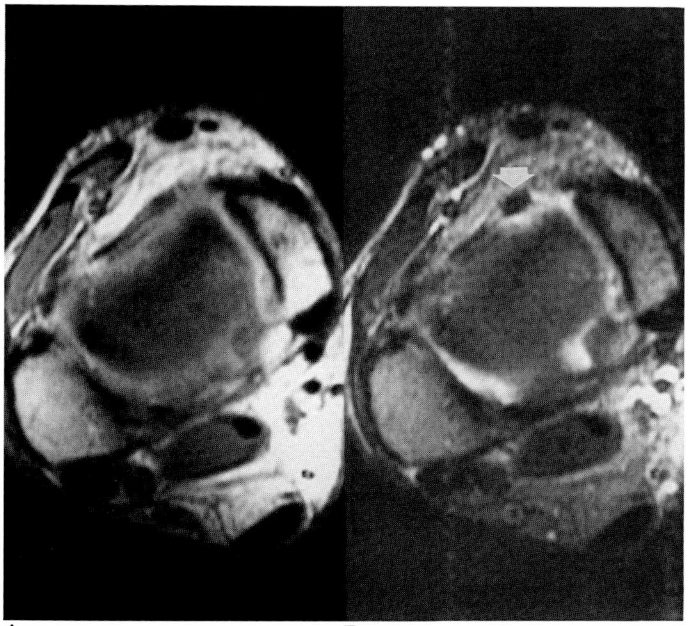

A **B**

FIGURE 15-1

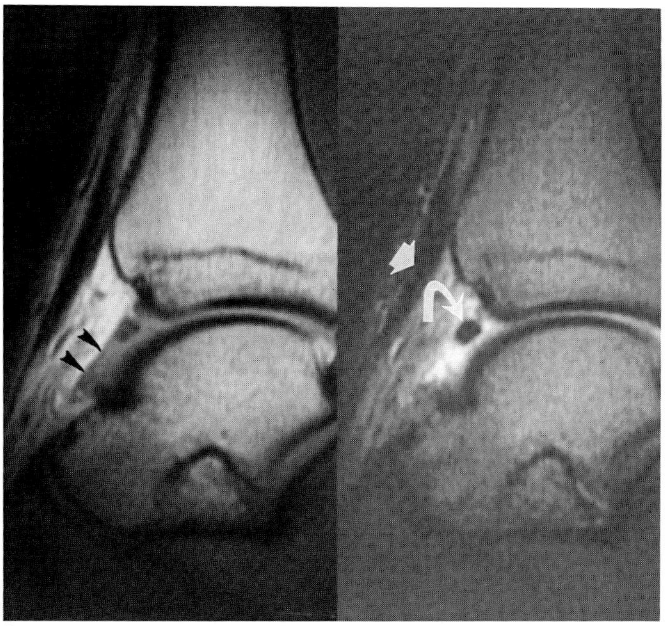

A **B**

FIGURE 15-2

DISCUSSION: Along the anterior joint line is a focal area of decreased signal that becomes more hypointense on T2-weighted imaging (curved white arrow in Fig. 15-2*B*). This hypointensity stands out against a background of joint fluid, which is hyperintense on the T2-weighted imaging and isointense on proton-density imaging. The effusion (paired arrowheads in Fig. 15-2*A*) completely surrounds this hypointense region, and the interface of the joint fluid (which is intermediate on spin-density imaging) corresponds to the anterior extent of the joint capsule, distended and easily separable from the more hyperintense anterior fat.

The tibialis anterior tendon is identified as a hypointense linear band (white arrow in Fig. 15-2*B*). The differential diagnosis of focal hypointensity includes calcium or bone, iron, gas, and flow. The lesion's shape and its progressive hypointensity with T2 weighting are compatible with calcification. Calcifications sometimes appear hyperintense on T1-weighted imaging, particularly posthemorrhagic calcification or synovial chondromas.

DIAGNOSIS: The patient has a calcific loose joint body.

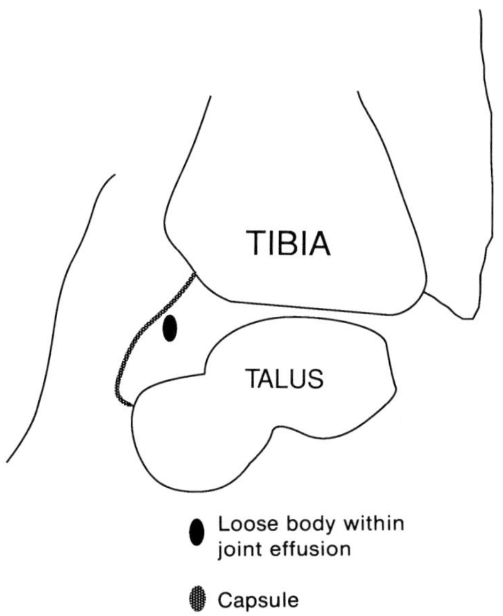

FIGURE 15-3

CASE 16

Differential Diagnosis of Chronic Ankle Pain

HISTORY: The MR images in this study show a spectrum of bone injuries in patients aged 35 to 37 years who sustained trauma in the 2 months preceding study and whose conventional radiographs were normal. Identify and diagnose the various injuries. (Figs. 16-1 through 16-3: sagittal multiformat (two-on-one) T1-weighted images, multiecho proton-density images, and T2-weighted images, respectively.)

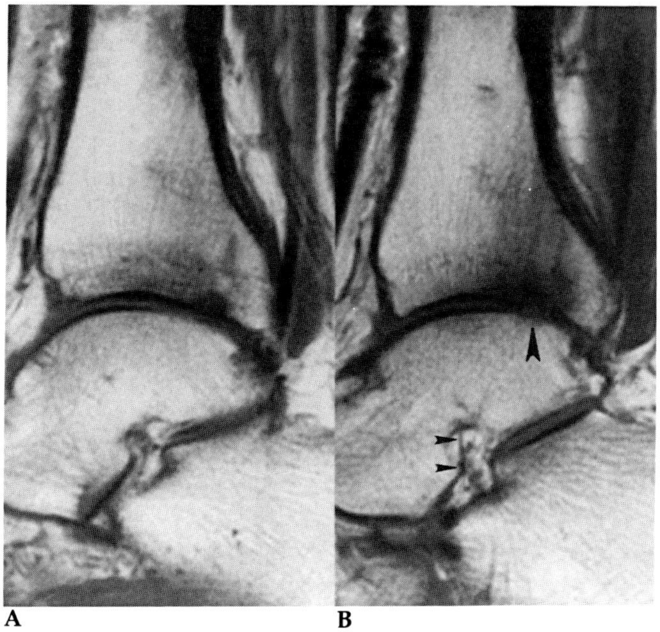

FIGURE 16-1

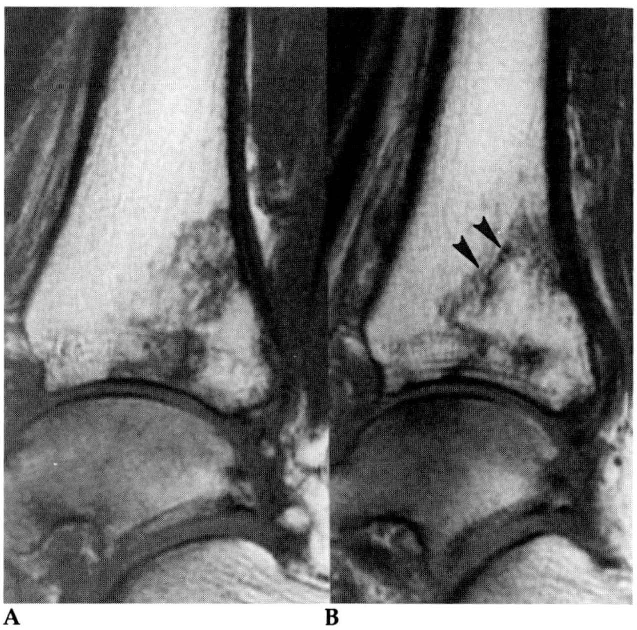

FIGURE 16-2

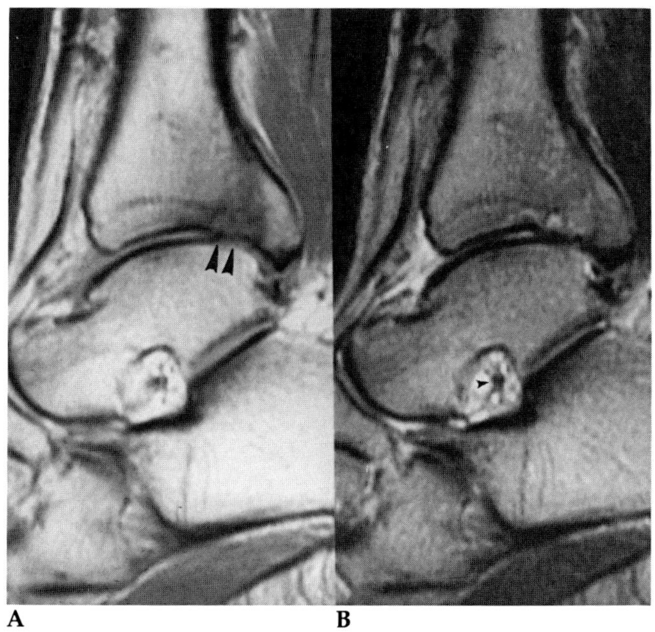

FIGURE 16-3

DISCUSSION: In Figure 16-1 the subarticular tibial surface demonstrates diffuse signal hypointensity that is poorly defined but without identifiable lines of stress or macrofracture. The appearance is typical of bone contusion. The posterior talus demonstrates subtle irregularity; however, there is interruption of the normally smooth, overlying intermediate signal intensity hyaline cartilage (single arrowhead in Fig. 16-1*B*). The findings are typical of transchondral fracture or defect. In this instance, the injury to the cartilage is far more extensive than that which occurs in the underlying talar bone. Therefore, osteochondral fracture would be a misnomer.

In Figure 16-2, the talus is of diffuse T1 signal hypointensity, poorly marginated, and not associated with microfracture or macrofracture lines. The hyaline cartilage is smooth, gray, and homogeneous, overlying the contused or edematous hypointense talus. The tibia, in contrast to Figure 16-1, has a nondisplaced microfracture line that was inapparent on plain radiographs. These latter findings (paired arrowheads in Fig. 16-2*B*) are typical of stress or microfracture.

In Figure 16-3 the normal posterior hyaline cartilage is interrupted and effaced (paired arrowheads in Fig. 16-3*A*). Irregularity of the overlying posterior tibial cortex and deeper medullary bone T2 signal hyperintensity demarcate a subchondral fracture or defect. Therefore, this lesion would qualify as a true osteochondral fracture, injury, and defect.

DIAGNOSIS: Shown are examples of transchondral fracture, osteochondral fracture, bone contusions or bruises, and stress fractures.

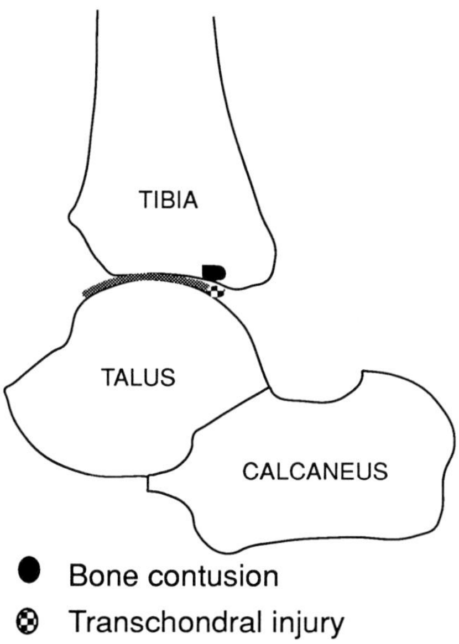

FIGURE 16-4

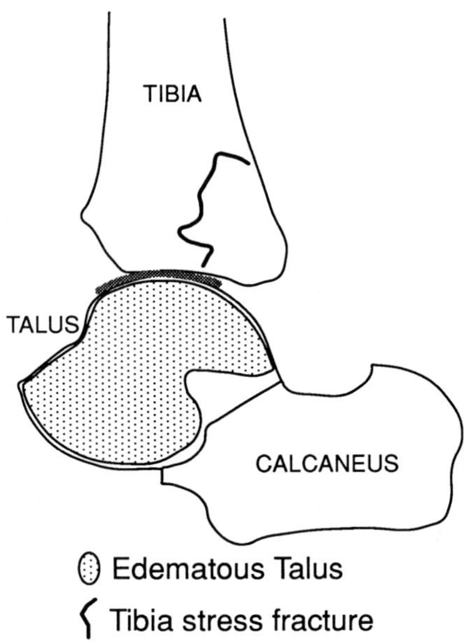

FIGURE 16-5

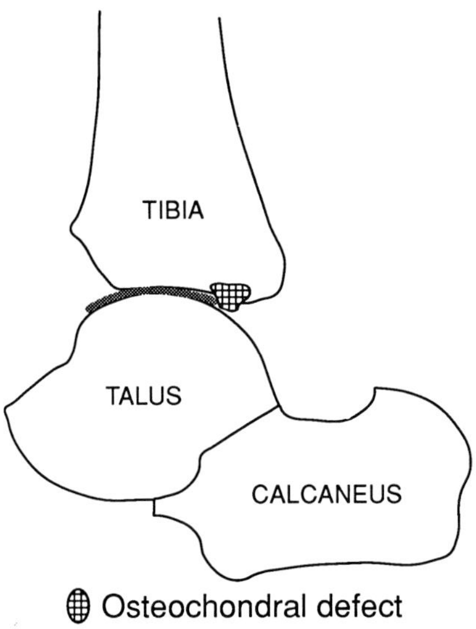

FIGURE 16-6

CASE 17

Differential Diagnosis of Heel Pain

HISTORY: Two cases are compared in this file. A 39-year-old man presented with pain in the heel and lower calf region, tenderness, and pain exacerbated on plantar flexion. The second patient was a 31-year-old woman with similar but less pronounced symptoms. What is the MRI diagnosis? (Patient 1—Fig. 17-1: sagittal T1-weighted MR image. Patient 2—Fig. 17-2: sagittal T1-weighted image, and Fig. 17-3: multiformat (two-on-one), multiecho proton-density (*A*) and T2-weighted MR images.)

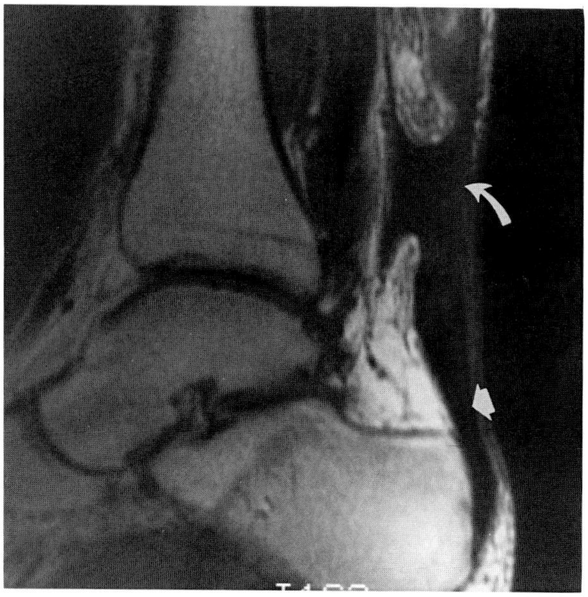

FIGURE 17-1

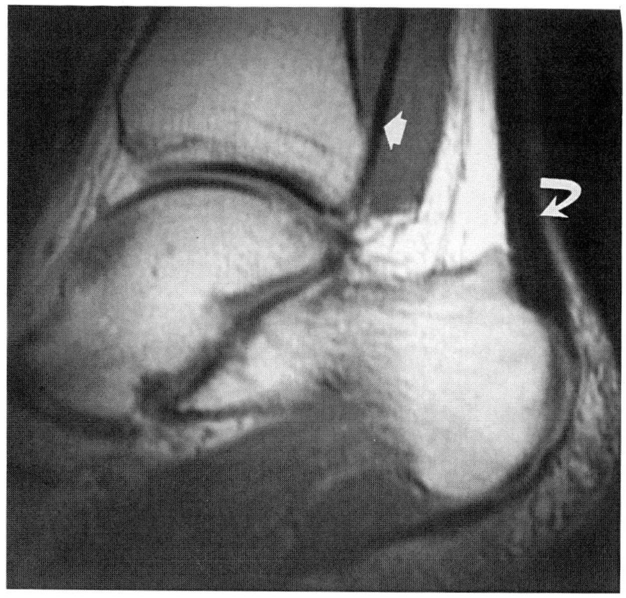

FIGURE 17-2

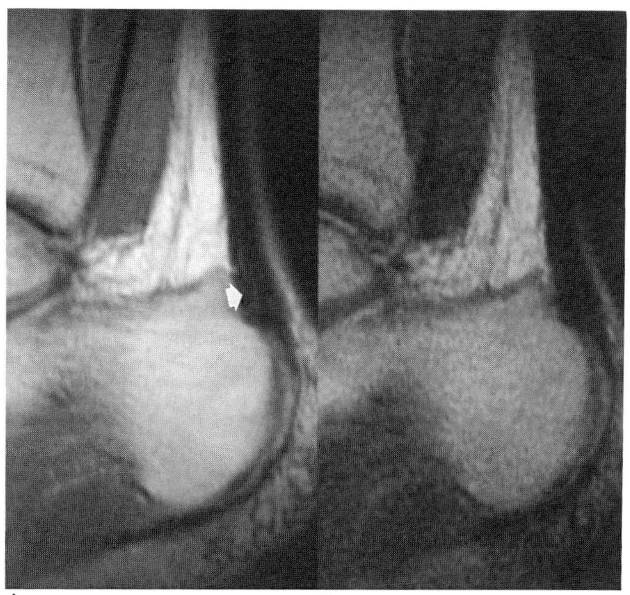

A **B**

FIGURE 17-3

DISCUSSION

PATIENT 1: The Achilles tendon is visualized as a hypointense black band that runs from the posterior calcaneal tubercle and extends as a thin sheet of hypointense signal toward the calf. The normal subcutaneous fat is interrupted by diffuse intermediate signal intensity edema. In addition, the hypointense tendon comes to an abrupt halt and is replaced by an area of intermediate signal intensity (curved white arrow in Fig. 17-1) that represents acute blood and edema. The fact that the tendinous anatomy cannot be traced through this intermediate signal intensity pseudomass, and that its proximal end cannot be identified, is diagnostic of complete tendinous transection. The distal portion of the tendon is identified (short white arrow in Fig. 17-1).

We assess the Achilles tendon with either a circular wraparound coil or tandem axial pair, 4 to 6 inches in diameter. The foot is held in a neutral position, since overflexion may produce false tendon thickening. Axial and sagittal multiecho proton-density and T2-weighted imaging with small fields of view (<16.0 cm) is critical to achieving appropriate resolution so that partial and complete tears are separable. However, two- or three-dimensional fast scan imaging is exquisitely sensitive for demonstrating subtle intrasubstance signal alterations.

Most Achilles tendon ruptures occur within 4.0 cm of the tendinous insertion on the calcaneal tubercle. Men are affected more often than women in a ratio of 4 : 1. This portion of the tendon tends to be less vascular, and the fibers cross anteriorly from lateral to medial aspects, but posteriorly from medial to lateral aspects. Factors predisposing to Achilles tendon rupture include prior steroid injection, rheumatoid arthritis, gout, and chronic renal failure. Sports-related injury or rupture of the Achilles tendon occurs with sudden pronation of the foot, particularly in athletes who overtrain by running on rough or uneven terrain.

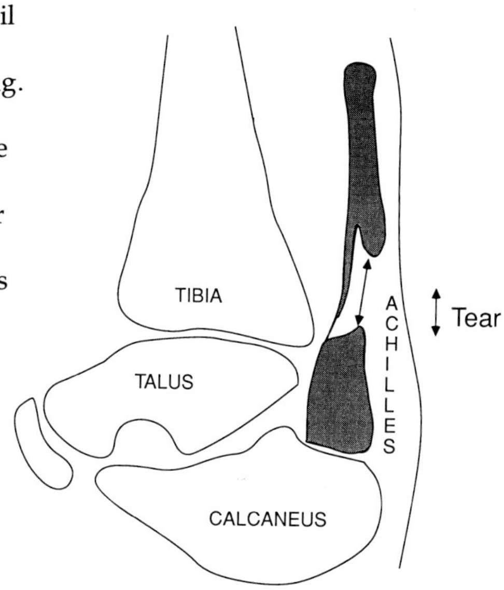

FIGURE 17-4

PATIENT 2: The Achilles tendon (curved white arrow in Fig. 17-2) on MRI is homogeneously hypointense; therefore, any increase in signal intensity should be considered abnormal. Linear striated intratendinous signal without tendon retraction (white arrow in Fig. 17-3*A*) is indicative of tendinitis.

Masses of blood that replace the normal tendon signal with some tendon contiguity represent partial tear. Complete transection is diagnosed when complete discontiguity is present; retraction may coexist. Sometimes the gastrocnemius muscle may retract into the proximal calf and is mistaken for a tumor. Because the tendon has no true synovial sheath, edema and hemorrhage are not well confined and often extend anteriorly into the paratenon.

The treatment of Achilles tendon rupture varies with the extent of transection. High-grade lesions may be treated with surgical excision and repair; however, the rate of rerupture is $2\frac{1}{2}$ times that seen with conservative repair. Tendinitis is treated with stretching, reduction in athletic training, orthotics, and antiinflammatory agents.

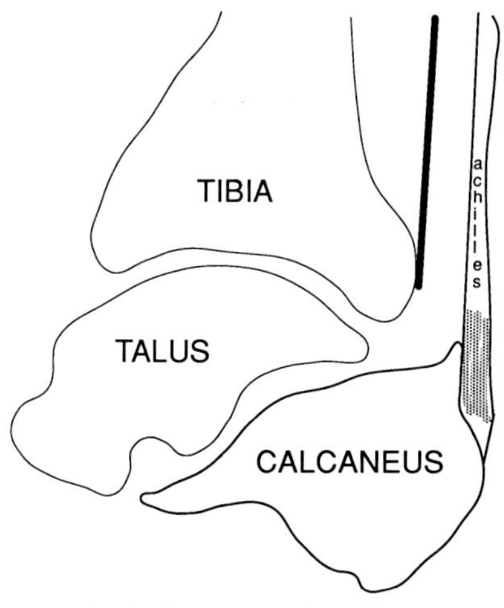

FIGURE 17-5

DIAGNOSIS: The first patient has complete Achilles tendon rupture; the second has Achilles tendinitis.

CASE 18

Differential Diagnosis of Acute Heel Pain

HISTORY: Two related cases are analyzed in this file. A 25-year-old ballet dancer presented with severe pain on plantar flexion, particularly when dancing with her toes pointed. She was referred to confirm a diagnosis of acute Achilles tendon tear. The second patient was a 34-year-old man with a questionable mass and pain behind the distal tibia and ankle joint. Achilles tendon rupture was suspected clinically. What are the MRI diagnoses? (Patient 1—Fig. 18-1: sagittal contiguous multiformat (two-on-one) T1-weighted images, and Fig. 18-2: axial T1-weighted image. Patient 2—Fig. 18-3: sagittal multiformat (two-on-one), multiecho proton-density (*A*) and T2-weighted (*B*) MR images.)

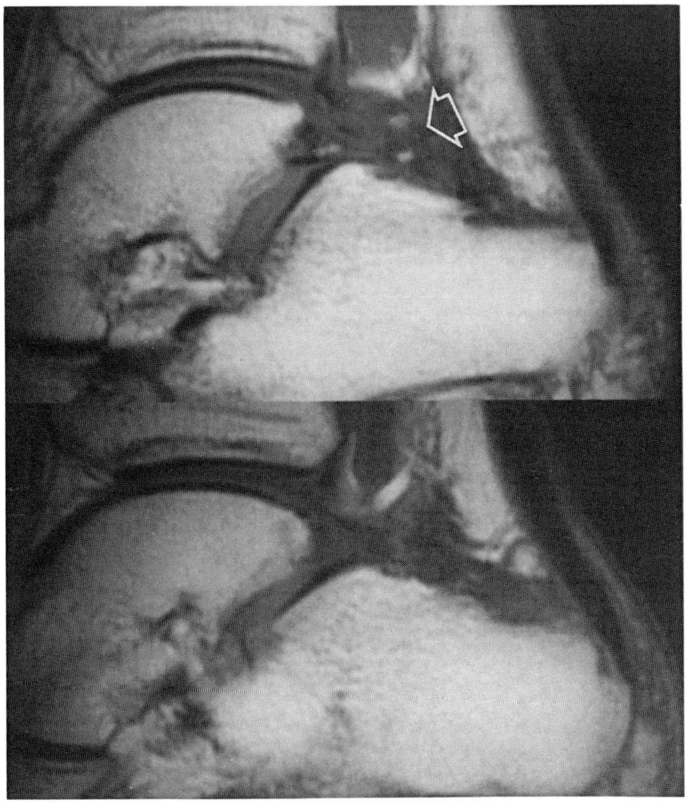

A

B

FIGURE 18-1

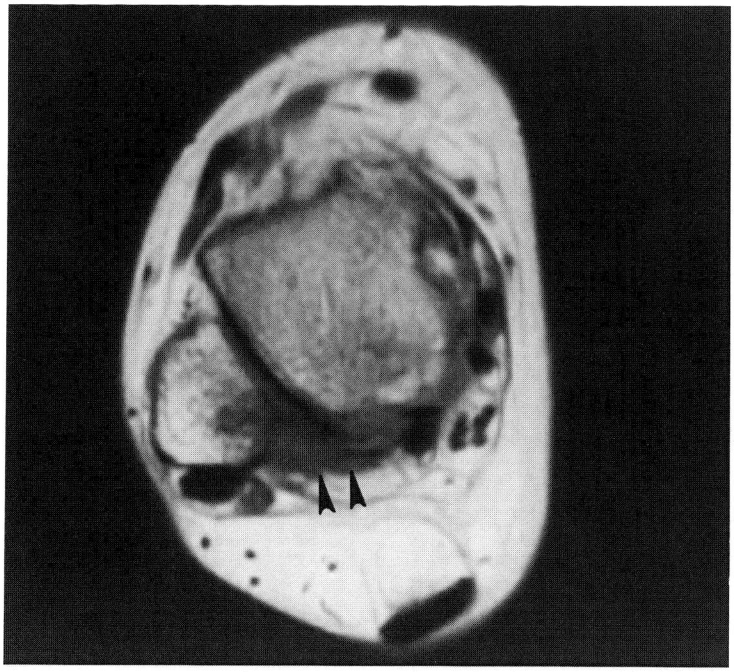

FIGURE 18-2

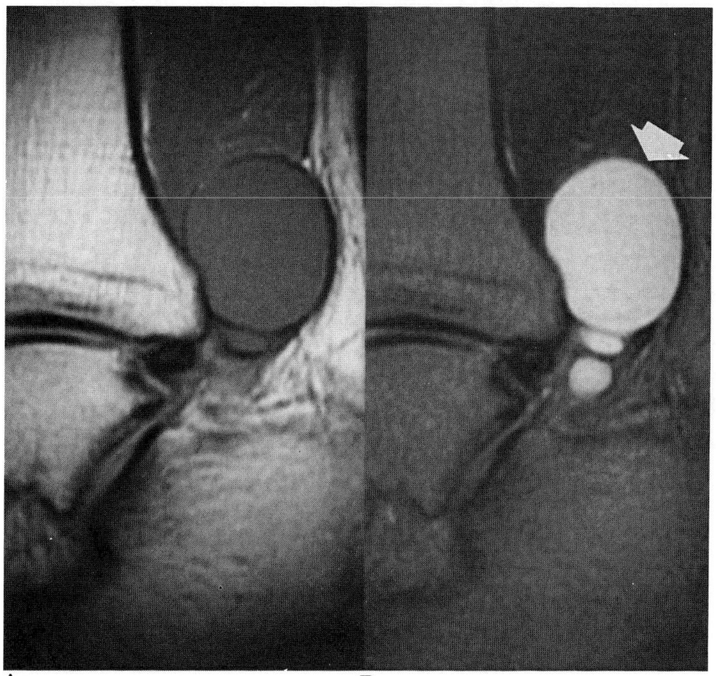

A **B**

FIGURE 18-3

DISCUSSION

PATIENT 1: In Figure 18-1, the sagittal contiguous T1-weighted images, the Achilles tendon is visualized as a thick, hypointense, homogeneous black band. Its insertion along the calcaneal tubercle is smooth and uninterrupted. However, deep to the tendon and just posterior to the tibiotalar interface is an inhomogeneous area of intermediate, mixed increased and decreased signal intensity (open arrow in Fig. 18-1*A*). This is the anatomic distribution of the posterior talofibular ligament.

The actual ligament itself cannot be identified, because of edema and hemorrhage at the injury site. The normal myofascial and fat planes are interrupted. In addition, peroneus longus and brevis tendinitis was discovered. In the axial projection, thickening of the posterior talofibular ligament (paired arrowheads in Fig. 18-2) confirms the diagnosis of ligamentous injury.

PATIENT 2: A well-circumscribed, smooth, homogeneous mass is apparent that is of low signal intensity on the sagittal T1-weighted image and high signal intensity on the T2-weighted image (arrow in Fig. 18-3*B*). The mass appears multiloculated and does not produce edema in the adjacent muscular soft tissues or bone. The anatomy just posterior to the tibia's posterior malleolus is obscured by the mass and by inhomogeneous foci of signal hypo- and hyperintensity. This is the anatomic location of the posterior tibiofibular ligament. The common ganglion actually develops as a result of myxoid degeneration and cystic softening of connective tissue of a joint capsule or tendon sheath. It tends to wrap around the tendon sheath. The ganglion contents are gelatinous and hypointense on T1 and hyperintense on T2 images.

Other myxoid soft tissue masses such as myxoid liposarcoma tend to have high signal on T1- and on T2-weighted images. Bursitis would have an identical signal intensity, but this would be an atypical location. Tenosynovitis would have a similar signal intensity but the signal pattern would be diffuse, poorly marginated, not masslike, and would extend directly along the tendon sheath.

Pigmented villonodular synovitis may produce rounded fluidlike signal masses, but these are inhomogeneous, cross joint spaces, are associated with bone or joint destruction, and exhibit hypointense T2 hemosiderin-laden nodules. Synovial sarcoma frequently arises near, but not from, the synovium of joint capsules, bursa, or tendon sheaths. These lesions are hypointense on T1-weighted imaging (but not as hypointense as seen in this case), markedly inhomogeneous, and hyperintense on T2-weighted images. Only 12% of synovial sarcomas occur in the foot.

DIAGNOSIS: The first patient has a normal Achilles tendon with a posterior talofibular ligamentous injury. The second patient has posterior tibiofibular ligament disruption and a common ganglion.

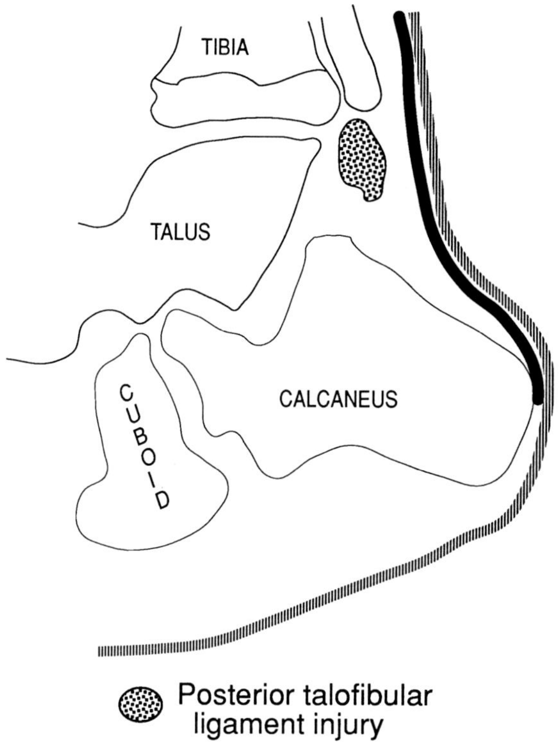

FIGURE 18-4

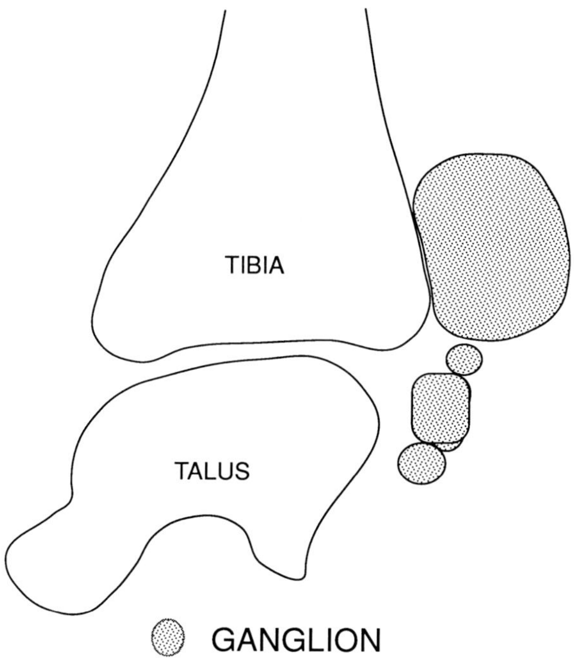

FIGURE 18-5

CASE 19

Differential Diagnosis of Acute Ankle Pain

HISTORY: A 35-year-old man with sickle cell disease sought medical attention for severe pain in the ankle and distal leg. The patient had a temperature of 102°F. What is the MRI diagnosis? (Fig. 19-1: anteroposterior radiograph of the left ankle. Fig. 19-2: coronal multiformat (two-on-one) T1-weighted (*A*) and T2-weighted (*B*) MR images.)

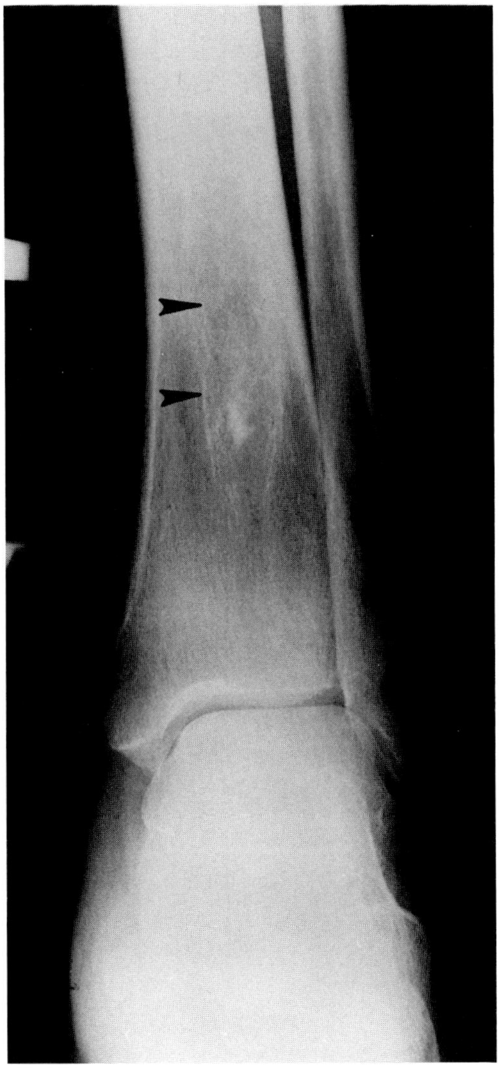

FIGURE 19-1

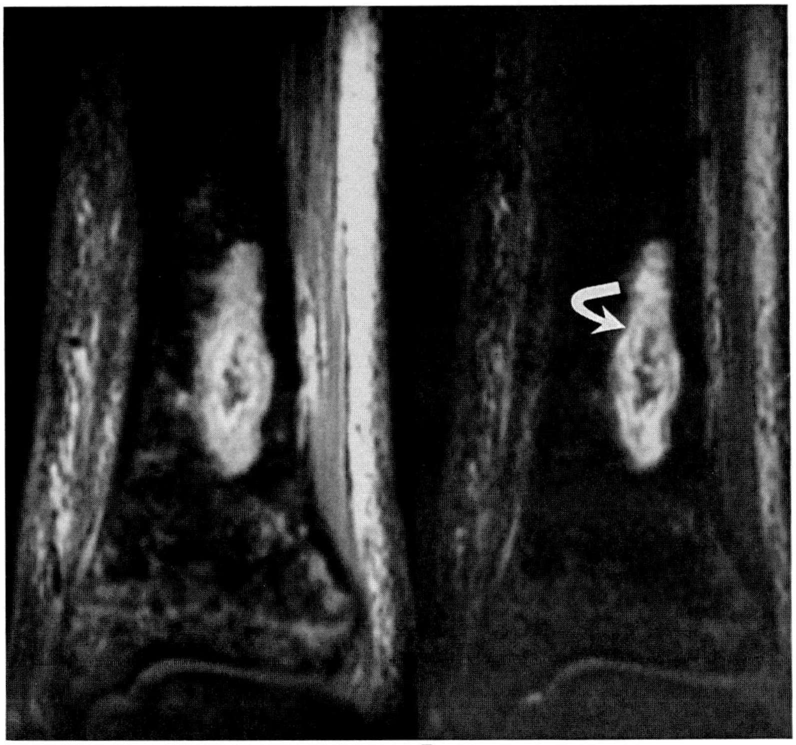

A B

FIGURE 19-2

DISCUSSION: The differential diagnosis of bone pain in the clinical setting of sickle cell disease includes infection and infarction. For a 35-year-old patient, the signal of the tibia is markedly decreased and quite inhomogeneous. The signal decrease is due to overproduction of red cells and an increase in the ratio of red marrow to yellow marrow as a result of peripheral hemolysis. This has been referred to as reconverted marrow.

Wherever red marrow exists (hemolytic anemia, pediatric population, red cell overproduction), the medullary bone signal will diminish. This case illustrates how important conventional radiographs are in the interpretation of musculoskeletal MR images. With conventional radiography, it becomes apparent that the lesion represents infarction. It appears well marginated and centrally sclerotic with a sclerotic rim (arrowheads in Fig. 19-1). An irregularly shaped hyperintense lesion is present on the T1-weighted image that becomes brighter on the T2-weighted image (curved white arrow in Fig. 19-2*B*) with a hypointense center. The hypointense center represents calcification. The facts that this lesion is so well circumscribed on MR, particularly on conventional radiographs, with little in the way of edema or periosteal reaction, and that the signal is hyperintense on both T1- and on T2-weighted imaging support a hemorrhagic component.

DIAGNOSIS: The patient has a hemorrhagic bone infarction.

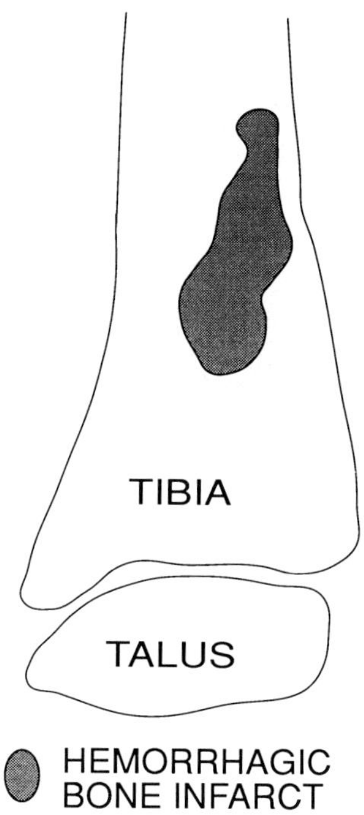

FIGURE 19-3

CASE 20

Differential Diagnosis of Chronic Lower Extremity Pain

HISTORY: A 40-year-old man presented with remote lower extremity trauma and chronic lower extremity pain, without tenderness or swelling. Images from a second case are shown for comparison. What is the MRI diagnosis? (Fig. 20-1: coronal T1-weighted MR image. Fig. 20-2: axial multiformat (two-on-one), multiecho proton-density (*A*) and T2-weighted images (*B*). For comparison—Fig. 20-3: lateral radiograph. Fig. 20-4: coronal multiformat (two-on-one) proton-density (*A*) and T2-weighted (*B*) MR images.)

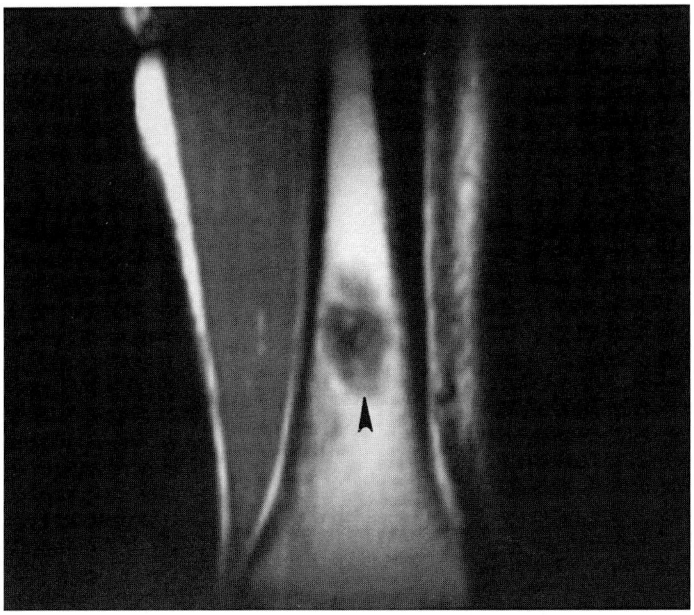

FIGURE 20-1

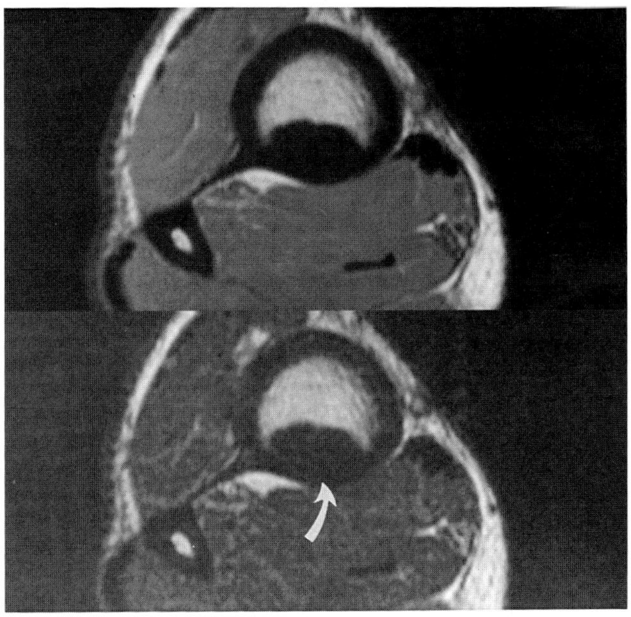

A

B

FIGURE 20-2

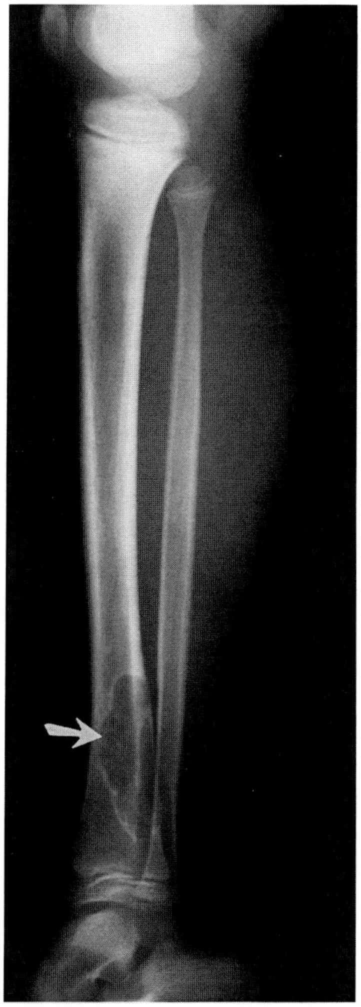

FIGURE 20-3

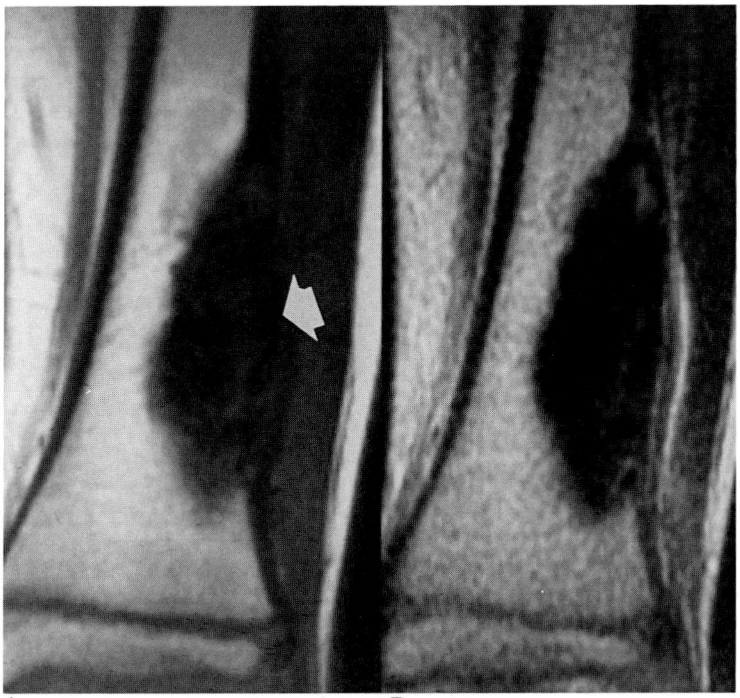

A B

FIGURE 20-4

DISCUSSION: Fibrous cortical defects and nonossifying fibromas are the most common fibrous lesions of bone. As nonosteogenic lytic lesions, they are more commonly seen in children and adolescents than in adults, in boys more often than girls, and have a predilection for the distal femur and tibia.

The lesions are asymptomatic in 30% of cases, eccentric, confined to the cortex of the long bone of the growth plate, and on conventional radiography appear marginated by thin sclerosis. When large, they may encroach on the medullary cavity. Margins are typically scalloped. When these lesions heal spontaneously, they may persist as a sclerotic, eccentric patch and should not be biopsied.

In the healed phase, the MRI appearance is that of a well-demarcated hypointense region without medullary bone or soft tissue edema, unless fracture is present and markedly hypointense on both T1-, spin-density, and T2-weighted imaging (arrowhead in Fig. 20-1, curved white arrow in Fig. 20-2*B*). Nonossifying fibromas or fibroxanthomas before they heal or sclerose may appear scalloped, well demarcated, and hypointense on T1 weighting and quite hyperintense on T2 weighting, with a dark fibrous rim (see case 93 in Chapter 2, The Knee). However, when xanthomatous elements predominate, the lesions are hyperintense on T1 and either intermediate or hyperintense on T2. The differential diagnosis includes the following:

1. Ossifying fibroma or Sissons' lesion: hypointense on T1, hyperintense on T2, tending to affect the tibia and humerus, and pathologically containing fibrous tissue with spindle cells and calcified cementum-like spherules.
2. Osteofibrous dysplasia (Kempson–Campanacci lesion): first or second decades of life; affecting the anterior tibia and fibula; frequently intercortical, osteolytic, eccentric, scalloped with sclerotic borders; and producing anterior bowing at the long bones. These lesions are also hypointense on T1 and hyperintense on T2.
3. Fibrous dysplasia: occurring at any age when monostotic and in the first to third decades of life when polyostotic; pathologically, woven bone in a loose connected tissue stroma; hypointensity on T1 not as pronounced as in nonossifying fibroma, ossifying fibroma, or osteofibrous dysplasia.

The comparison case shows a lesion that appears cystic on plain radiographs (arrow in Fig. 20-3) but is hypointense on the coronal sequences (arrow in Fig. 20-4*A*). We have referred to this hypointense fibrous signal in the setting of a lytic lesion on plain radiography as the fibrous type of nonossifying fibroma.

DIAGNOSIS: The patient has a nonossifying fibroma or fibroxanthoma.

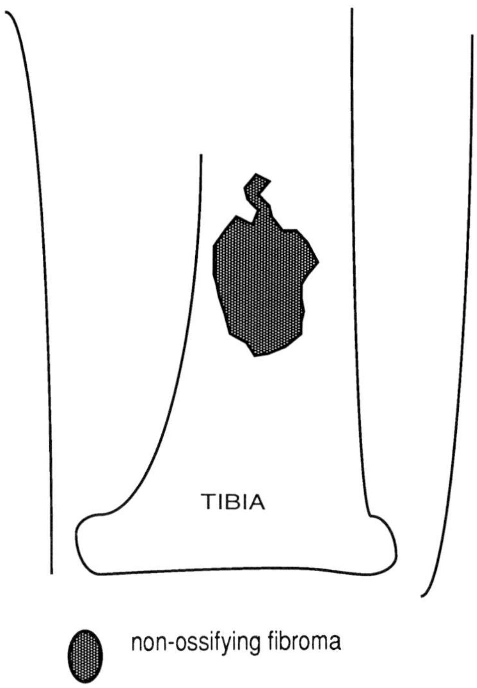

FIGURE 20-5

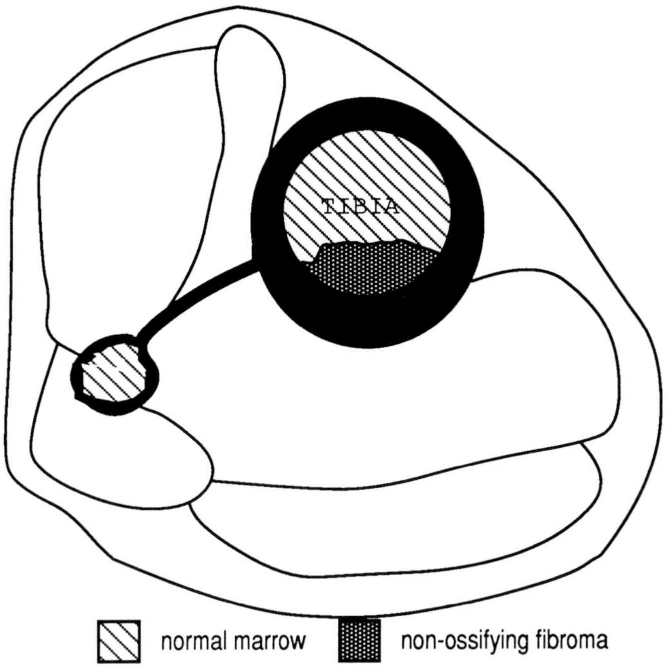

FIGURE 20-6

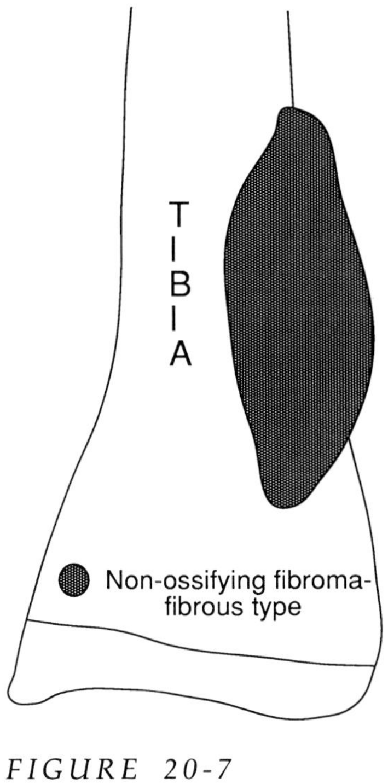

FIGURE 20-7

PART V

Elbow, Forearm, Wrist, Hand, and Miscellaneous Disorders

CASE 1

Differential Diagnosis of Wrist Pain

HISTORY: A 30-year-old baseball pitcher hyperextended his left wrist while sliding into third base. He experienced pain along the ulnar aspect of the wrist for 4 days after the injury. What is the MRI diagnosis? (Fig. 1-1: coronal multiformat (two-on-one) T1-weighted MR images of the left wrist. Fig. 1-2: fast scan gradient-echo MR images of the left wrist. Fig. 1-3: coronal fast scan gradient-echo MR image of the right wrist of another patient, shown for comparison.)

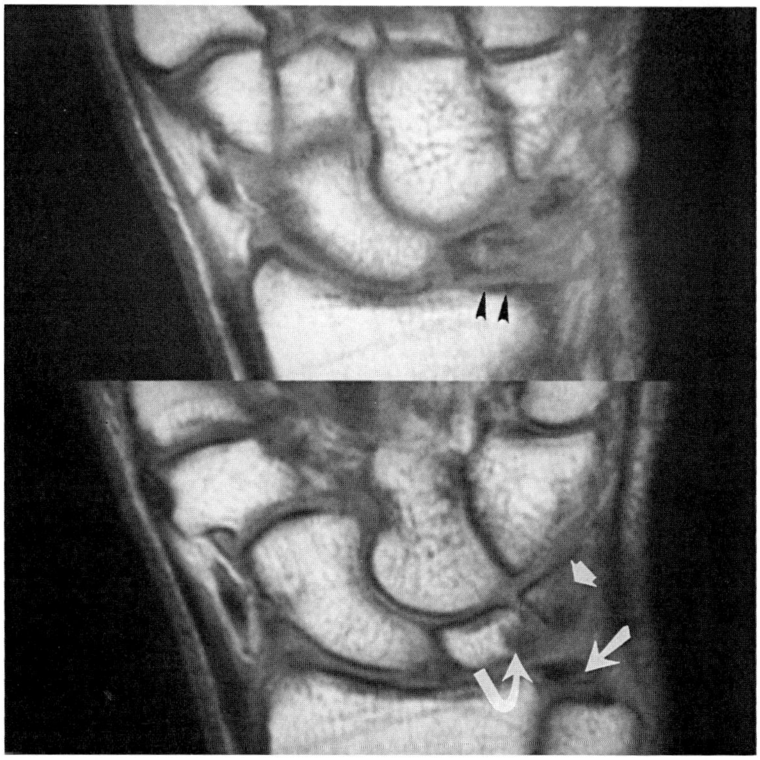

A

B

FIGURE 1-1

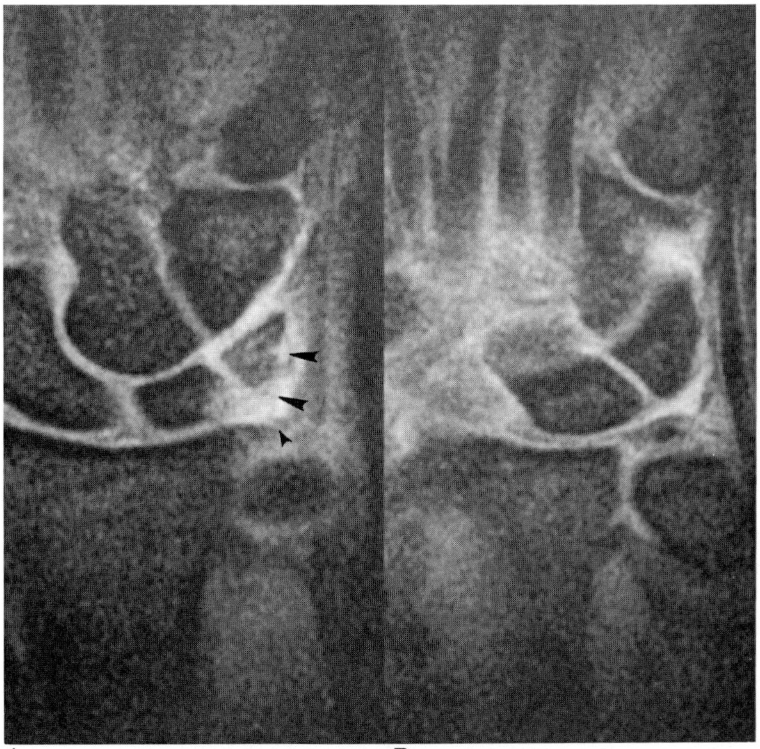

A B

FIGURE 1-2

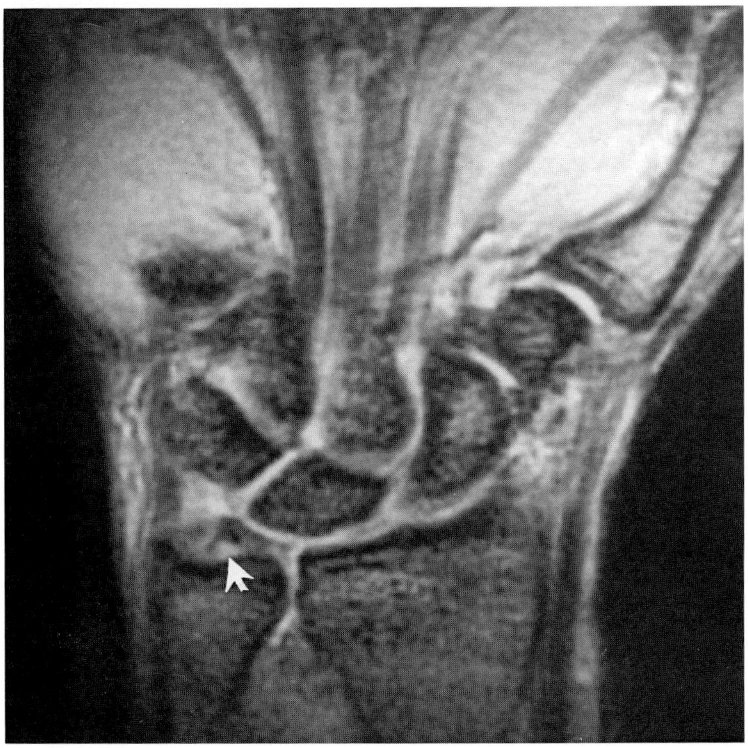

FIGURE 1-3

DISCUSSION: Areas of edema are intermediate in signal intensity on the T1-weighted images and hyperintense on the gradient-echo images. Involved are the triquetrum (short white arrow in Fig. 1-1*B*) and the lunate (curved white arrow in Fig. 1-1*B*). Edema in the triquetral bone and soft tissues just proximal to it is apparent on the fast scan image (black arrowheads in Fig. 1-2*A*). This area of signal alteration encroaches on the more proximal triangular fibrocartilage on both the T1-weighted (paired black arrowheads in Fig. 1-1*A*) and fast scan images (small white arrowhead). A subtle area of linear signal hyperintensity traverses the base of the triangular fibrocartilage (white arrow in Fig. 1-1*B*).

The findings are compatible with a contusion (bruise) of the triquetrum (short white arrow in Fig. 1-1*B*) and a focal osteochondral fracture of the triquetrum (short black arrowhead in Fig. 1-2*A*) and lunate (curved white arrow in Fig. 1-1*B*). Injury to the triangular fibrocartilage is implied by its diminished size, poor visibility, and intracartilaginous signal alteration. The triangular fibrocartilage is demarcated in the accompanying diagram (Fig. 1-4) and is better seen in the comparison case (Fig. 1-3), where it appears as a triangular hypointense structure that contains a focal hyperintense tear at its base (white arrow).

The triangular fibrocartilage is analogous to the meniscus of the knee in that it supports the ulnar–carpal interface and prevents compressive forces from producing osteochondral damage. The intercarpal hyaline cartilage is analogous to the femorotibial hyaline cartilage in the knee. The triangular fibrocartilage provides stabilization of the radioulnar joint along with the dorsal and volar radioulnar ligaments, the ulnar collateral ligament, and the extensor carpi ulnaris tendon.

Most tears of the triangular fibrocartilage occur at the ulnar–lunate interface; however, tears on the radial side or at the tapered tip of the triangular fibrocartilage occur in athletes. These are best imaged with a dedicated wrist coil that immobilizes the wrist and fingers in a "guillotine-type" fixation apparatus. Multiecho spin-echo images are usually too noisy and lengthy to achieve the degree of spatial resolution desired. Fields of view of 10 cm or less are recommended for wrist imaging.

The coronal plane is best suited for evaluation of the triangular fibrocartilage. We used both the bone-sensitive T1 sequence with the water-sensitive gradient-echo fast scan sequence to optimize contrast detection within both bone and cartilage. Another option is to use T1 fast scans and T2 appearing fast scans (gradient-echo or steady-state free precession) in conjunction with 1- or 1.5-mm volume acquisitions.

Injuries to the triangular fibrocartilage and surrounding anatomy may be evaluated with wrist arthrography utilizing a triple phase injection technique. The compartments injected include the radioscaphoid joint, the scaphocapitate joint (midcarpal injection), and the radioulnar joint. Congenital defects of the triangular fibrocartilage may exist in 20% to 50% of normal subjects and may produce false positive results on arthrography. Therefore, absence of edema or fluidlike signal in surrounding tissues on MRI may make MRI more specific in the diagnosis of injury to the triangular fibrocartilage.

DIAGNOSIS: The patient has a bone contusion of the triquetrum and osteochondral lunatotriquetral fractures, two examples of injuries to the triangular fibrocartilage.

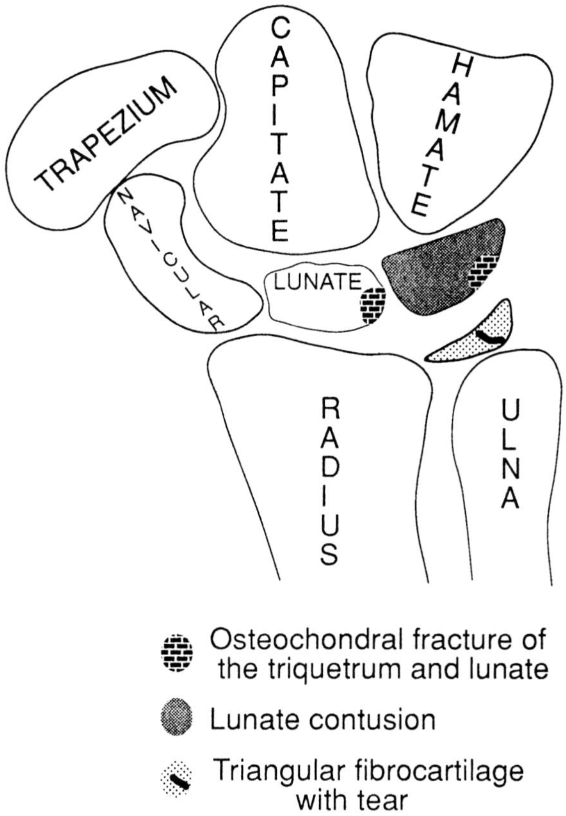

FIGURE 1-4

CASE 2

Differential Diagnosis of Wrist Pain

HISTORY: A 35-year-old man presented with a history of wrist pain for many years and mild tenderness over the dorsum of the right wrist. What is the MRI diagnosis? (Fig. 2-1: coronal T1-weighted MR image. Fig. 2-2: sagittal T1-weighted MR image.)

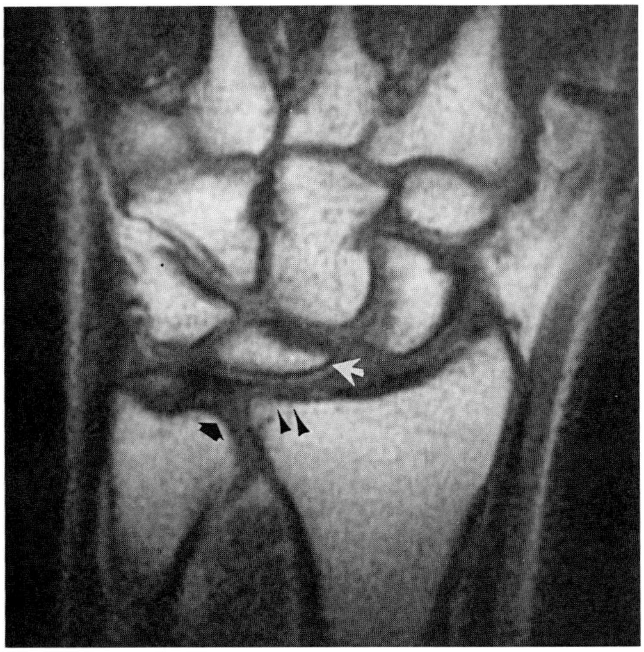

FIGURE 2-1

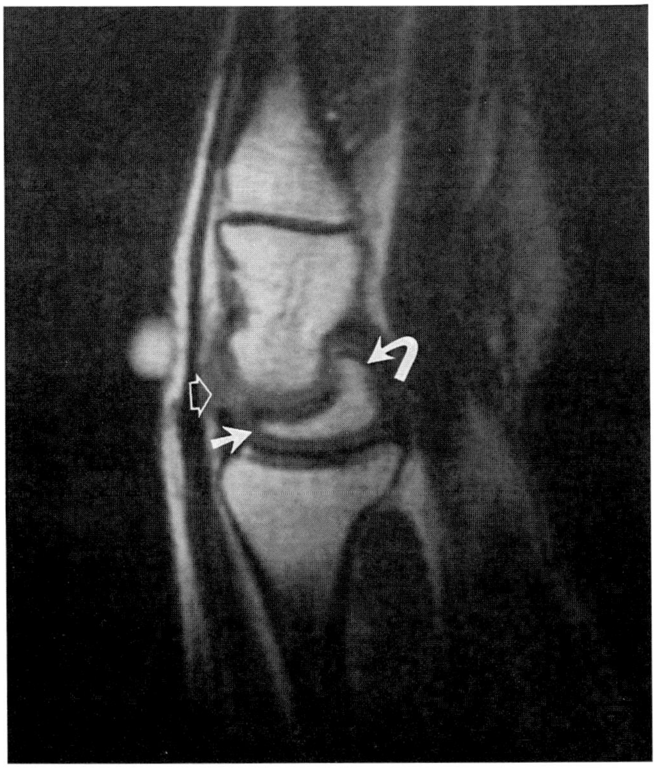

FIGURE 2-2

DISCUSSION: The lunate is hypoplastic along its dorsoradial margin (straight white arrows in both figures), which may account for the history of longstanding pain for many years. In addition, the radiolunatocapitate line is interrupted with anterior lunate subluxation (curved white arrow in Fig. 2-2). Projected dorsal to the capitate is an area of intermediate signal intensity that represents pannus and granulation tissue secondary to interruption of the dorsal capsule and radioscapholunate ligament (clear arrow in Fig. 2-2).

Conventional tomography and radiography have long been used to assess bone position, size, shape, and orientation after injury; however, both two-dimensional and volumetric data acquisition allow tomographic sectional assessment of the skeleton in any projection, including oblique views. MRI can demonstrate ligaments, tendons, and soft tissue in far greater detail than any conventional radiographic modality.

Disruption of the capitolunate joint is the hallmark of perilunate dislocation. As in this case, the proximal portion of the capitate lies dorsal to the lunate, in contrast to a volar perilunate dislocation, where the capitate lies volar to the lunate. The lunate tilts in volar fashion; this should not be misconstrued as volar lunate dislocation. In some cases, neither the lunate nor the capitate is centered over the radius; the lunate is anteriorly positioned while the capitate has a dorsal orientation. This is known as a dorsal midcarpal dislocation.

Two other features of this case are worthy of note: (1) negative ulnar variance, and (2) dorsal intercalated instability (DISI). The relative positions of the articular surfaces of the medial aspects of the radius and ulna represent ulnar variance. The distal ulna in this case (black arrow in Fig. 2-1) lies proximal to the radius (paired arrowheads in Fig. 2-1) in the frontal projection, so-called negative ulnar variance. Normally, the radius receives 80 percent of the axial loading forces of the forearm through its relationship with the lateral carpus. The ulna, via the triangular fibrocartilage complex, carries 20 percent of axial loading forces. The existing abnormalities and ulnar variance can result in Kienböck's disease, distal radial fractures, triangular fibrocartilage injuries, and ulnocarpal impingement syndrome. Positive ulnar variance is associated with triangular fibrocartilage tears and degeneration and ulnolunate impingement syndrome. Negative ulnar variance is associated with Kienböck's disease in as much as 80 percent of cases.

DORSAL DISI: The weakest link between the radius and proximal carpal row is the radioscapholunate ligament (clear arrow in Fig. 2-2) as injured in this case. The weakest link between the radius and distal carpal row is the radioscaphocapitate ligament. The strongest ligament in the wrist is the scapholunate interosseous ligament. Most prominent ligamentous elasticity is noted in the radioscaphoid ligament. Of all the volar intracapsular ligaments, the radiotriquetral is the strongest. Carpal dislocations and instability can vary in extent and type, since ligaments can tear completely, partially, or become lax due to partial failure. When patients have scapholunate dissociation (notice the wide gap between the lunate and the navicular in Figs. 2-1, 2-3, and 2-4), the scaphoid can no longer counteract the lunate's bias toward dorsiflexion or the influence on dorsiflexion of the triquetrum on the lunate. Therefore, the lunate may collapse into a dorsiflexed position with proximal capitate migration and associated wrist shortening, as seen on the sagittal MRI (Fig. 2-2). Scapholunate dissociation may occur with or without DISI. With DISI, the colinear relationship of the radius, lunate and capitate is lost, and results in a Z-like or crooked configuration. Volar rotation of the scaphoid may occur (not shown).

An important point to remember is that the lunate in ulnar deviation dorsiflexes and exhibits volar shift. The capitate usually remains centered with the radius. However, with true DISI the capitate assumes a dorsal position relative to the center of the radius in the sagittal projection, as seen in Figure 2-2, and the lunate exhibits volar shift, both of which fail to occur with simple ulnar deviation of the hand in a patient who is normal.

DIAGNOSIS: The patient has hypoplasia of the lunate with perilunate dislocation, DISI, and negative ulnar variance.

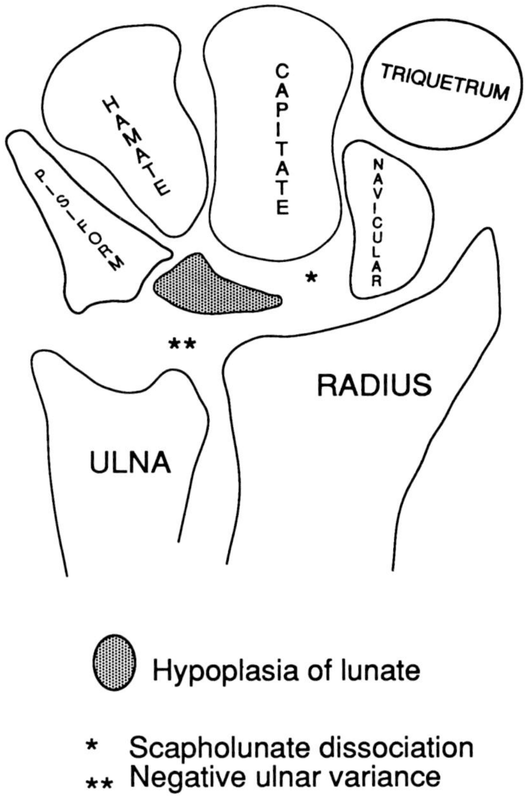

FIGURE 2-3

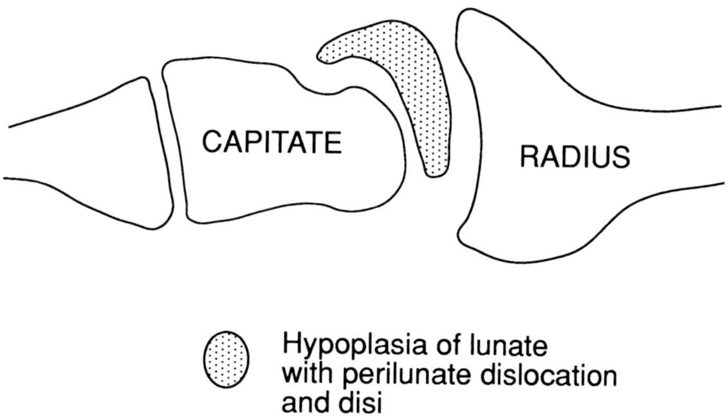

FIGURE 2-4

CASE 3

Differential Diagnosis of Wrist Pain

HISTORY: A 14-year-old boy presented with chronic wrist pain 1 year after a traumatic incident that resulted in a lunate fracture. What is the MRI diagnosis? (Fig. 3-1: coronal T1-weighted MR image.)

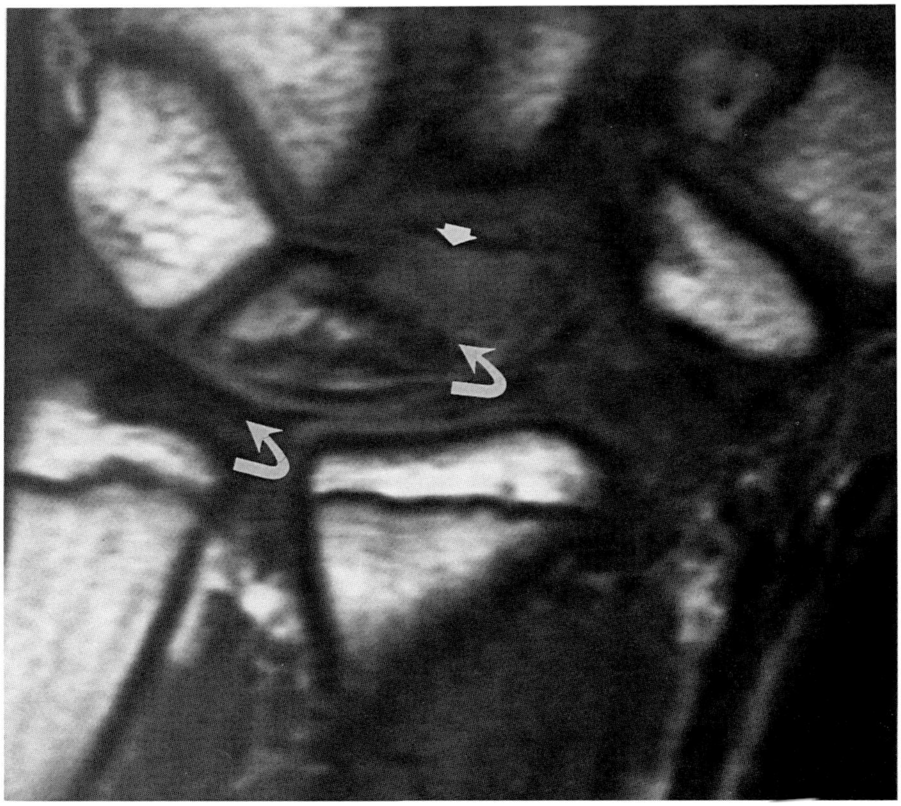

FIGURE 3-1

DISCUSSION: In the lunate is a distal area of signal hypointensity (short arrow), and between two lunate fragments is an area or cleft of signal hypointensity (distal curved arrow). Incidentally identified is a triangular area of hypointensity, the triangular fibrocartilage.

Lunatomalacia or Kienböck's disease usually results from an axial compression force that may be trivial or may result in transverse macrofracture. However, Kienböck's disease associated with lunate or perilunate subluxation is rare. Signal hypointensity on T1-weighted imaging that persists and is diffuse is the hallmark of the disease. Signal changes on MRI may or may not be associated with sclerosis on conventional radiographs.

Fibrous union demonstrated on MRI can often be differentiated from other types of malunion in that nonunion and pseudarthrosis result in T1 signal hypointensity and T2 or fast scan signal hyperintensity. However, fibrous union or malunion is associated with persistent signal hypointensity on all pulse sequences.

DIAGNOSIS: The patient has lunatonecrosis with fibrous nonunion.

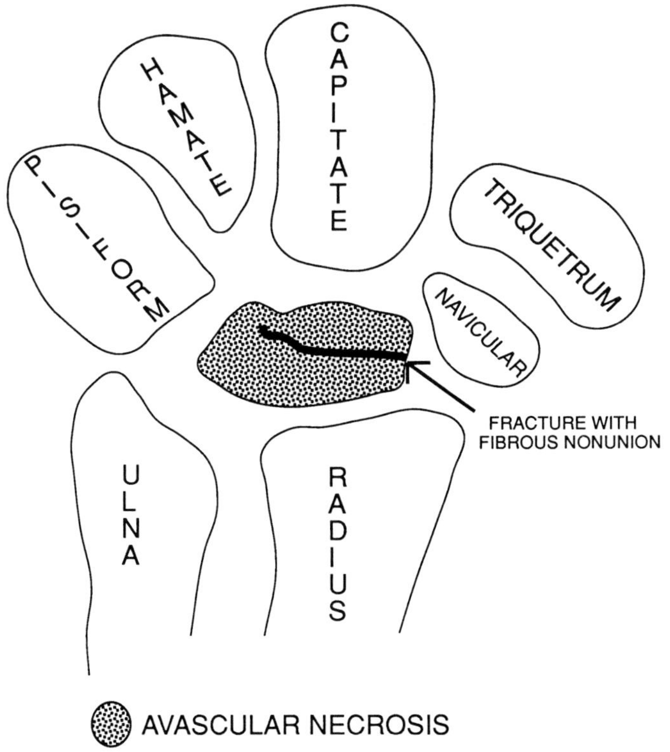

FIGURE 3-2

CASE 4

Differential Diagnosis of Wrist Pain

HISTORY: A 52-year-old woman presented with pain, tingling, and numbness in the wrist and thenar eminence of the hand. The symptoms were exacerbated by cleaning or dusting for prolonged periods. What is the MRI diagnosis? (Fig. 4-1: axial fast scan gradient-echo MR image, TR/TE 100/14 msec, 20° flip angle.)

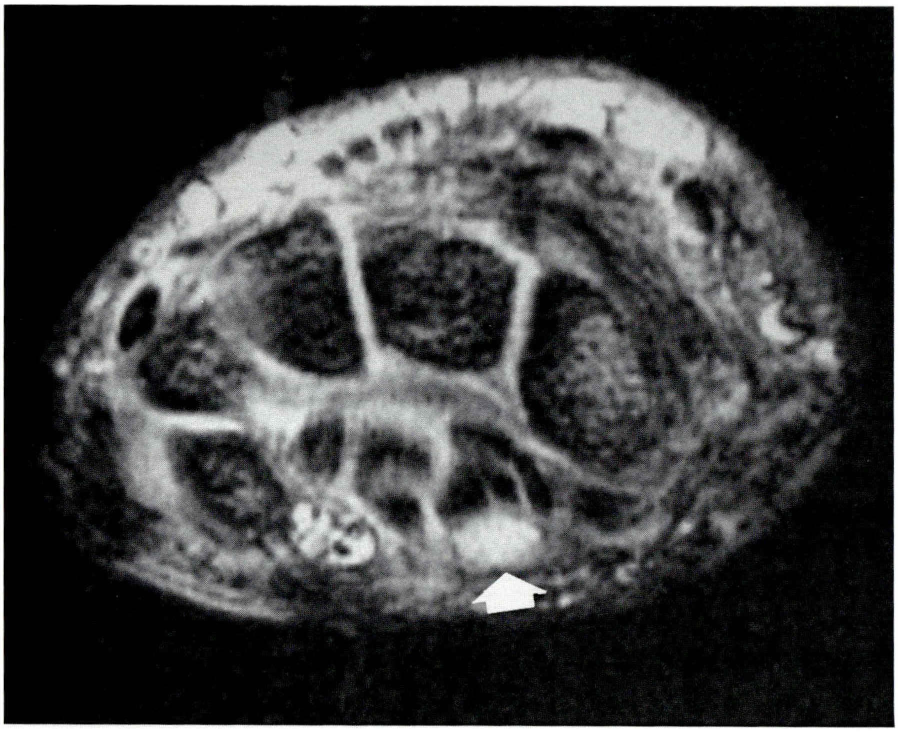

FIGURE 4-1

DISCUSSION: The median nerve (white arrow) appears swollen and exhibits signal hyperintensity. It is surrounded by the hypointense signal of the flexor digitorum superficialis and profundus tendons. Normal nerves are of intermediate signal intensity on T1-weighted and proton-density imaging. With T2 weighting the signal intensity is intermediate to minimally increased on spin-echo and fast scan gradient-echo images respectively, but marked signal hyperintensity should not be present.

The patient's clinical complaints are typical of carpal tunnel syndrome. Idiopathic carpal tunnel syndrome may occur secondary to fibrosis, edema, thickening, or arthritis. The MRI findings may vary and may include the following:

1. A vertical or elliptical median nerve in the dorsovolar direction, due to a tight or small carpal tunnel space, with flexor tendon swelling, so-called carpal tunnel stenosis.
2. Segmental or diffuse swelling of the median nerve proximal to the tunnel or inside it.
3. Irregular nerve shape with surrounding areas of hypointense fibrosis.

Simple median nerve neuritis has the identical MRI appearance to this case and can be seen after retinacular release for idiopathic carpal tunnel syndrome. The utility of MRI in evaluation of the median nerve lies not in the diagnosis of idiopathic carpal tunnel disease but in the exclusion of secondary carpal tunnel syndrome when the presenting symptoms are atypical or severe.

DIAGNOSIS: The patient has carpal tunnel syndrome with median nerve edema and neuritis.

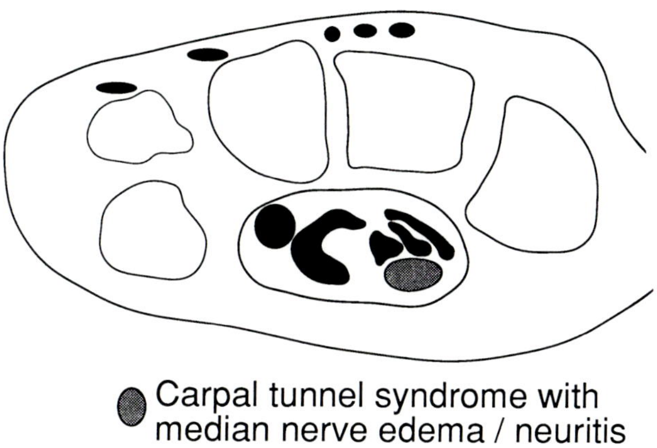

FIGURE 4-2

CASE 5

Differential Diagnosis of Chronic Elbow Pain

HISTORY: A 19-year-old Olympic diver underwent radiologic evaluation for chronic elbow pain exacerbated by extension and hyperextension during water entry from the high diving platform. What is the MRI diagnosis? (Fig. 5-1: conventional anteroposterior radiograph. Fig. 5-2: sagittal multiecho proton-density (*A*) and T2-weighted (*B*) MR images. Fig. 5-3: coronal T1-weighted MR image. Figs. 5-4 and 5-5: coronal T2-weighted images.)

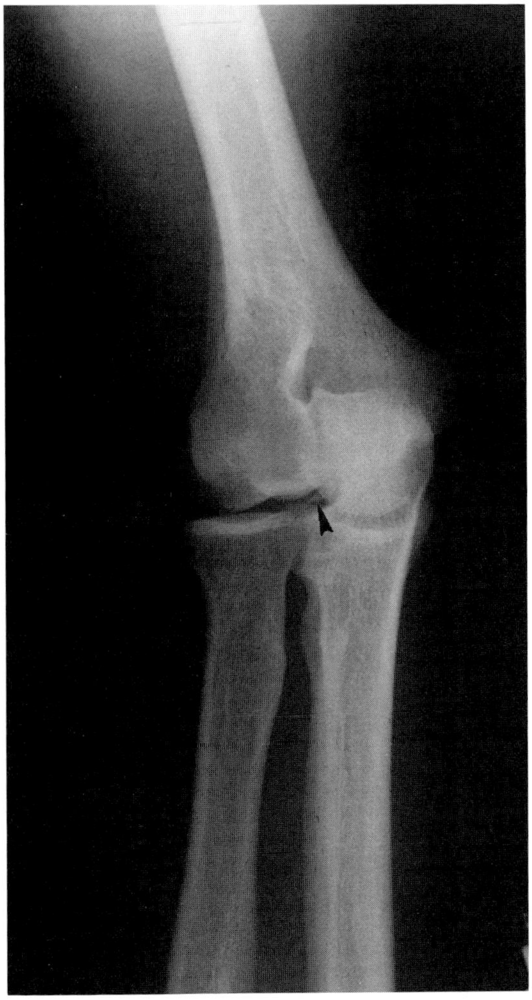

FIGURE 5-1

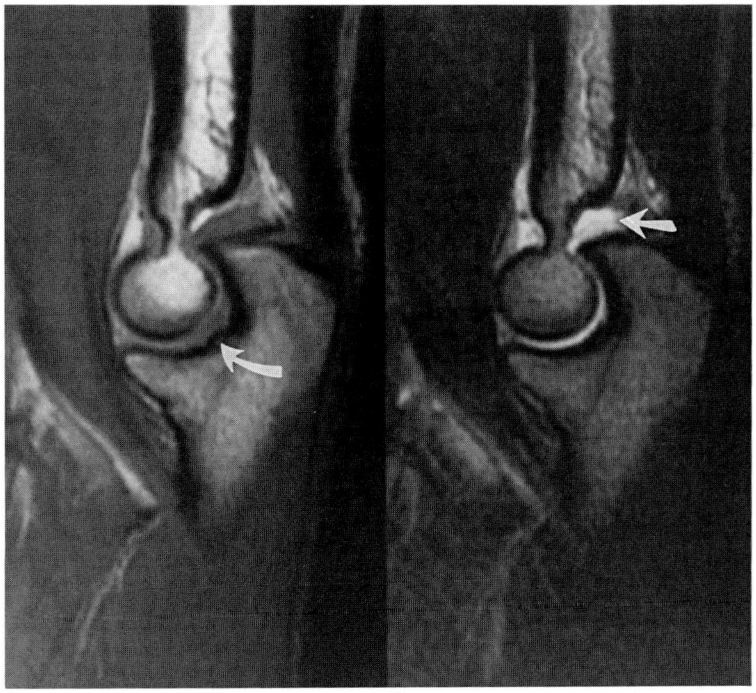

A **B**

FIGURE 5-2

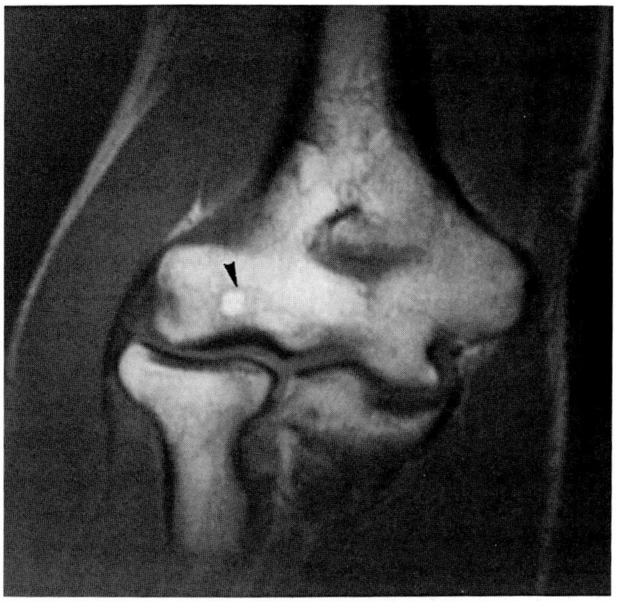

FIGURE 5-3

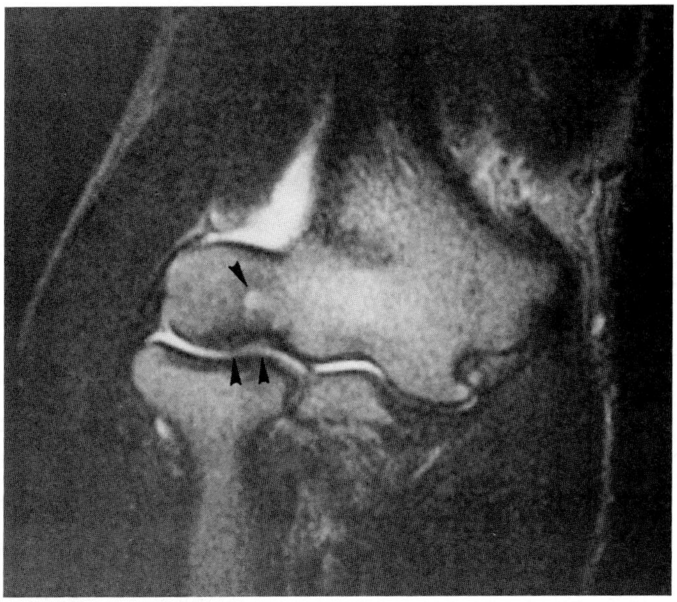

FIGURE 5-4

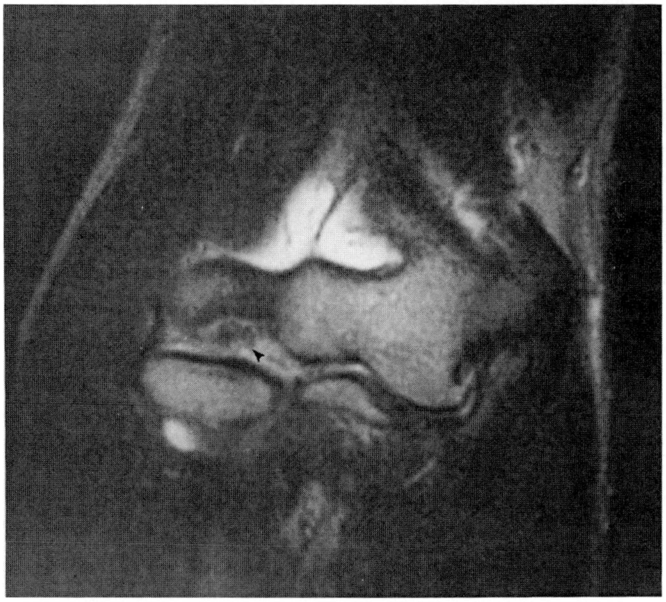

FIGURE 5-5

DISCUSSION: The plain radiograph shows a calcific loose body (arrowhead in Fig. 5-1) that is not visible on the MR images. The sagittal images show areas of cortical irregularity (curved white arrow in Fig. 5-2*A*) and an associated joint effusion (white arrow in Fig. 5-2*B*). On the coronal T1-weighted images, an area of focal bone repair in the medullary bone (arrowhead in Figs. 5-3 and 5-4) is suggested by a punctate area of fat signal. This signifies the presence of prior trauma or an irritative focus that stimulates this signal alteration and histologic effect.

Along the radiocapitellar interface is a focal area of signal hypointensity that is well marginated and associated with cortical irregularity (paired arrowheads in Fig. 5-4). Nominal amounts of increased signal intensity are present in the adjacent joint space.

Figure 5-5, a coronal image, shows a definite area of sequestered osteocartilaginous hypointense signal. Coupled with the patient's age, the findings are typical in location and signal of osteochondritis dissecans, a lesion that is usually traumatic in origin and associated with throwing and racquet sports. The lesions may be confined to cartilage or bone, or may involve both. Any component may be nondisplaced, displaced, or migrated (loose body). The ratio of capitellar to radial head involvement from transchondral injury is 9:1. Repetitive valgus overload of the radiocapitellar joint may lead to irregularity of the capitellum and subsequent hypertrophic bone or spur formation in the adjacent radial head. Pain, swelling, and limited range of motion with catching and locking are not atypical. Once bony hypertrophic changes occur, they are difficult to reverse or correct.

Persons subjected to chronic compressive forces on the radiocapitellar interface simultaneously experience distractive forces on the medial side of the elbow joint. A traction spur from the coronoid tubercle may then develop. Stress produced by the ulnar collateral ligament is the supposed mechanism for this phenomenon.

Ulnar collateral ligament tears do occur in adults, particularly in baseball players or pitchers. However, they are less common in children, as ligamentous and joint laxity allows most of the valgus stresses to be placed on the flexor muscle group that attaches to the medial epicondyle. Thus, the term "Little League elbow" has been applied to medial epicondylar avulsion in adolescents.

Osteochondrosis occurs in patients under the age of 12 and has been referred to as Panner's disease. These patients rarely have limited range of motion, and the capitellum ossification center appears fragmented but may be of normal signal intensity on MRI in the first 3 to 5 months of symptoms. The condition is usually self-limited.

DIAGNOSIS: The patient has osteochondral capitellar injury with osteochondral and cortical loose bodies.

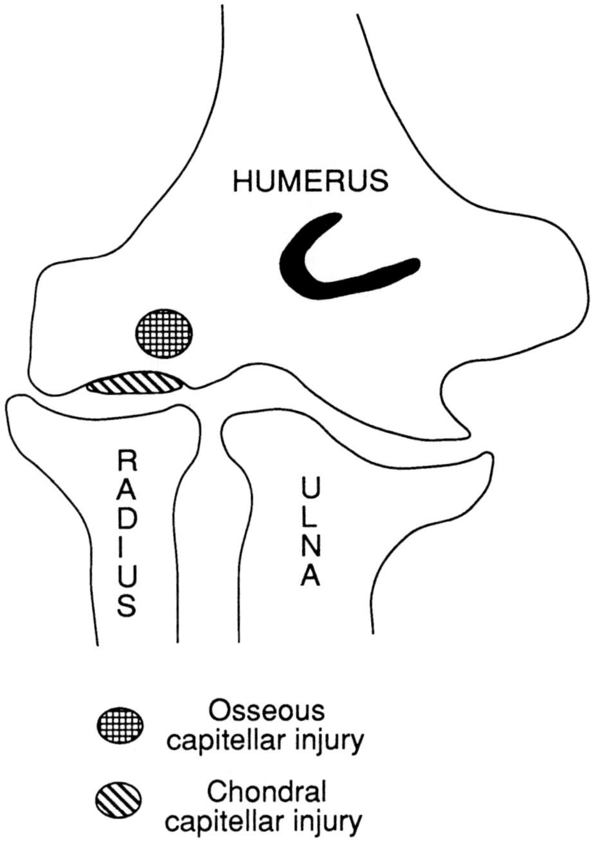

FIGURE 5-6

CASE 6

Differential Diagnosis of Wrist Injury

HISTORY: A 39-year-old woman presented with inability to extend her fifth digit. What is the MRI diagnosis? (Fig. 6-1: sagittal T1-weighted MR image, TR/TE 700/20 msec, 256 × 128 pixel matrix, 4 excitations, 5.0-mm sections, 10.0-cm FOV.)

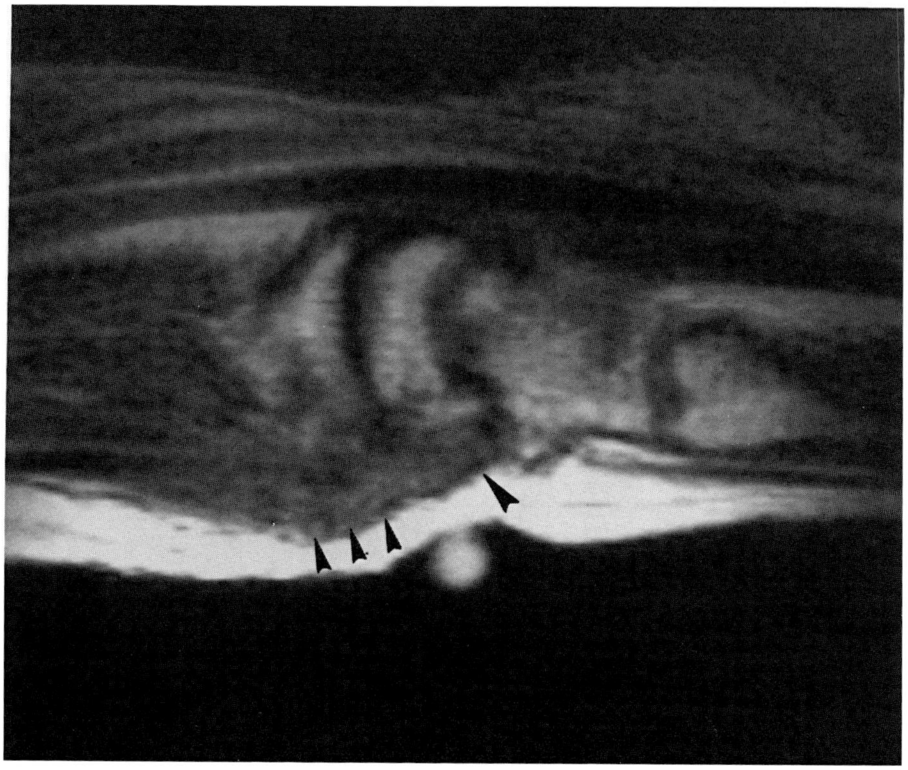

FIGURE 6-1

DISCUSSION: Near the midsaggital plane are visualized linear, hypointense fibers of the extensor digiti minimi that are discontiguous and interrupted by an area of intermediate signal intensity (triple black arrowheads) that represents scar and granulation tissue. The linear hypointense tendon fibers are identified distally (single arrowhead). The anatomic discontiguity is compatible with complete tendon rupture. Isolated rupture of this tendon complex would account for the patient's inability to extend the digit.

Depending on the outcome and age of this tendon rupture, one might see granulation tissue, fibrous tissue, hemorrhage, or edema. Granulation tissue is isointense on T1 weighting and isointense to hyperintense on T2 weighting. Fibrous tissue is hypointense on both T1 and T2 weighting. Hemorrhage has variable hyperintensity on T1 weighting and is usually hyperintense on T2 weighting in the soft tissues. Edema is hyperintense on T2-weighted images.

DIAGNOSIS: The patient has extensor digiti minimi transection.

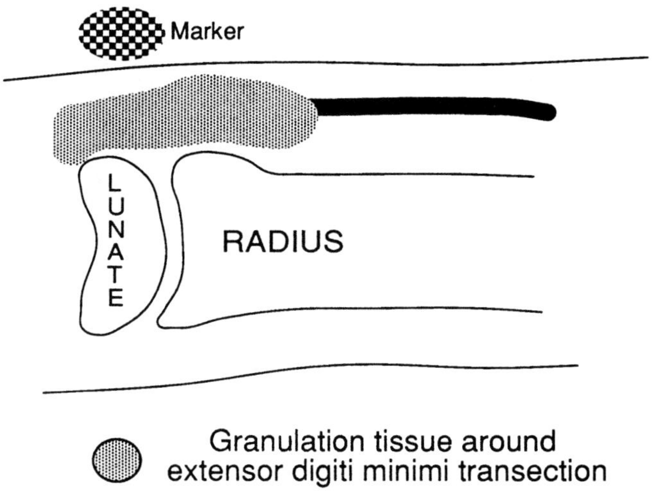

FIGURE 6-2

CASE 7

Differential Diagnosis of Soft Tissue Masses about the Wrist and Forearm

HISTORY: A 38-year-old man presented with acute pain and a palpable mass in the distal forearm. The pain was most noticeable when the patient swung a baseball bat. What is the MRI diagnosis? (Fig. 7-1: sagittal (through the brachioradialis tendon) multiformat (four-on-one), multiecho proton-density (*A,C*) and T2-weighted (*B,D*) MR images, TR/TE 1,500/40, 80 msec, 12.0-cm FOV, 128 × 256 pixel matrix, 5.0-mm sections, 2 excitations.)

A **B**

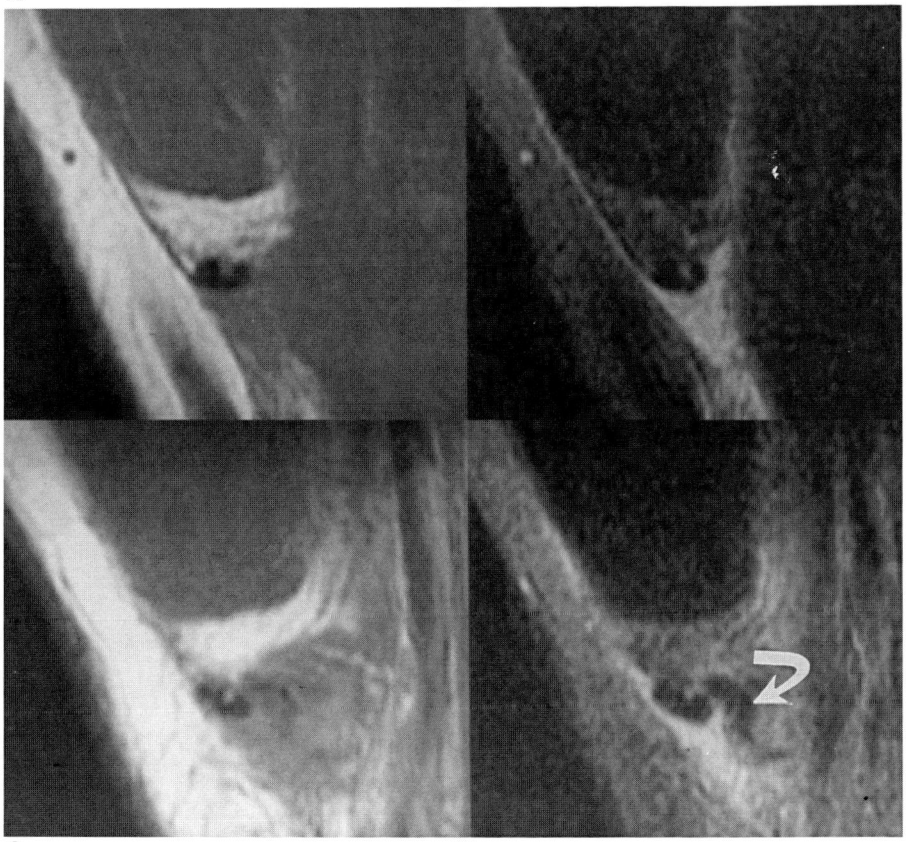

C **D**

FIGURE 7-1

DISCUSSION: The sagittal MR images were obtained through the distal tendon of the brachioradialis muscle. The tendon is not straight but tortuous (arrow in *D*) and is surrounded by hyperintense edema or acute hemorrhage. The normal tendinous insertion is straight. The tendon is diagramed in Figure 7-2.

In the assessment of ligamentous and tendinous anatomy, sections of 5.0 mm or less, fields of view of 16.0 cm or less, and matrices of 192 × 256 pixels or greater are used to improve edge detail and spatial resolution. Tendon injury may be partial, with intratendinous signal alteration; complete, as in this case, with tendon retraction; or may be surrounded by edema, hemorrhage, or ganglion formation.

The brachioradialis avulses far less frequently than the biceps brachii. A flexion injury, often with forced supination, results in a loud snap and a painful, palpable mass distal and medial to the antecubital fossa. This lesion may be confused with biceps muscle rupture since a palpable mass is present on flexion, the so-called "Popeye" sign of biceps tear. Unlike biceps muscle tear, few cases of degenerative disease inducing brachioradialis rupture have been reported. Brachioradialis tears have been noted with increasing frequency in the competitive weightlifters, bodybuilders, and gymnasts.

DIAGNOSIS: The patient has a complete brachioradialis tendon rupture.

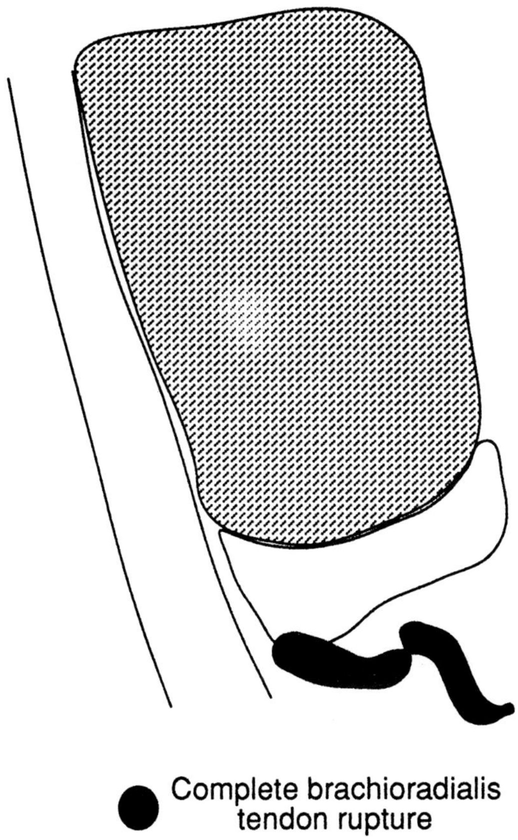

FIGURE 7-2

CASE 8

Differential Diagnosis of Soft Tissue Masses about the Hand and Arm

HISTORY: A 72-year-old woman presented with inability to extend the fifth digit and a palpable soft tissue nodule on the dorsum of the hand. What is the MRI diagnosis? (Fig. 8-1: axial multiecho proton-density (*A*) and T2-weighted (*B*) MR images.)

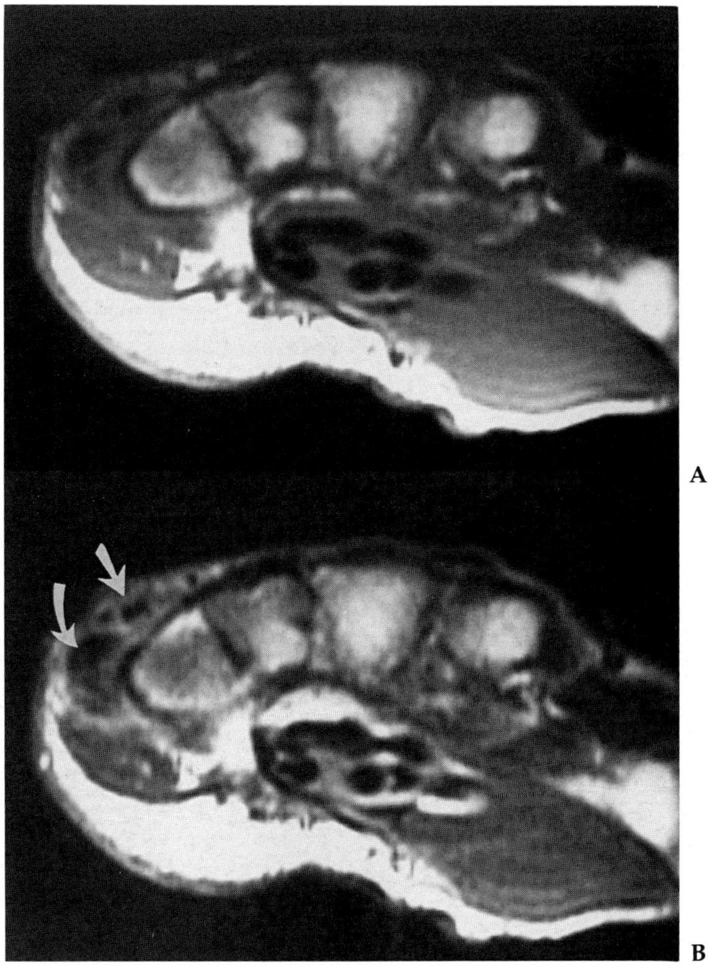

FIGURE 8-1

DISCUSSION: Along the dorsoulnar aspect of the hand is a round area of hypointensity (straight white arrow in Fig. 8-1*B*), the normal extensor digiti minimi tendon. The normal medially positioned rounded hypointensity of the extensor carpi ulnaris has been replaced by or enlarged by an area of mixed hypo- and isointense signal (curved white arrow in Fig. 8-1*B*). The extensor carpi ulnaris runs in a separate compartment of the extensor retinaculum in a groove formed between the styloid process and the ulnar head. It inserts at the base of the fifth metacarpal. The extensor digiti minimi along with the extensor indices accompany the extensor digitorum communis to the index and small fingers. However, the extensor digiti minimi travels in its own fibro-osseous tunnel medial to the extensor digitorum communis and extensor indices.

Tendon injury may be complete or incomplete and may be associated with edema, hemorrhage, or even ganglion formation. Granulation tissue (see case 7) or fibrosis may occur at a site of chronic or remote tendon rupture. The fact that this pseudomass becomes more conspicuous and more hypointense on the T2-weighted image suggests its hemorrhagic nature and confirms the presence of an injury to the tendon anatomy in this region. The sagittal view (not provided) would further assist the interpretor in confirming the presence of complete or incomplete rupture.

DIAGNOSIS: The patient has an injury of the extensor carpi ulnaris tendon.

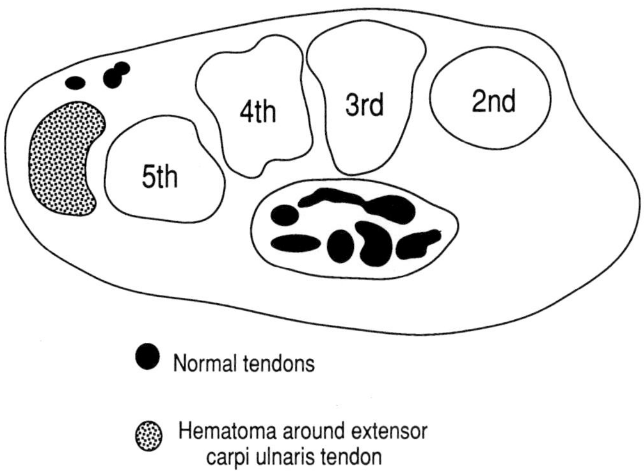

FIGURE 8-2

CASE 9

Differential Diagnosis of Soft Tissue Masses about the Hand and Arm

HISTORY: A 33-year-old woman presented with pain in the index finger and a palpable doughy consistency along the dorsum of the second digit. What is the MRI diagnosis? (Fig. 9-1: axial multiecho proton-density (*A*) and T2-weighted MR images at the level of the proximal phalangeal interface. Fig. 9-2: similar images at the level of the metacarpal heads.)

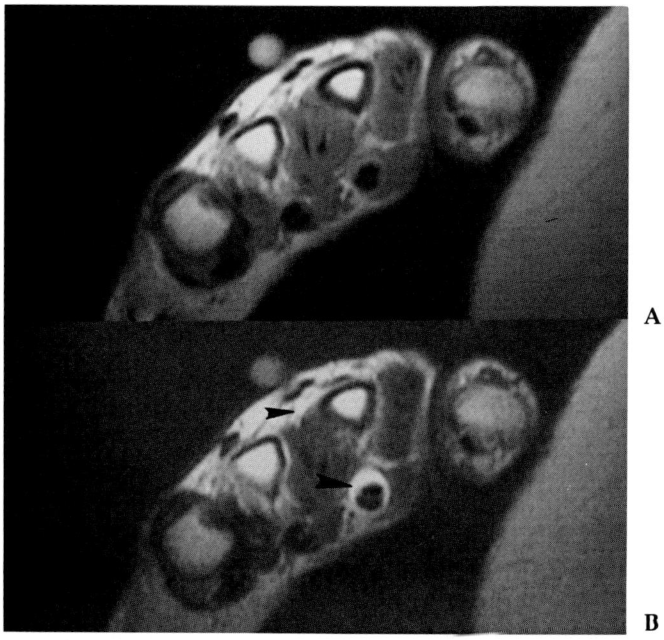

FIGURE 9-1

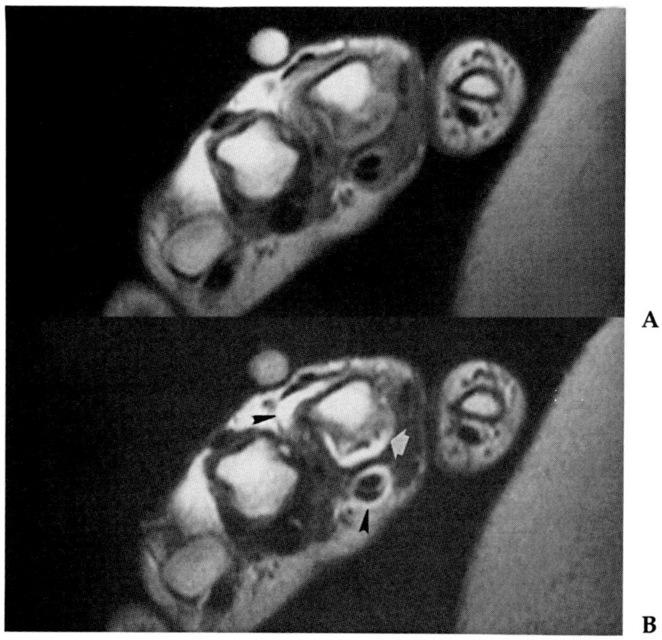

FIGURE 9-2

DISCUSSION: Areas of fluid signal or edema that are isointense on proton-density images and hyperintense in T2-weighted images surround the extensor and flexor tendons (arrowheads in Figs. 9-1*B* and 9-2*B*) as well as the joint capsule (short white arrow in Fig. 9-2*B*). The findings are pathognomonic of capsular inflammation and tenosynovitis. In a young woman without a history of trauma, rheumatoid arthritis is the most likely diagnosis. Tenosynovitis and arthropathy of any etiology could produce this same appearance.

With rheumatoid arthritis, regardless of the joint, the following findings predominate:

1. synovial redundancy and capsular thickening, most easily seen as signal hyperintensity on T2-weighted imaging;
2. increased joint fluid;
3. tendon or peritendinous hyperintense T2 edema;
4. autodigestion and reduction in size of hyaline and fibrocartilage; and
5. a late or end-stage change consisting of subchondral irregular hypointensity in the medullary bone.

DIAGNOSIS: The patient has rheumatoid arthritis with secondary capsulitis and tenosynovitis.

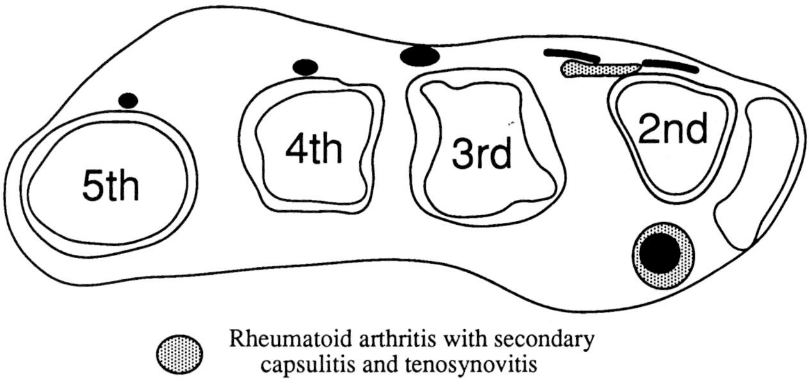

FIGURE 9-3

CASE 10

Differential Diagnosis of Soft Tissue Masses about the Wrist, Hand, and Arm

HISTORY: A 21-year-old woman presented with arm pain, heat tenderness, a soft tissue mass, and palpable thrill. What is the MRI diagnosis? (Figs. 10-1 and 10-2: respectively axial and sagittal T1-weighted MR images obtained with a surface coil. The remaining images, from a different patient, are shown for comparison. Fig. 10-3: sagittal T1-weighted image. Fig. 10-4: axial multiformat, multiecho proton-density (*A*) and T2-weighted (*B*) images.)

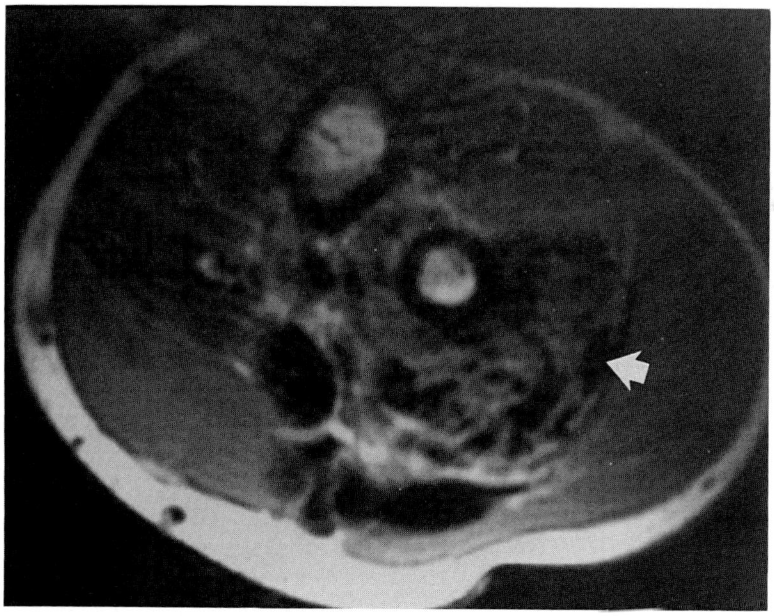

FIGURE 10-1

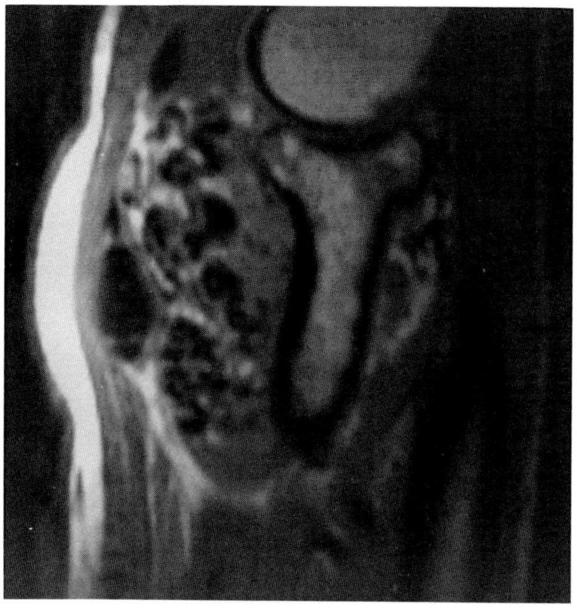

FIGURE 10-2

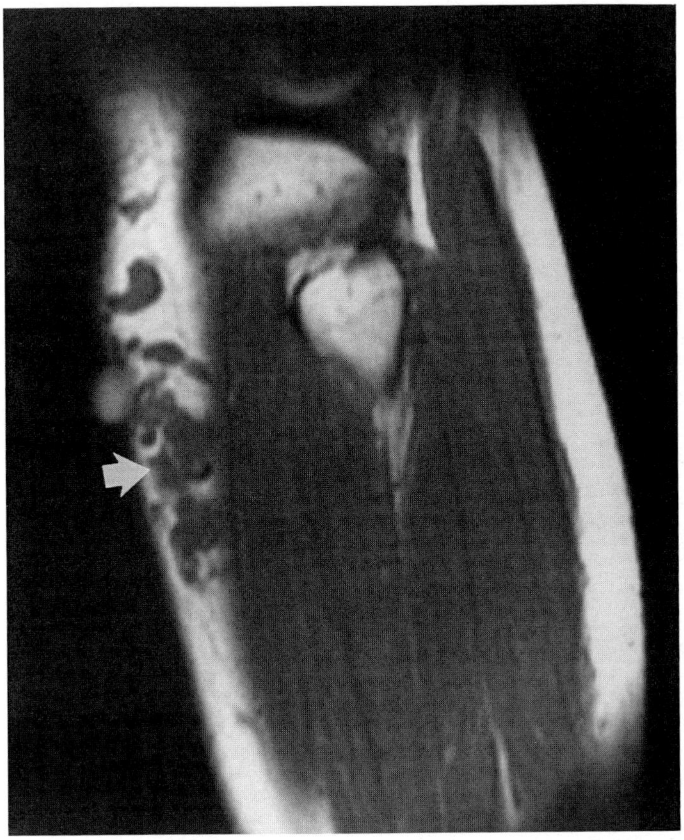

FIGURE 10-3

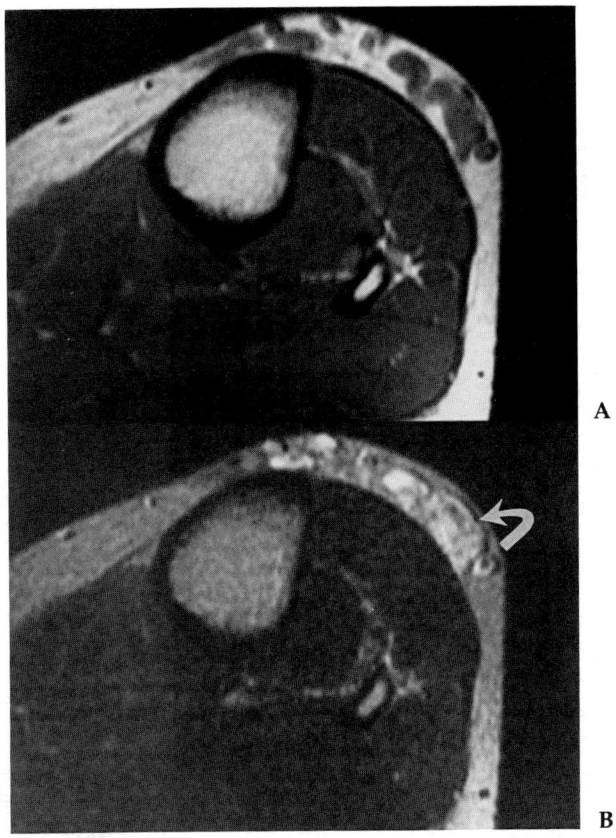

FIGURE 10-4

DISCUSSION: Throughout both the muscular compartment as well as the subcutaneous compartment are wormian or gyriform foci of signal void (arrow in Fig. 10-1) compatible with a lesion that has produced flow-related signal void. Unlike hemangiomas, the incidence of signal void on both T1- and T2-weighted imaging in arteriovenous malformations is higher due to faster flow rates. Arteriovenous malformations tend to be more invasive and deeper in location.

Flow-related signal void is most conspicuous when long echo times, long repetition times, high flow rates, turbulent flow, and thin sections are present. The vascular signal will appear quite hyperintense with most fast scan or gradient-echo imaging techniques and with spin-echo imaging that employs even echoes, short repetition times, short echo times, high field strength scanners, and thicker sections (weaker gradients).

MRI is used preoperatively to assess the extent of vascular malformations and to decide whether surgical intervention is possible. If nonferromagnetic coils or nonmetallic occlusive devices are employed, MRI can be used to assess progression or regression of vascular disease.

Unlike the rarer arteriovenous malformations, vascular malformations of the hemangioma type are the most common congenital abnormality in humans. All vascular tumors are considered hamartomas rather than true neoplasms. These benign growths consist of increased numbers of vascular channels, an overgrowth of endothelial lining cells with adipose tissue, fibrous tissue, smooth muscle, and, rarely, bone. Peripheral hemangioma, capillary hemangioma, cavernous hemangioma, arteriovenous malformation, venous malformation, hamartoma, and angiolipoma belong to the spectrum of vascular malformations that occur in the body.

Extremity hemangiomas may produce regional gigantism and may have adverse psychological effects. Hemangioma treatment consists of argon laser therapy with or without preoperative embolization. Most large hemangiomas are not resectable. MRI findings consist of serpiginous or gyriform foci of intermediate or increased signal intensity on T1-weighted images (arrow in Fig. 10-3) and T2-weighted images (curved white arrow in Fig. 10-4) due to section entry flow effects, in-plane flow effects, and even-echo rephasing. Such section entry phenomena are visualized in the subcutaneous fat on this patient's calf. The flow rates will determine whether even-echo rephasing and bright T2 signal are visualized on the second echo image. Focal inhomogeneity in or around the lesion may represent fibrosis, fat, thrombosis, or calcification. Calcification is best seen on fast scan or T2-weighted imaging as focal areas of hypointense signal that may be impossible to differentiate from flow void. Therefore, correlation with conventional radiographs is critical.

The hypointense signal of phleboliths is most easily contrasted with the hyperintense signal of even-echo rephasing on T2-weighted images. A longitudinal sagittal or coronal and an axial T1-weighted image are obtained to document lesion extent, in conjunction with a multi-echo spin density and T2 image set in one plane. The major utility of MRI is in the determination of feasibility of surgical intervention and argon laser therapy and in the establishment of limb salvage.

DIAGNOSIS: The patient has an arteriovenous malformation in the forearm and a lower extremity hemangioma.

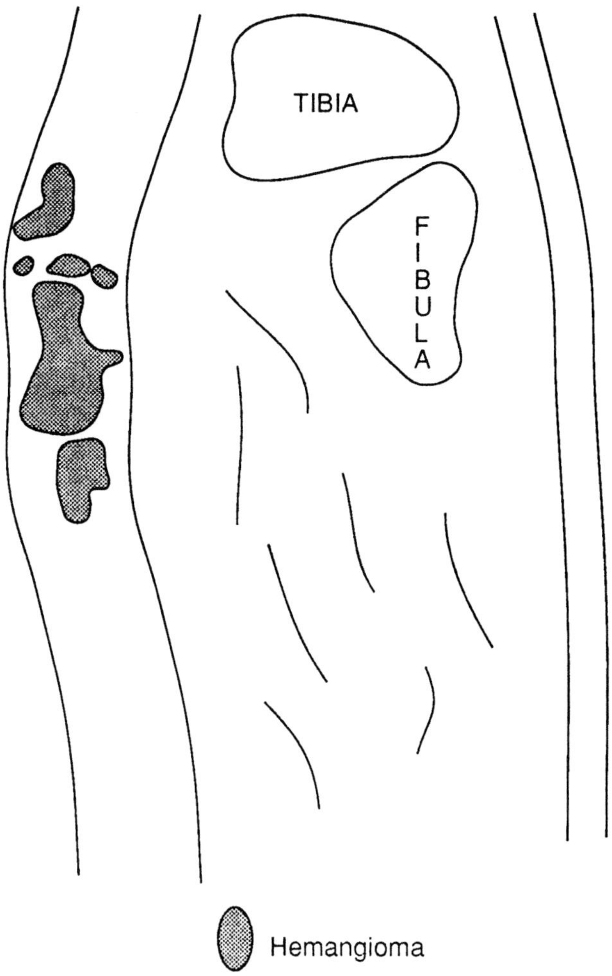

FIGURE 10-5

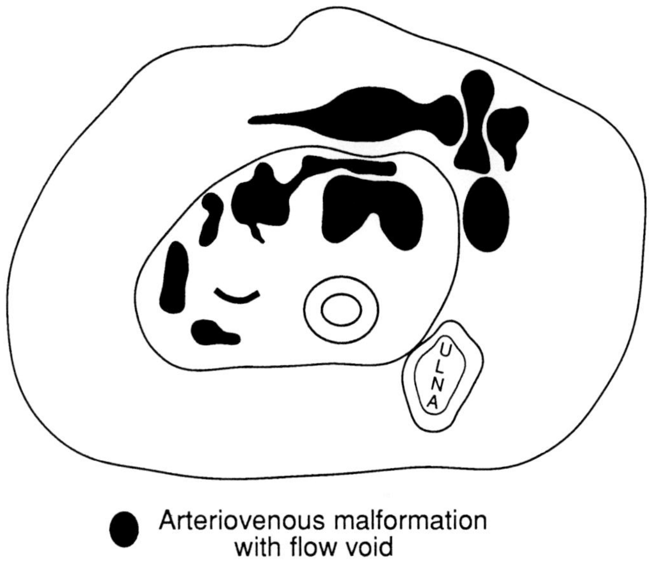

FIGURE 10-6

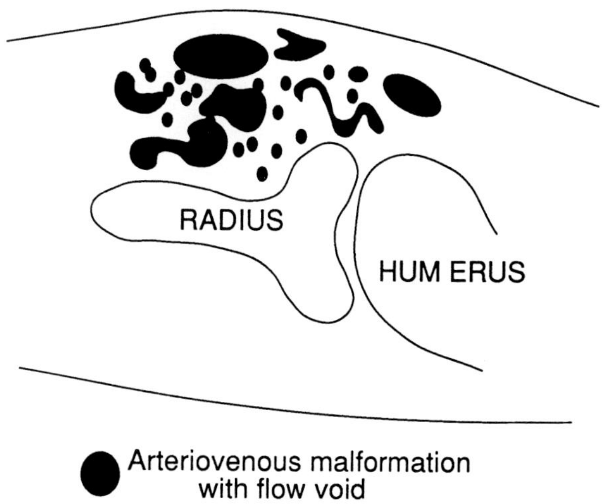

FIGURE 10-7

CASE 11

Differential Diagnosis of Soft Tissue Masses

HISTORY: A 50-year-old man presented with anterior chest pain. He had been evaluated by a cardiologist for possible angina and subsequently by a chiropractor and an orthopaedic surgeon for possible costochondritis. What is the MRI diagnosis? (Figs. 11-1 and 11-2: respectively sagittal and axial T1-weighted MR images obtained with a body coil, TR/TE 600/20 msec, 42.0-cm FOV, 128 × 256 pixel matrix, 10.0-mm sections, 4 excitations.)

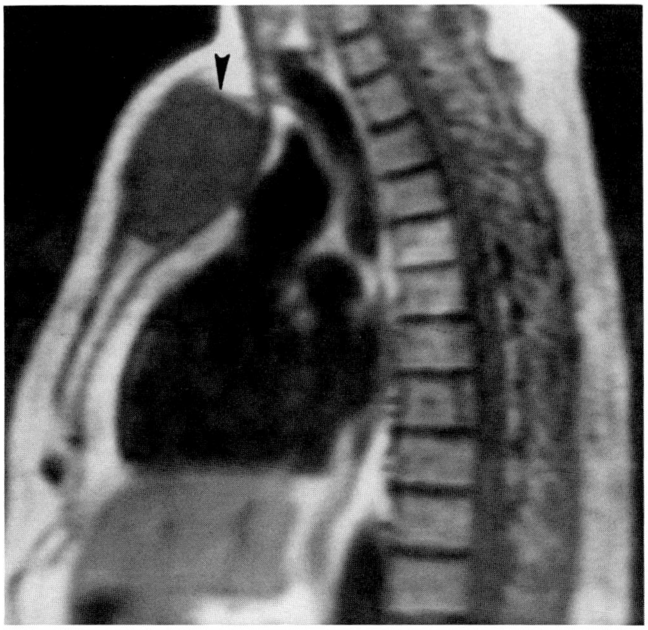

FIGURE 11-1

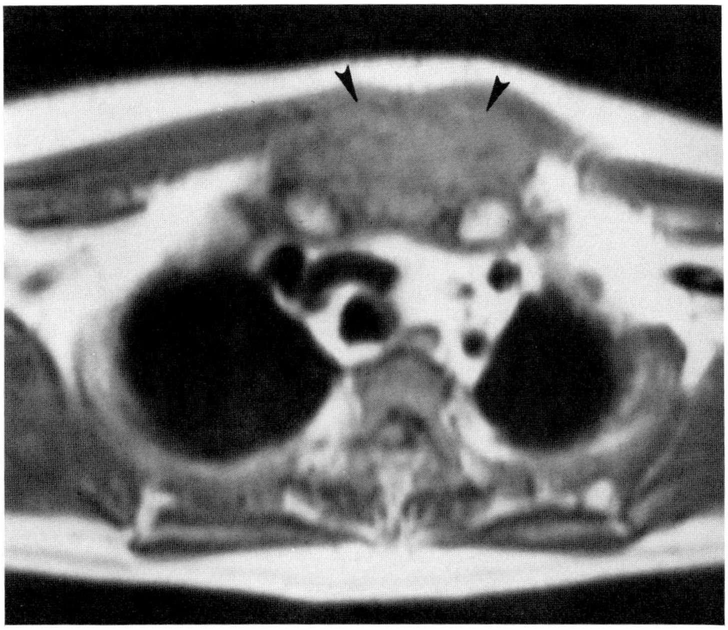

FIGURE 11-2

DISCUSSION: An expansile soft tissue mass (arrowheads in Figs. 11-1 and 11-2) has completely replaced the sternum, but the signal intensity of the mass is not that of water, which would appear more hypointense on T1-weighted imaging. The signal intensity indicates that the mass is a solid lesion. Expansile masses of the sternum include three entities: chondrosarcoma, plasmacytoma or myeloma variants, and aneurysmal bone cysts, in descending order of frequency.

Aneurysmal bone cysts tend to exhibit hemorrhagic or hyperintense signal on T1-weighted imaging and are more hypointense on T1-weighted imaging when hemorrhage does not accompany the lesion. Chondrosarcoma, the most common expansile mass in this location, is extremely inhomogeneous and often exhibits hypointense calcification or matrix formation. A solid homogeneous side mass is most likely to represent a plasmocytoma or plasmasarcoma or immunoblastic sarcoma.

Myeloma, the systemic manifestation of plasma cell dyscrasia, produces poorly defined, mild signal hypointensity within the marrow, particularly in the spine. Often the bright end-plate signal is spared on T1-weighted imaging, and multilevel vertebral body collapse is present. Focal plasmacytomas are hyperintense on T2-weighted imaging and can mimic complex cystic lesions. Often these lesions are initially so well-circumscribed that they mimic benign bone tumors on conventional radiography and MRI.

DIAGNOSIS: The patient has a plasmasarcoma of the sternum.

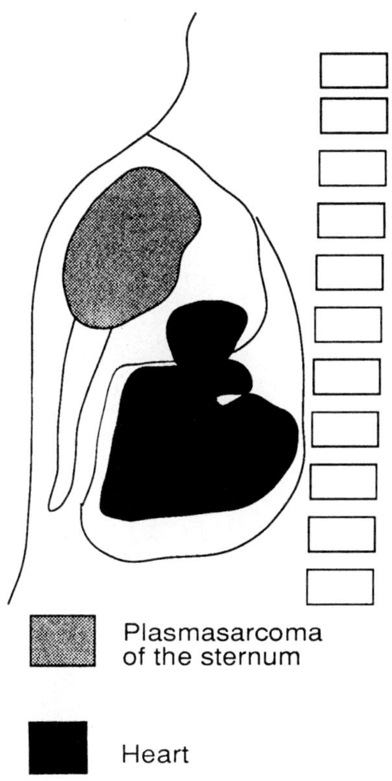

FIGURE 11-3

CASE 12

Differential Diagnosis of Soft Tissue Masses about the Wrist and Forearm

HISTORY: A 40-year-old woman presented with pain in the forearm of 3 months and no history of trauma. She had had severe gallstone pancreatitis 4 months earlier. What is the MRI diagnosis? (Fig. 12-1: axial multiformat (two-on-one), multiecho proton-density (*A*) and T2-weighted (*B*) MR images. Fig. 12-2: sagittal T1-weighted (*A*) and T2-weighted (*B*) MR images.)

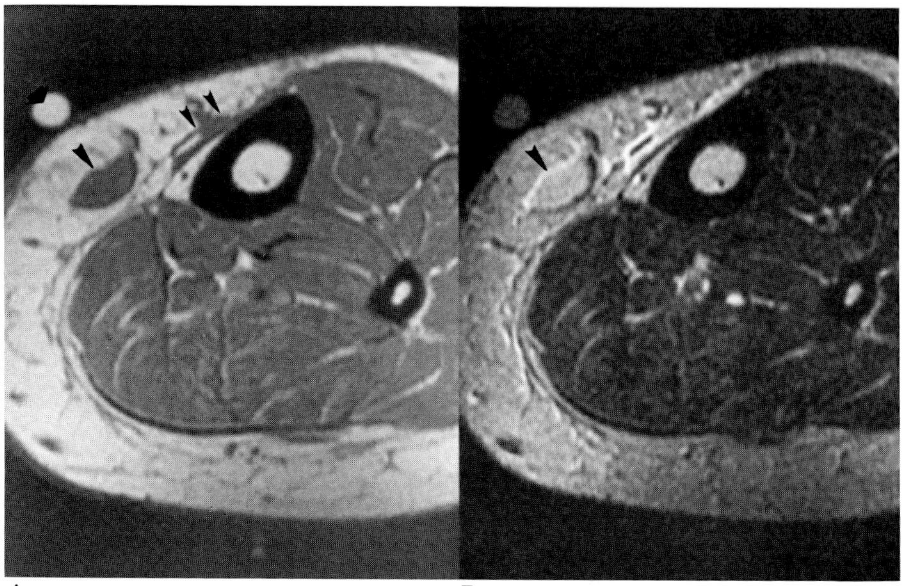

A B

FIGURE 12-1

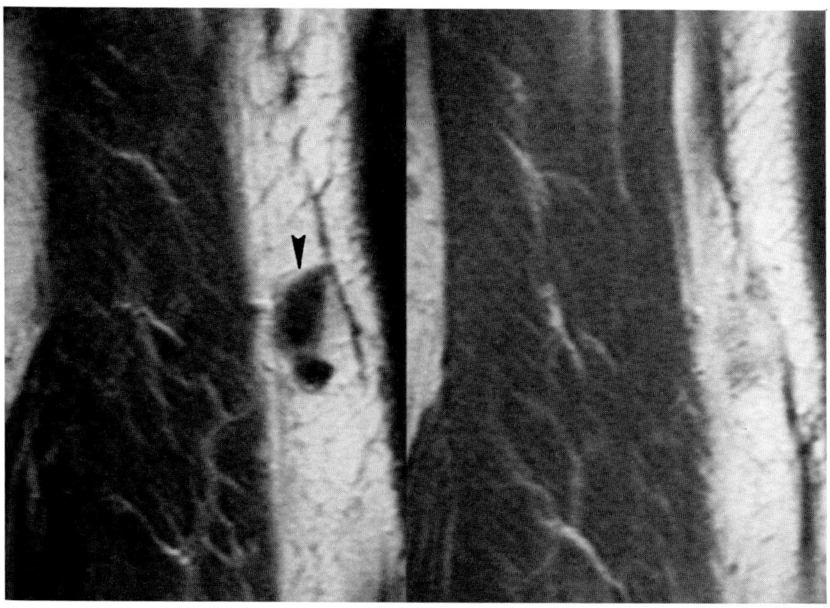

A B

FIGURE 12-2

DISCUSSION: Areas that appear hypointense on T1 weighting, isointense on proton-density weighting, and hyperintense on T2 weighting (single arrowheads in Figs. 12-1*A* and *B* and 12-2*A*) are present in the subcutaneous space of the forearm with extension (paired arrowheads in Fig. 12-1*A*) over the cortical surface of the radius. The bones and underlying muscular compartment are spared, and the degree of mass effect (in relation to lesion size) is nominal. A gelatin capsule (arrow in Fig. 12-1*A*) has been used to localize the patient's pain.

Fat necrosis or panniculitis is the most likely explanation for the MRI findings and clinical presentation in this case. Fat necrosis may occur de novo. Secondary causes include pancreatitis, trauma, Weber-Christian disease, vasculitis, and inflammatory bowel disease. Large areas of fat necrosis may be painful and initially may result in cyst formation (large arrowhead). Eventually these areas will progress to hypointense scar and/or retraction. Involvement of the underlying muscular or skeletal compartment, as evidenced by hyperintense T2 signal, precludes the diagnosis of simple fat necrosis, and neoplasia must then be excluded. Most nontraumatic systemic causes of fat necrosis are multifocal and have a propensity to involve the lower extremity. Idiopathic fat necrosis may occur in any body part.

DIAGNOSIS: The patient has fat necrosis of the forearm.

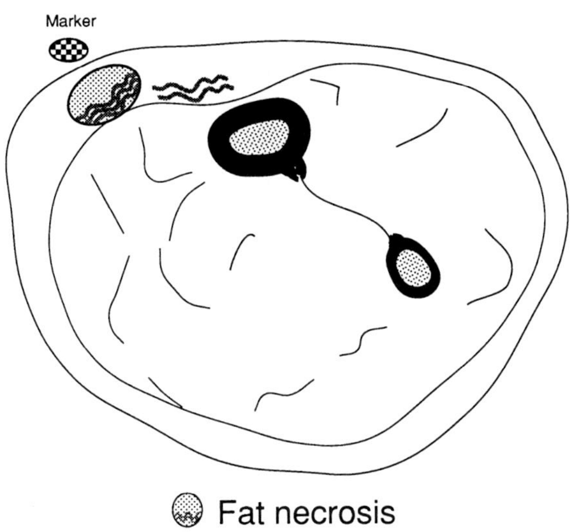

FIGURE 12-3

CASE 13

Differential Diagnosis of Soft Tissue Masses of the Hand and Forearm

HISTORY: The first patient described in this study was a 15-year-old boy with a soft tissue mass along the dorsum of the fourth digit. The mass was firm and nontender. The second patient, a 24-year-old man, presented with a mildly tender mass in the forearm. He lifted weights and exercised vigorously. What is the MRI diagnosis in each case? (Patient 1—Figs. 13-1 and 13-2: respectively coronal and axial T1-weighted MR images. Fig. 13-3: multiformat, multiecho proton-density (*A*) and T2-weighted (*B*) images. Patient 2—Figs. 13-4 and 13-5: axial non-contrast-enhanced T1-weighted images obtained respectively in March and May of the same year.)

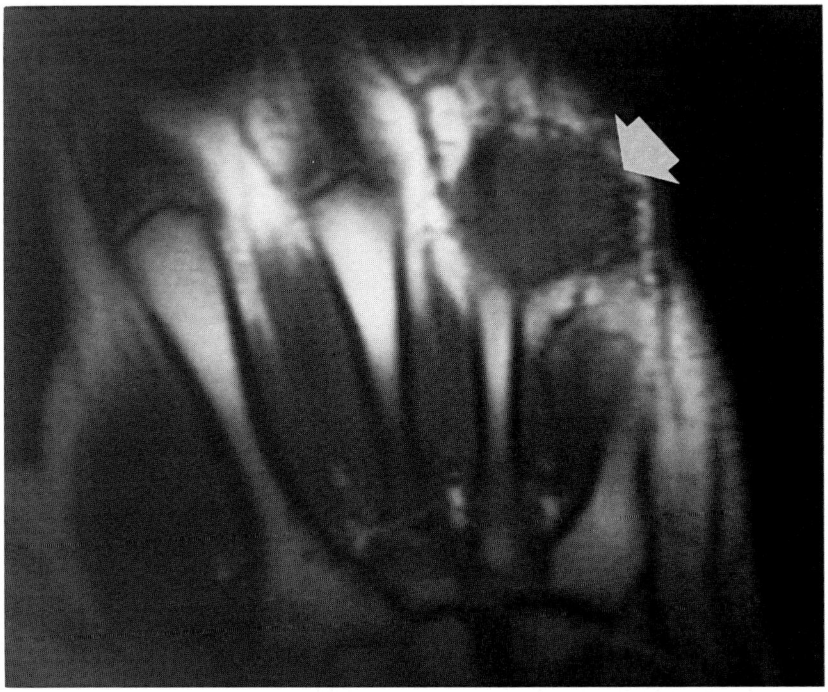

FIGURE 13-1

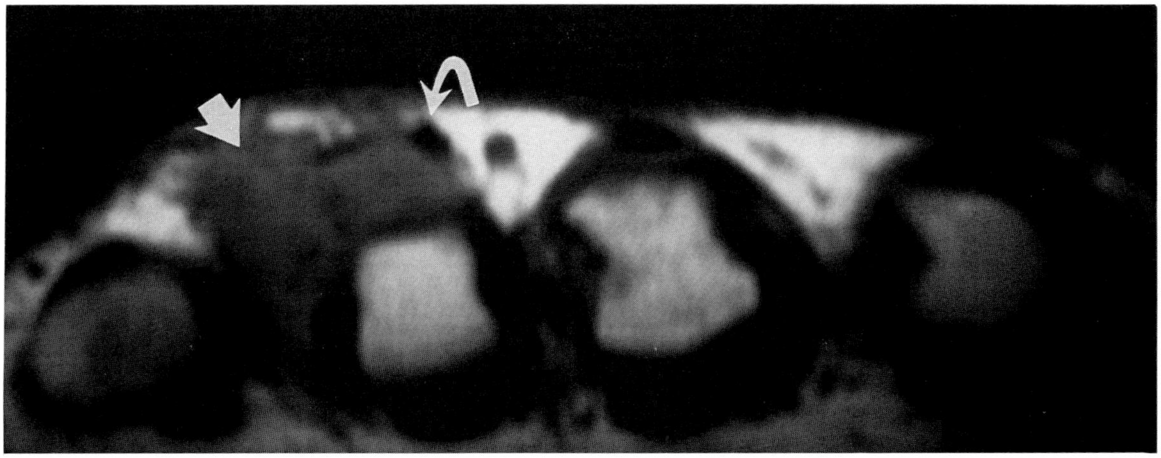

FIGURE 13-2

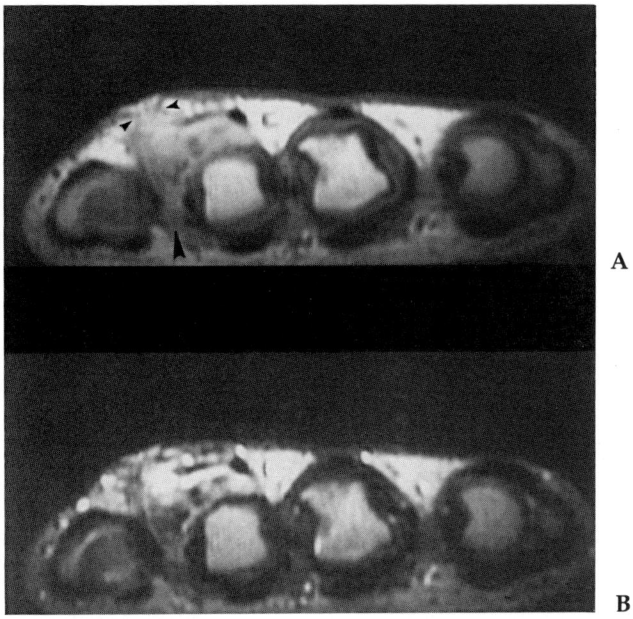

FIGURE 13-3

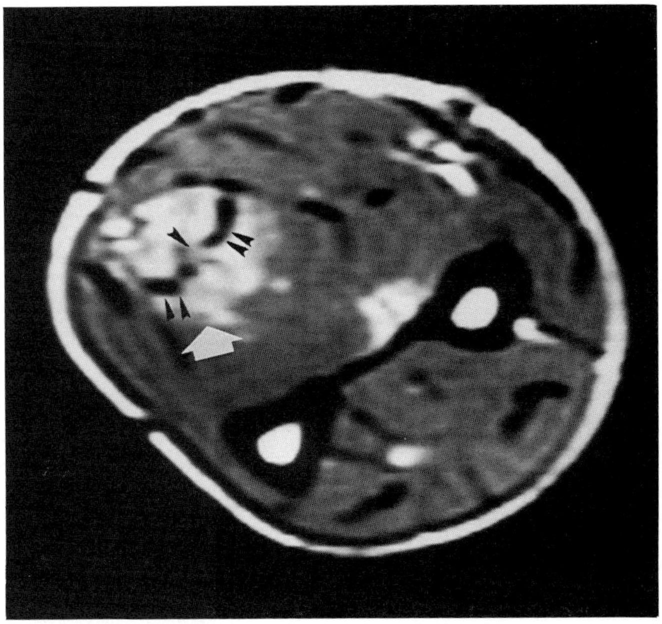

FIGURE 13-4

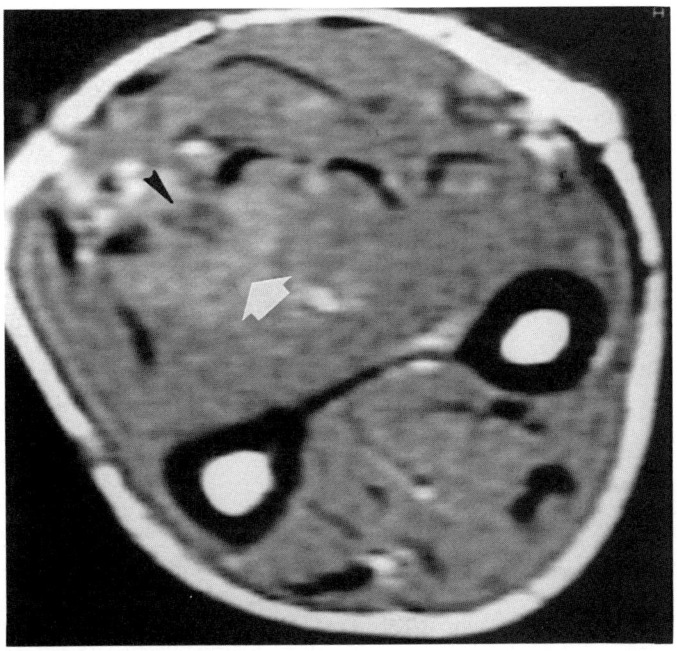

FIGURE 13-5

DISCUSSION

PATIENT 1: At the level of the fourth metacarpal head is a soft tissue mass (white arrow in Fig. 13-2) growing underneath the hypointense extensor tendons (curved white arrow in Fig. 13-2), invading the cortical bone but sparing the hyperintense medullary bone, and involving the adjacent soft tissues and subcutaneous hyperintense fat. The mass extends into the volar surface of the hand through the interosseous web (arrowhead in Fig. 13-3*A*). The mass also grows underneath the isointense dermis (small arrowheads in Fig. 13-3*A*). The signal of the mass is inhomogeneous on T2 imaging and is mildly increased in intensity.

A soft tissue mass relatively sparing bone with aggressive growth characteristics and little signal increase on T2-weighted imaging is most typical of a soft tissue sarcoma. Sarcomatous lesions to consider in this distribution include malignant fibrous histiocytoma, malignant epithelioid, and spindle cell sarcoma, of which synovial sarcoma is a subtype. Soft part sarcomas, soft tissue osteogenic or chondroid sarcomas, and rhabdomyosarcomas are rarer in this location.

Soft part sarcomas usually occur in adults in the 20- to 40-year-old age range. This neoplasm has a propensity to involve the thigh. Epithelioid sarcoma is a tumor of subcutaneous tissue, fascia, or tendons. Two thirds of these tumors occur in the upper extremities and often involve the hand. The median age of involvement is 29 years, and growth along fascia and tendinous structures in nodular fashion is typical. Occasionally involvement of pretibial tendons and soft tissues has been noted in the lower extremity.

Synovial sarcoma is a rare tumor arising near but not necessarily from synovium, bursa, or tendon sheaths. This neoplasm tends to arise in extremities, and more than 50% of cases occur in adults aged 20 to 40 years (the median age of involvement is 35). The lesions tend to be more hyperintense than other sarcomas on MRI. Most involve the lower extremity, with the thigh, knee, and upper leg predominating. Less than 7% involve the hand. Since the mass is of water density on other imaging modalities, it is not surprising that the signal of the mass is quite high on T2-weighted imaging.

Soft tissue or tendon sheath osteogenic or chondrosarcomas are extremely rare lesions and exhibit calcification and matrix formation, not present on the conventional radiographs (not shown) in this case, and are extremely rare in the hand. Rhabdomyosarcoma occurs in children but is unusual in the hand and does not grow along tendon sheaths. Malignant fibrous histiocytoma is uncommon in the upper extremity (less than 25%) and is a tumor of late adulthood. These tend to have intermediate or slightly hyperintense T2 signal with brighter signal being seen in larger neoplasms.

PATIENT 2: The soft tissue mass (white arrow in Fig. 13-4) in the forearm has hyperintense T1 signal, suggesting hemorrhage. The absence of a trauma history and nominal tenderness worried the clinicians. An important finding that initially went unrecognized was splaying of the hypointense fascial interface (paired arrowheads) by an intermediate signal intensity nodule (arrowhead). We refer to this as the "fascial retraction sign" and have observed it in numerous soft tissue neoplasms of the extremities.

A biopsy was interpreted as nodular fasciitis with hemorrhage. Follow-up MRI performed 2 months later showed loss and resolution of the hyperintense hemorrhagic signal, but the mass was now larger (white arrow in Fig. 13-5). The nodule (arrowhead in Fig. 13-5) was also larger and further splayed the epimysial fascial bundles apart, an ominous sign. Further biopsy suggested nodular fasciitis with hemorrhage; however, specimen review at multiple outside institutions confirmed the diagnosis of epithelioid sarcoma that had bled.

DIAGNOSIS: The first patient has epithelioid sarcoma of the hand, proven on two-digit resection. The second patient has epithelioid sarcoma with hemorrhage of the forearm.

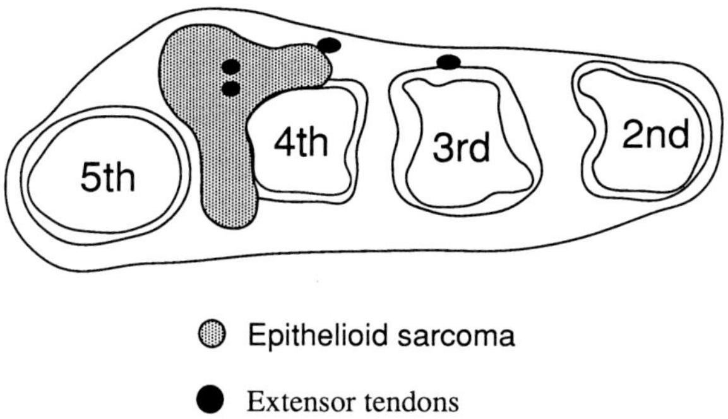

FIGURE 13-6

CASE 14

Differential Diagnosis of Soft Tissue Masses about the Hand and Elbow

HISTORY: The first patient in this study was a 72-year-old woman with a palpable mass over the hypothenar eminence of 1 year's duration. The second patient was a 10-year-old boy. What is the MRI diagnosis in each case? (Patient 1—Fig. 14-1: coronal T1-weighted MR image. Patient 2—Fig. 14-2: coronal T1-weighted MR image.)

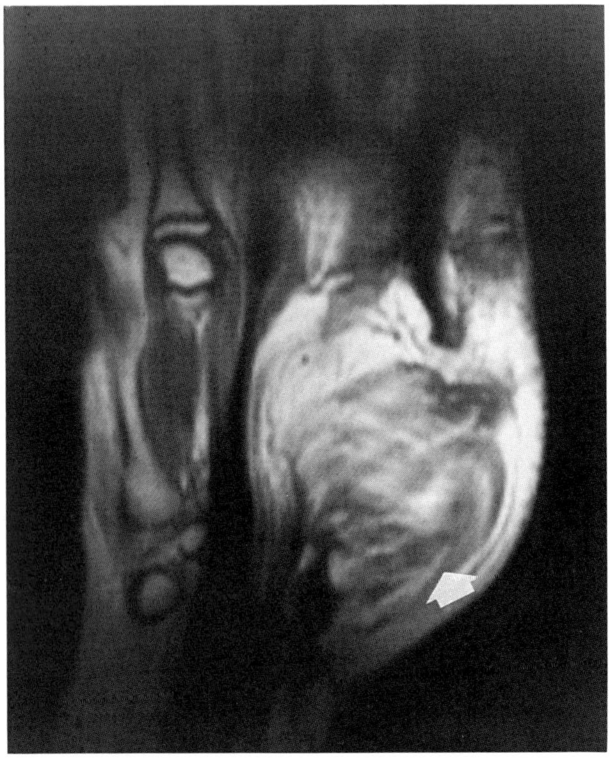

FIGURE 14-1

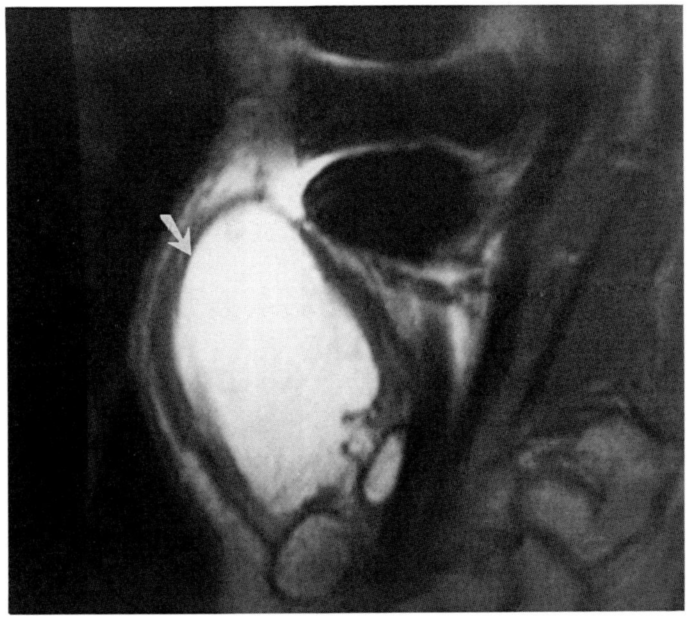

FIGURE 14-2

DISCUSSION

PATIENT 1: A homogeneous mass in the thenar eminence (white arrow in Fig. 14-1) is well circumscribed, exhibits sharp margins, is multilobulated, and does not appear to invade adjacent medullary bone. Lesion signal homogeneity supports a benign etiology. The signal intensity matches that of a known tissue, the subcutaneous fat, and is therefore pathognomonic of lipoma.

PATIENT 2: Liposarcoma may have intermediate signal intensity streaks intermixed with fat signal, or may present as a myxoid variant with mild hyperintensity on T1 weighting and marked hyperintensity on T2 weighting (see case 13 in Chapter 3, The Hip). The poorer the differentiation of lipid-containing tumors, the less it sustains the MRI appearance of pure fat, which is hyperintense on T1 weighting and hypointense on T2 weighting.

DIAGNOSIS: The first patient has a lipoma of the hypothenar eminence; the second patient has a liposarcoma.

CASE 15

Differential Diagnosis of Soft Tissue Masses about the Hand and Arm

HISTORY: A 38-year-old man presented with a palpable, firm, soft tissue mass in the distal arm. What is the MRI diagnosis? (Fig. 15-1: sagittal T1-weighted MR image of the left arm.)

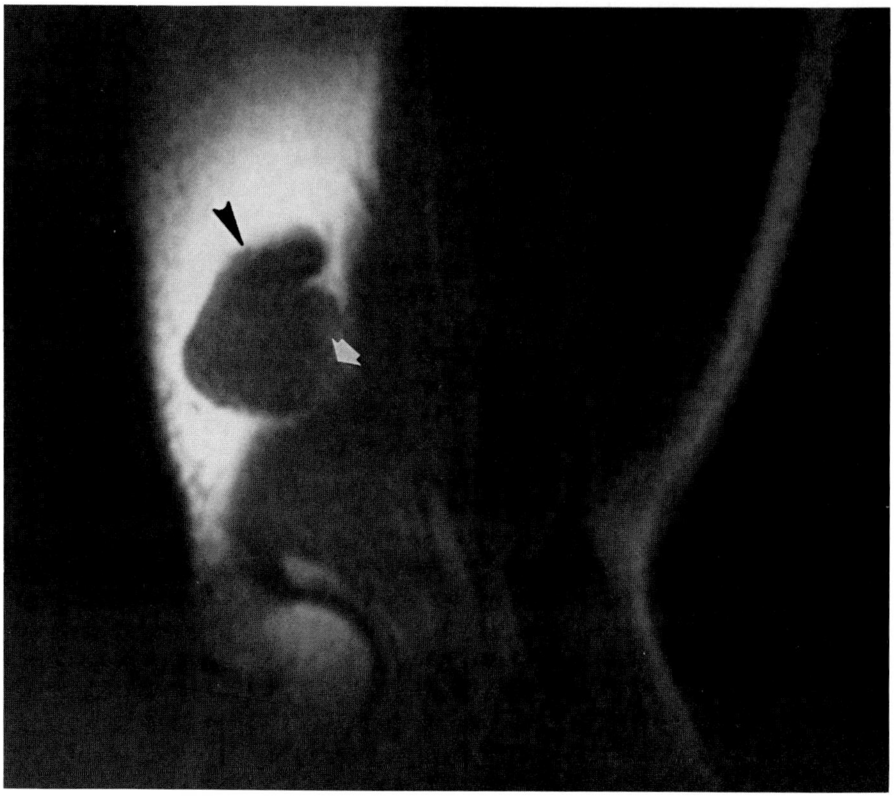

FIGURE 15-1

DISCUSSION: A homogeneous well-circumscribed mass (arrowhead in Fig. 15-1) lies in the subcutaneous fat, has waterlike signal, and is multilobulated. The mass has homogeneous signal and circumscribes an adjacent extensor tendon (white arrow), which appears to run through the mass and allows a specific diagnosis to be made. The findings are pathognomonic of peritendinous ganglion.

A mass with waterlike signal that is hypointense on T1 weighting and hyperintense on T2 weighting is typically seen in a periarticular or peritendinous location. Myxoid softening and degeneration of tissue about a joint capsule or tendon is the supposed mechanism of development of these lesions.

DIAGNOSIS: The patient has a soft tissue peritendinous ganglion.

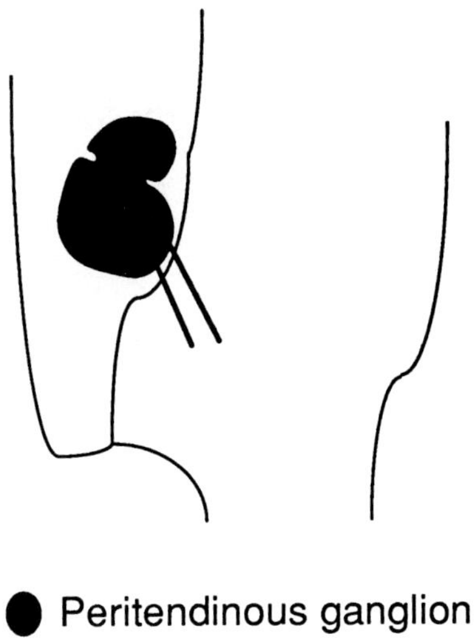

FIGURE 15-2

CASE 16

Differential Diagnosis of Soft Tissue Masses about the Hand and Arm

HISTORY: A 59-year-old woman reported progressive difficulty playing golf due to gradual flexion deformity and radial deviation of the hand. The patient noticed a firm area in her forearm for 3 weeks that she thought began 1 day after a golf game when she experienced discomfort. What is the MRI diagnosis? (Fig. 16-1: axial multiformat (two-on-one), multiecho proton-density (*A*) and T2-weighted (*B*) MR images.)

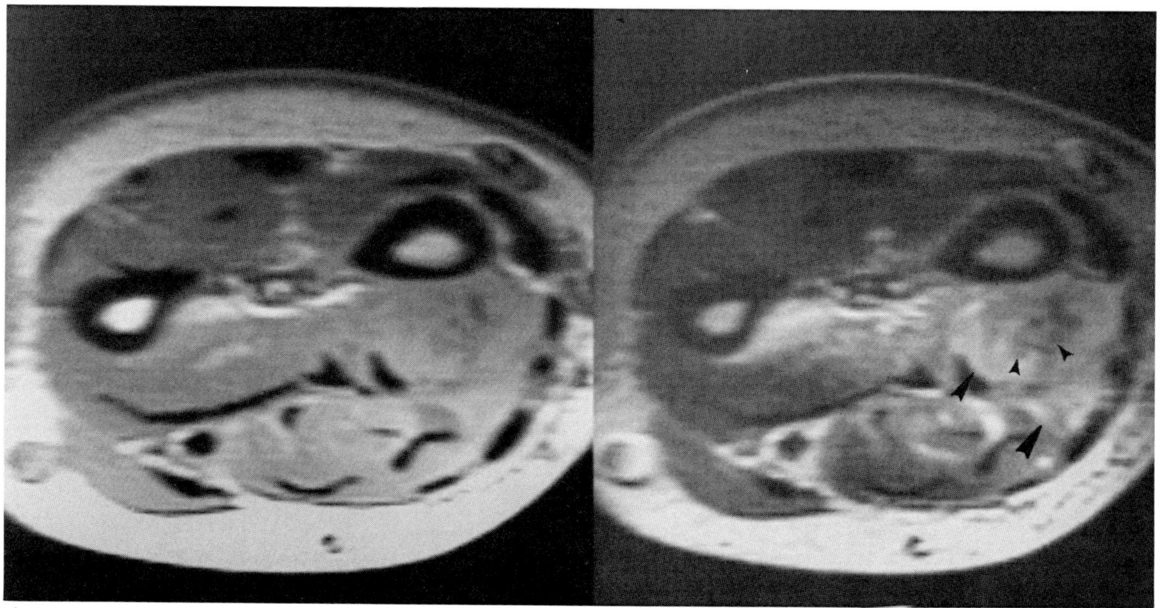

A **B**

FIGURE 16-1

DISCUSSION: Because of the history of progressive deformity, the tendinous anatomy of the forearm is of interest. With a history of flexion and radial deviation, the flexor carpi radialis should be investigated. Normally it appears as a linear hypointense black band in the sagittal projection but as a rounded, hypointense area in the axial projection. Within this band is an intermediate signal intensity nodule (small arrowheads in Fig. 16-1*B*).

Engulfing the displaced tendon (intermediate-sized arrowhead in Fig. 16-1*B*) is a large soft tissue mass, easily visualized in the axial projection. The mass has a hypointense center (paired arrowheads in Fig. 16-1*B*) but is surrounded by diffuse hyperintense myofascial edema (large arrowhead). Although sarcoma is a definite consideration in view of the signal intensity on the T2 images, an intratendinous location of a sarcoma is very rare. Most sarcomas and diseases that affect tendons and their sheaths grow around the tendons rather than directly inside them. Two lesions that may exhibit this growth pattern are epithelioid sarcoma, synovial sarcoma, and giant cell tumor of the tendon sheath. An intratendinous mass coupled with surrounding soft tissue mass and associated edema implies lesion aggressiveness.

DIAGNOSIS: The patient has metastatic adenocarcinoma from an unknown primary.

INDEX

Page numbers in *italics* indicate figures.

ISBN 0-397-51105-1